Case Studies in Sex Therapy

CASE STUDIES IN SEX THERAPY

Edited by

RAYMOND C. ROSEN
SANDRA R. LEIBLUM

THE GUILFORD PRESS
New York   London

© 1995 The Guilford Press
A Division of Guilford Publications, Inc.
72 Spring Street, New York, NY 10012

Printed in the United States of America

This book is printed on acid-free paper.

Last digit is print number: 9 8 7 6 5 4 3

Library of Congress Cataloging-in-Publication Data

Case studies in sex therapy / edited by Raymond C. Rosen, Sandra R.
  Leiblum.
       p.   cm.
  Includes bibliographical references and index.
  ISBN 0-89862-848-2
  1. Sex therapy—Case studies.   I. Rosen, Raymond, 1946–
II. Leiblum, Sandra Risa.
  RC557.C37   1995
  616.85'830651—dc20   94-49590
                                                           CIP

This book is dedicated to our patients.
Their trust and confidences have touched us deeply.

Contributors

Stanley E. Althof, Ph.D., Department of Urology, Case Western Reserve University School of Medicine, Cleveland, Ohio; and Center for Marital and Sexual Health, Beachwood, Ohio

Bernard Apfelbaum, Ph.D., Berkeley Sex Therapy Group, Berkeley, California

J. Gayle Beck, Ph.D., Department of Psychology, State University of New York at Buffalo, Buffalo, New York

Lois H. Blum, M.M.H., Department of Psychiatry and Behavioral Sciences, Johns Hopkins University School of Medicine, Baltimore, Maryland

Eli Coleman, Ph.D., Program in Human Sexuality and Department of Family Practice and Community Health, University of Minnesota Medical School, Minneapolis, Minnesota

Peter J. Fagan, Ph.D., Department of Psychiatry and Behavioral Sciences, Johns Hopkins University School of Medicine, Baltimore, Maryland

Julia R. Heiman, Ph.D., Department of Psychiatry and Behavioral Medicine, University of Washington School of Medicine, Seattle, Washington

Helen Singer Kaplan, M.D., Ph.D., Human Sexuality Program, New York Hospital–Cornell University Medical Center, New York, New York

Carol L. Lassen, Ph.D., private practice, Denver, Colorado; and Department of Psychiatry, University of Colorado Medical School, Denver, Colorado

Arnold A. Lazarus, Ph.D., Graduate School of Applied and Professional Psychology, Rutgers University, Piscataway, New Jersey

Sandra R. Leiblum, Ph.D., Department of Psychiatry, UMDNJ–Robert Wood Johnson Medical School, Piscataway, New Jersey

Stephen B. Levine, M.D., Department of Psychiatry, Case Western Reserve University School of Medicine, Cleveland, Ohio

Harold I. Lief, M.D., Department of Psychiatry, University of Pennsylvania, Philadelphia, Pennsylvania

Joseph LoPiccolo, Ph.D., Department of Psychology, University of Missouri–Columbia, Columbia, Missouri

Barry W. McCarthy, Ph.D., Department of Psychology, American University, Washington, DC

Sharon G. Nathan, Ph.D., M.P.H., Department of Psychiatry, Cornell University Medical College, New York, New York

Margaret Nichols, Ph.D., Institute for Personal Growth, Highland Park, New Jersey

S. Michael Plaut, Ph.D., Department of Psychiatry, University of Maryland School of Medicine, Baltimore, Maryland

Cathryn G. Pridal, Ph.D., Department of Psychology, University of Missouri–Columbia, Columbia, Missouri

Candace B. Risen, L.I.S.W., Department of Psychiatry, Case Western Reserve University School of Medicine, Cleveland, Ohio; and Center for Marital and Sexual Health, Beachwood, Ohio

Domeena C. Renshaw, M.D., Department of Psychiatry and Sexual Dysfunction Clinic, Loyola University Chicago, Maywood, Illinois

Raymond C. Rosen, Ph.D., Department of Psychiatry, UMDNJ–Robert Wood Johnson Medical School, Piscataway, New Jersey

Leslie R. Schover, Ph.D., Center for Sexual Function and Department of Urology, Cleveland Clinic Foundation, Cleveland, Ohio

John P. Wincze, Ph.D., Department of Psychology/Psychiatry, Brown University/VA Medical Center, Providence, Rhode Island

Bernie Zilbergeld, Ph.D., private practice, Oakland, California; and Center for Sexual Health, San Jose, California

Preface

As practicing clinicians, we are often struck by the wide gulf that separates theory and practice in the field of sex therapy. In fact, whereas treatment interventions and techniques have proliferated in recent years, limited progress has occurred in our understanding of the nature and etiology of most sexual dysfunctions. Despite the potpourri of new psychological, pharmacological, and mechanical options available, many of the cases currently presenting for treatment are highly challenging from both a conceptual and clinical standpoint. Simple cases of premature ejaculation or anorgasmia are increasingly rare, and have been largely superseded by chronic desire or arousal difficulties, frequently in combination with medical, intrapsychic, or interpersonal concomitants. At the same time, we have noted a growing trend toward multidisciplinary and theoretically eclectic approaches to treatment, which are inadequately reflected in the existing treatment literature.

How are these issues managed in actual clinical practice? Has the practice of sex therapy changed significantly since the early days of Masters and Johnson (1970) and Kaplan (1974)? The present volume of case studies is intended, primarily, to illustrate the enormous breadth and variety of current clinical approaches to sexual disorders. Despite the fact that all of our contributors are highly experienced and knowledgeable sex therapists, the differences in both theoretical orientation and clinical approach are often striking. Whereas some authors routinely use medical or pharmacological approaches in treatment, others view such interventions cautiously and use them infrequently. For some authors, intrapsychic or personality dynamics are central to treatment, while others focus more intensively on interpersonal or relationship issues. By presenting a series of in-depth case studies, we hope to illustrate the rich diversity of clinical approaches in current sex therapy practice.

The present book represents the fourth volume in our series on contemporary issues in sex therapy. Other volumes are *Sexual Desire Disorders* (Leiblum & Rosen, 1988), *Principles and Practice of Sex Therapy: Update for the 1990s* (Leiblum & Rosen, 1989), and *Erectile Disorders: Assessment and Treatment* (Rosen & Leiblum, 1992). While our previous books have focused on specific topics or general approaches to sex therapy, the present volume is intended to portray the "nuts and bolts" or clinical reality of sex therapy practice. By means of detailed case descriptions and clinical commentaries, our contributors vividly illuminate some of the major issues that arise in treatment, such as relapse and resistance to change, the role of the uncooperative partner, and psychiatric concomitants of sexual dysfunction. We hope this book will complement our other volumes in providing readers with a more intensive and case-based approach to formulation and treatment. Conceptual and theoretical issues are also highlighted through the accompanying clinical commentaries and detailed case discussions.

How were cases selected for inclusion? Generally speaking, our contributors were given wide latitude in the choice of clinical problems or treatment interventions to be presented. We encouraged our authors to select *typical* cases, however, which exemplified the type of practice and theoretical orientation of the writer. No constraints were placed on the outcome of the case, and it is interesting to note that several authors chose to present less-than-successful outcomes. In addition to demonstrating the "ego strength" of the individual contributors, these cases offer provocative and challenging examples of the current limits of sex therapy treatment. It is noteworthy that most cases of unsuccessful outcome fell into the categories of hypoactive or hyperactive sexual desire. These problems remain among the most challenging and perplexing disorders presenting for sex therapy treatment.

A particular issue of concern in the present volume was the need to safeguard the privacy and confidentiality of the individuals and couples described. Each author was strongly advised to remove or disguise all identifying information, such as the name, age, occupation, or ethnic origin of the patient/client. Some, but not all, authors chose additionally to obtain written consent from their clients/patients before submitting their chapters for publication. During the editorial process, each chapter was carefully screened for possible breaches of confidentiality, and appropriate steps were taken, where necessary, to further disguise or alter the information presented. In this manner, we believe that the rights of patients to confidentiality and anonymity have been afforded suitable protection, while recognizing the need for professionals to communicate their ideas and experiences in the clinical arena.

We are especially gratified with the list of contributors to the current volume. Included are several of the major pioneers of the field, such as Helen Singer Kaplan, Harold I. Lief, Joseph LoPiccolo, and Arnold A. Lazarus, as well as a distinguished list of "master clinicians," such as Bernard Apfelbaum, Julia R. Heiman, Leslie R. Schover, Stanley E. Althof, and Bernie Zilbergeld. All of our authors have made significant contributions in at least one area of the field, and their influence has been enormous in determining the shape and form of sex therapy today. In addition to the detailed and thought-provoking case descriptions they provided, we are also grateful to our authors for their sincerity and openness in discussing the limitations of current clinical practice. It is rare to have the work of so many talented and creative individuals represented in a single volume, and we are deeply appreciative of the time and effort involved.

Finally, our sincere thanks are due once again to our publisher, confidant, and friend, Seymour Weingarten. He has loyally supported and advised us on many writing projects over the past decade and a half, and we are very grateful for his support. Our editor, Judith Grauman, has also provided many valuable suggestions and ideas, in addition to her outstanding editorial contributions. As always, we are most grateful for the loyal support of friends and family, especially Linda Rosen, Joshua Rosen, Michael Rosen, Jonathan Leiblum Kassen, and Frank Brickel.

RAYMOND C. ROSEN
SANDRA R. LEIBLUM

REFERENCES

Kaplan, H. S. (1974). *The new sex therapy*. New York: Brunner/Mazel.

Leiblum, S. R., & Rosen, R. C. (Eds.). (1988). *Sexual desire disorders*. New York: Guilford Press.

Leiblum, S. R., & Rosen, R. C. (Eds.). (1989). *Principles and practice of sex therapy* (2nd ed.): *Update for the 1990s*. New York: Guilford Press.

Masters, W. H., & Johnson, V. E. (1970). *Human sexual inadequacy*. Boston: Little, Brown.

Rosen, R. C., & Leiblum, S. R. (Eds.). (1992). *Erectile disorders: Assessment and treatment*. New York: Guilford Press.

Contents

Introduction

The Changing Focus of Sex Therapy

RAYMOND C. ROSEN
SANDRA R. LEIBLUM

INTRODUCTION

At the time of publication of *Human Sexual Inadequacy* (Masters & Johnson, 1970), anorgasmia in women and rapid ejaculation in men were the sexual disorders of greatest visibility in therapy clinics across the United States and abroad. Among those seeking help, the majority tended to be young (i.e., under 40 years of age) and well educated and had come of age in the 1960s. These individuals sought, and were encouraged to seek, high levels of sexual gratification for both themselves and their partners. Sustaining this interest was an explosion of self-help manuals and popular press articles, which offered a barrage of techniques and advice for enhancing sexual satisfaction, including longer-lasting erections and ejaculatory control for men and orgasmic competence for women (e.g., Barbach, 1975; Heiman, LoPiccolo, & LoPiccolo, 1976; Zilbergeld, 1978). Sex therapy in the 1970s tended to be structured along the straightforward lines proposed by Masters and Johnson (1970), including conjoint cotherapy and brief, problem-focused approaches to treatment. Treatment outcome was generally positive, and a sense of optimism and confidence was widely evident (Leiblum & Pervin, 1980).

In the past decade, the range of problems addressed by sex therapists has broadened considerably, as have the types and variety of treatment interventions employed. With the growing complexity and chronicity of problems encountered, brief behavioral interventions, or "14-day cures," have become increasingly rare, as medical treatments and longer-term individual and couple therapy approaches now predominate. Mechanical, pharmacological, and surgical procedures have proliferated, along with the development of multidimensional assessment algorithms, systems-interactional clinical formulations, and cognitive-behavioral approaches to treatment (Rosen, Leiblum, & Spector, 1994; Wincze & Carey, 1991). The chapters in this book attest to the enormous breadth and variety of diagnostic and treatment approaches currently in use.

A major change in the patient population seeking services has become apparent in the past decade (Schover & Leiblum, 1994). As the number of sexually naive and inexperienced individuals referred for treatment has declined, older patients and those with more complex or chronic sexual difficulties are more frequently seen. Among older men, for example, the problem of erectile failure is especially prevalent and troubling. According to the recent Massachusetts Male Aging Study (Feldman, Goldstein, Hatzichristou, Krane, & McKinlay, 1994), a random sample survey of 1,700 men age 40 to 70 years, the incidence of severe erectile disorder ("complete impotence") tripled from 5% to 15% in male subjects between the ages of 40 and 70. The combined prevalence of mild, moderate, and severe cases of erectile disorder in this study was 52%. Chronic illness and prescription drug use were frequent concomitants of erectile dysfunction, particularly in the older age group. Unfortunately, the impact of erectile difficulties on partner satisfaction was not assessed.

Sexual desire disorders have similarly increased in frequency and significance in recent years. In fact, hypoactive sexual desire (HSD) is a major focus of both the current volume and the field of sex therapy generally (Leiblum & Rosen, 1988; Rosen & Leiblum, 1995). Historically, hypoactive or inhibited sexual desire was first identified as a discrete or separate clinical entity by Lief (1977) and Kaplan (1977). Both authors emphasized the widespread prevalence of HSD in males and females and the relative resistance to treatment with traditional sex therapy approaches. Kaplan's (1977) formulation was based on her triphasic model of the sexual response cycle, which differentiated among desire, excitement, and orgasm phases, and which replaced the earlier four-stage model of Masters and Johnson (1966). In the revised third edition (DSM-III-R; American Psychistric Association, 1987) and the fourth edition (DSM-IV; American Psychiatric Association, 1994) of the *Diagnostic and Statistical Manual of Mental Disorders*, the term "inhibited" was replaced by the more phenomenologically based term "hypoactive," to underscore the possible biological etiology of some cases of sexual apathy. In the interim, hypoactive desire has come to be recognized as a frequent sexual complaint, with prevalence rates ranging from

15% of adult males (Nathan, 1986) to 30–40% of females applying for sexual counseling (Hawton, Catalan, Martin, & Fagg, 1986).

Low sexual desire presents a major therapuetic challenge in current sex therapy. Treatment is frequently protracted over months, or even years, and the resulting outcome is often uncertain (Rosen & Leiblum, 1995). In some instances, short-term interventions can be used effectively, as illustrated, by Cathryn G. Pridal and Joseph LoPiccolo (Chapter 7), Bernard Apfelbaum (Chapter 1), and J. Gayle Beck (Chapter 2) in the current volume. For others, however, intensive, long-term therapy is required, and drug or hormonal treatments are increasingly combined with individual and/or couple therapy. Harold I. Lief (Chapter 6, this volume) provides an excellent in-depth illustration of this current trend. Finally, low desire in homosexual or lesbian couples can present special concerns or difficulties for the clinician, as described by Margaret Nichols (Chapter 9, this volume).

Most recently, we have noted a significant increase in the number of individuals referred for evaluation or treatment of hypersexuality, or "sexual addiction." In part, the interest in sexual compulsivity or addiction has been fueled by intense media coverage of highly visible professionals, such as teachers, priests, and physicians, who are accused of engaging in sexual acts and behaviors that strongly violate social and professional standards. Concurrently, there has been dramatic growth in the availability of self-help or 12-step groups for so-called sexually addicted or compulsive individuals. It has also been proposed that the current focus on hypersexuality is, in part, a "backlash" to the sexual freedom movement of the 1960s and 1970s (Levine & Troiden, 1988). Along with societalwide concern about sexual "addiction" in adults, a parallel trend has been observed in the recent tendency to pathologize sexual behavior in children (Becker, 1994; Okami, 1992). Current diagnostic and treatment dilemmas are illustrated by Eli Coleman (Chapter 19), Sharon G. Nathan (Chapter 20), Candace B. Risen and Stanley E. Althof (Chapter 21), and John P. Wincze (Chapter 22) in the final section of this volume.

ETIOLOGY AND DIAGNOSIS

In contrast to the earlier emphasis on psychogenic factors and performance anxiety, medical or organic determinants are currently a major focus of attention in sex therapy. This trend is most clearly evident in the literature on male erectile disorder, although attempts have also been made to investigate physiological causes of low desire (Rosen & Leiblum,

1995) and premature ejaculation (Assalian, 1994). Although less attention has been devoted, overall, to the role of organic causes in female
dysfunction, Leslie R. Schover (Chapter 17, this volume) discusses the
possible contribution of organic factors in female dysfunction.

At a psychological level, a major shift has taken place toward more
complex or "postmodern" formulations of sexual dysfunction (LoPiccolo,
1992; Rosen et al., 1994). Early sexual trauma or abuse has been identified as a key determinant in many instances, as shown dramatically by
Julia R. Heiman (Chapter 12, this volume). In this chapter, early incest
experiences played a critical role in the development of the client's sexual
and relationship script, and a ritual "healing ceremony" was necessary
to effect a successful outcome. Although less common, sexual abuse
experiences in males can also play a major role, as described by Barry
W. McCarthy (Chapter 8, this volume). The resulting guilt and shame
experienced by male victims of abuse are graphically illustrated in this
case.

Personality style and relationship conflicts are additional dimensions
of interest, as patients with a history of obsessive–compulsive or depressive personality disorders are frequently encountered (Donahey &
Carroll, 1993). Similarly, many couples present with a history of trust
and intimacy problems, conflicts over power and control, and a lack of
physical attraction (Leiblum & Rosen, 1991). As described by Pridal and
LoPiccolo (Chapter 7, this volume), sexual dysfunction needs to be considered always from the perspective of potential homeostatic mechanisms
in the relationship. Stephen B. Levine (Chapter 5, this volume) similarly
emphasizes the subtle and complex interplay between intrapsychic and
interpersonal determinants of sexual dysfunction, and Apfelbaum (Chapter 1, this volume) notes the pervasive influence of "response anxiety."
Clearly, our etiological models and clinical formulations have expanded
greatly in the past two decades.

In contrast, relatively few changes have occurred in the diagnosis
and classification of sexual dysfunctions (e.g., DSM-IV). As in the previous classification system (DSM-III-R), psychosexual disorders are divided into four major categories (1) sexual desire disorders, including
HSD and sexual aversion disorder; (2) sexual arousal disorders, including
female sexual arousal and male erectile disorder; (3) orgasmic disorders,
including female orgasmic disorder (anorgasmia), male orgasmic disorder
(retarded ejaculation), and premature ejaculation; and (4) sexual pain
disorders, including dyspareunia (painful intercourse) and vaginismus.

The current system (DSM-IV) emphasizes the clinical criterion of
"marked distress or interpersonal difficulty" in defining the various disorders. This dimension is particularly significant in the definition of HSD,
which is now qualified by the need for both the judgment of the clini-

cian and the level of subjective or interpersonal distress associated with the disorder. The highly subjective and potentially arbitrary nature of the diagnosis is a major problem for both research and clinical practice (Rosen & Leiblum, 1995). Additionally, the current classification system fails to include common desire disorders, such as desire discrepancy disorder and sexual compulsion or hyperactive desire (Coleman, 1991). Omission of the latter category is particularly controversial at present.

TREATMENT FORMAT AND INTERVENTIONS

As the case studies in this volume attest, the format of sex therapy has become increasingly flexible and individualistic in the past decade. Whereas most therapists subscribed at one time to the "dual therapy" and "conjoint counseling" format of the early Masters and Johnson (1970) model, it soon became apparent that conjoint therapy was costly and inefficient in the majority of cases. According to one recent review (Hawton, 1992), there is no consistent effect across studies of single versus dual sex therapist treatment formats. Most chapters in the current volume describe the use of individual or couple therapy approaches, which are generally conducted in a single therapist format.

Frequency of therapy contact was similarly assumed to be important, with weekly or biweekly sessions being viewed as optimal. However, most studies in this area have revealed little difference between couples treated on a weekly or biweekly basis, compared to those who had more frequent treatment sessions (e.g., Hawton, Catalan, & Fagg, 1991). The duration of therapy is also highly variable, and it is more likely nowadays to be determined by reimbursement practices and managed care policies rather than the therapist's concerns regarding efficacy or outcome. Treatment frequency and duration vary widely in the cases presented in the current volume and appear unrelated overall to treatment outcome.

Regarding specific treatments employed, as noted, the most significant trend has been toward increasing use of surgical, mechanical, or medical interventions. This trend can be traced back to the early 1980s, and the entry of vascular and urological surgeons, in large numbers, into the arena of male erectile disorder. According to Bancroft (1989), specialists in these areas were attracted to the field for two major reasons: (1) the need for marketing their skills in new fields as more traditional practice areas declined, and (2) the readiness of men with erectile failure to opt for medical rather than psychological solutions to their sexual difficulties.

The "medicalization" of sex therapy was also instigated by major advances in the area of penile vascular physiology. Four individuals in particular are credited with important discoveries in this area: Vaclav Michal (1982), a Czechoslovakian surgeon who pioneered the use of penile vascular surgery; Ronald Virag in Paris (Virag, Fryden, Legmans, & Virag, 1984) and Giles Brindley (1983) in London, who first identified the effects of intracavernosal administration of smooth muscle relaxants (e.g., papaverine and phentolamine); and the investigations of Tom Lue in the United States, who pioneered research in duplex ultrasound scanning procedures for assessment of erectile dysfunction (Lue, Hricak, & Tanagho, 1985).

Spurred by these developments, medical and surgical interventions for male erectile disorder have proliferated in the past decade (Rosen & Leiblum, 1992). Surgical implants in a wide range of models and types, intracorporal injection therapy, vacuum pump devices, oral medications, laser-based venous ligation procedures, and other technologically sophisticated interventions have attained prominence in recent years. As noted by Tiefer (1994), "No one in our field can have failed to notice that a medical juggernaut is sweeping over the definition, diagnosis, and treatment of men's erection problems" (p. 371). Regrettably, there is a lack of agreement concerning the proper matching of patients to procedures, and few controlled studies are available evaluating the long-term safety or efficacy of these approaches. Moreover, we have emphasized the risk of reinforcing cultural stereotypes regarding rigid erections as the *sine qua non* of sexual exchange (Rosen & Leiblum, 1992).

More popular than surgery, nowadays, in cases involving erectile failure has been the use of intracavernosal injection of smooth muscle relaxants, such as papaverine, phentolamine, and prostaglandin E_1. However, Althof and Turner (1992) note that injection therapy is accepted by only 40–50% of men who are referred for this treatment. Many men and their partners (as the case study by Peter J. Fagan and Lois H. Blum, Chapter 11, this volume, illustrates) are uncomfortable with the notion of self-injection, and the cost of such treatment is often high. Treatment side effects, such as fibrotic nodules, penile bruising, and abnormal liver function values, are not uncommon. Nevertheless, self-injection therapy remains popular and has the capacity to significantly enhance sexual functioning for individuals or couples who are motivated to use it (Althof et al., 1991).

Clinically, the chapters on erectile disorder in the present volume attest to the breadth and variety of treatment interventions currently in use. As indicated, there has been a major trend toward greater reliance on technological or mechanical solutions, such as the vacuum pump, intracorporal injections, and surgical implants. These interventions are now widely used in the treatment of both psychogenically and organically based erectile disorders (Wagner & Kaplan, 1993), despite a lack of adequate long-term evaluation of safety or efficacy. Mechanical solutions are highly appealing to both physicians and patients, each of whom may seek a "quick fix" in the face of chronic erectile difficulties and/or relationship conflicts. The wide variety of assessment and treatment methods currently in use has been fully described in a separate volume (Rosen & Leiblum, 1992). In the present book, case studies by Bernie Zilbergeld (Chapter 18), Fagan and Blum (Chapter 11), and S. Michael Plaut (Chapter 15) illustrate the complex choices and challenges of combining medical and psychological treatments for male erectile disorder.

Pharmacological approaches to the treatment of desire disorders—both hypoactive and hyperactive—are yet another component of this trend. Aphrodisiacal substances have been used throughout history for this purpose, and a wide variety of food stuffs and herbal remedies has been recommended. More recently, the role of various dopaminergic, adrenergic, and serotonergic agents have come under intense investigation. Initial research has been conducted with dopamine agonists in nonhuman species (Bitran & Hull, 1987; Everitt & Bancroft, 1991) and, more recently, with humans (Rosen, 1991; Rosen & Ashton, 1993). Interest has also centered on the potential prosexual effects of alpha-adrenergic antagonists such as yohimbine hydrochloride. As discussed by Coleman (Chapter 19, this volume), serotonergic agents are increasingly used in the treatment of hyperactive or compulsive sexual disorders.

Recently, several authors have advocated the use of serotonergic antidepressants, such as clomipramine (Anafranil), for the treatment of premature ejaculation (e.g., Althof, Levine, Corty, Risen, & Stern, 1994; Segraves, Saran. Segraves, & Maguire, 1993). In fact, Assalian (1988, 1994) has raised the question whether premature ejaculation should be classified as a psychogenic disorder based on these findings. Rather, he suggests, men with premature ejaculation suffer from a constitutional vulnerability, which manifests itself as a heightened level of autonomic (i.e., sympathetic) arousal, and which leads, in turn, to rapid or uncontrolled ejaculation. Empirical support for the use of clomipramine in this context comes from independent studies by Segraves et al. (1993) and Althof et al. (1994), both of whom report moderate effectiveness and improved sexual function in premature ejaculators and their partners. In Chapter 16 (this volume) by Raymond C. Rosen, pharmacological therapy (clomipramine) is combined with individual and couple therapy approaches in the treatment of premature ejaculation.

Despite the obvious appeal of pharmacological therapy, certain limitations are clearly evident. In general, it is not clear which patients should be offered treatment with which of these drugs, and what role prosexual drugs should play in the overall treatment plan. The effects of gender, age, and health status on treatment outcome have been insufficiently studied. There is little empirical basis for deciding which patients might benefit from a drug trial, and clinical guidelines are lacking for the choice of appropriate dosage levels and duration of use. Finally, the long-term side effects of prosexual drug use have not been adequately evaluated to date (Rosen & Ashton, 1993).

TREATMENT OUTCOME

As reported by Masters and Johnson (1970), overall success rates were remarkably high in their initial treatment program. Premature ejaculation, for example, had a failure rate of only 2.2%, and primary orgasmic dysfunction had a failure rate of 16.6%. No instances of treatment failure were reported with vaginismus. Masters and Johnson (1970) acknowledged that situational orgasmic inadequacy and secondary erectile dysfunction were more difficult problems to treat, but they claimed an overall failure rate of only 20% for all sexual dysfunctions combined. As time has passed, however, positive outcomes have become less predictable, and success rates now vary considerably, depending on the age, health status, and population studied. Outcome also depends on the specific dysfunction, type of intervention employed, and assessment methods used. Moreover, long-term maintenance and treatment follow-up are rarely conducted (Hawton, 1992).

Not surprisingly, treatment outcome has been most variable in the areas of HSD and male erectile disorder. In fact, few controlled studies have evaluated treatment effectiveness for low desire (Hawton, 1992; Rosen & Leiblum, 1995). Two early studies (Crowe, Gillan, & Golombok, 1981; Zimmer, 1987) compared the effectiveness of conventional sex therapy with or without marital therapy and relaxation training. Unfortunately, both studies were based on heterogeneous groups of subjects with varied sexual complaints, and no attempt was made to differentiate treatment effects in the low-desire patients. Neither study assessed long-term follow-up or provided adequate clinical assessment of treatment efficacy.

In a national survey of sex therapists conducted in the mid-1980s, Kilmann, Boland, Norton, and Caid (1986) reported that problems of desire required the greatest number of treatment sessions compared to other sexual dysfunctions, and that successful outcome was achieved in fewer than 50% of cases. We have noted a similar trend in our own outcome statistics (Rosen, Leiblum, & Hall, 1987). In the present volume, Levine (Chapter 5) and Lief (Chapter 6) report mixed results following long-term, intensive treatment, whereas more positive results are reported by Apfelbaum (Chapter 1), Arnold A. Lazarus (Chapter 4), Pridal and LoPiccolo (Chapter 7), and Beck (Chapter 2).

Treatment outcome is similarly uncertain in cases of hyperactive desire or sexual compulsion. In fact, there are no adequately controlled treatment outcome studies to date in this area. It is noteworthy that two of the four chapters on sexual addiction or compulsion in the present volume (Nathan, Chapter 20; Wincze, Chapter 22) reported negative outcomes, despite heroic efforts on the part of the therapists to engage their clients in the treatment process. More positive outcomes are reported in the case studies by Coleman (Chapter 19, this volume) and by Risen and Althof (Chapter 21, this volume), although extensive therapy contact was required in both instances.

In the area of male erectile disorder, surprisingly few controlled outcome studies have evaluated the efficacy or outcome of sex therapy treatment alone (Rosen et al., 1994; Schover & Leiblum, 1994). Masters and Johnson (1970), for example, reported an initial failure rate of 26.3% for couples undergoing conjoint sex therapy for secondary erectile failure, with an additional 5-year relapse rate of 11%. Results for men with primary erectile dysfunction were less encouraging, however, and it is noteworthy that no data were presented for cases involving organic erectile difficulties.

More recently, Hawton, Catalan, and Fagg (1992) evaluated treatment outcome in 36 couples seeking sex therapy because of the male partner's complaint of erectile dysfunction. All subjects were screened for a history of organic causes, and treatment consisted of approximately 12 sessions of sensate focus and graduated sexual stimulation techniques. Complete resolution of the erectile difficulty was achieved in 42% of cases, and a further 28% showed marked improvement with treatment. Thirty percent of couples showed little or no change. At 3-month follow-up, the proportion of couples with positive outcome had declined to 56%, although nine couples were unavailable for follow-up assessment. The quality of the couple's relationship and the degree of sexual receptivity of the partner were major predictors of outcome in this and other studies (see Leiblum & Rosen, 1991).

Among the chapters in the present book that focus on couple issues, Lazarus (Chapter 4) takes the position that relatively brief interventions or "carburetor adjustments" are sometimes called for. Certainly, it is both cost-effective and gratifying when such interventions are effective. In most instances, however, more intensive or longer-term therapy appears necessary. For example, Zilbergeld (Chapter 18, this volume) describes a case in which couple communication is lacking, and the female partner actively sabotages therapy via her critical and domineering attitude toward her spouse. Moderate improvement is ultimately achieved, although the case raises questions concerning the efficacy of conventional sex therapy techniques in such situations. In our experience, many sex therapy failures are associated with chronic or unresolved relationship issues, as illustrated most clearly in the case presented by Wincze (Chapter 22, this volume).

Female arousal and penetration difficulties (i.e., dyspareunia and vaginismus) are generally associated with positive therapy outcome (Hawton et al., 1986; Wincze & Carey, 1991). A broad array of treatment interventions may be required, however, as illustrated in this volume in the cases presented by Heiman (Chapter 12), Carol L. Lassen (Chapter 13), and Sandra R. Leiblum (Chapter 14). These cases also illustrate the wide variety of treatment issues and obstacles encountered in treating sexual disorders in women. These issues include, but are are not restricted to, a history of physical or sexual abuse, long-standing body image and self-esteem problems, religious orthodoxy, and sexual inhibitions and conflicts. As in the treatment of male erectile disorder, the quality of the partner relationship is a critical determinant of treatment outcome (Hawton, 1992; Leiblum, Pervin, & Campbell, 1989).

THE SOCIAL CONTEXT OF SEX THERAPY

The role of social and cultural factors in the definition, diagnosis, and treatment of sexual dysfunctions cannot be overstated. Societal mores constantly shape and influence our notions of sexual normality, as well as determining the goals and objectives of sexual interaction. At a professional level, the practice of sex therapy has been greatly influenced in recent years by the prevailing zeitgeist in other areas of medicine and psychology (Tiefer, 1994). This trend is clearly apparent, for example, in the current emphasis on sexual addiction or compulsion as the "sexual disorder of the 1990s." Despite the lack of diagnostic criteria or etiological models, increasing numbers of individuals are referred for pharmacological therapy (e.g., serotonin reuptake inhibitors) or 12-step group treatment approaches (Coleman, 1991).

The ever-present specter of AIDS has similarly shaped personal and professional behavior in innumerable ways. Both homosexual and heterosexual behavior patterns have been affected, as sexual choices and practices take on new meanings and significance. Writing earlier about "sex therapy in the age of AIDS" (Leiblum & Rosen, 1989), we noted the difficulty for professionals in balancing positive attitudinal messages about sexuality, as is traditionally the goal of sex therapy and education, with the current emphasis on sexual caution and concern. New ethical dilemmas have been raised as, for example, clients engage in unsafe sexual practices without the knowledge of a spouse or sexual partner. This issue is particularly salient in dealing with the sexually addictive or hypersexual individual, as in the case study presented by Nathan (Chapter 20, this volume).

Among the public at large, a more cautious attitude toward sexual exchange and experimentation has evolved over the past two decades (Laumann, Gagnon, Michael, & Michaels, 1994). In particular, rates of premarital and extramarital sex have shown a marked decline as couples strive increasingly to maintain sexual comfort and compatibility in long-term, committed relationships. Sexual experimentation, "open marriages," and "swinging singles" have all but disappeared from the contemporary sexual scene. This trend is apparent despite the continuing bombardment of sexual themes and images in the popular media. Not surprisingly, self-regulation of sexual behavior in this environment remains complex and problematic for many individuals.

In keeping with the conservative trend in society at large, the practice of sex therapy has become distinctly less risky or flamboyant in recent years. Several examples could be cited, including the virtual disappearance of "body sex therapists" or sex surrogates from routine clinical practice. In fact, none of the authors in the present volume even consider this option in the cases presented. Although arguments can still be made for the use of sexual surrogates in certain situations, there is a strong trend away from the use of this intervention. Similarly, we have noted a marked decline in the use of explicit visual erotica, sexual attitude reassessment programs, and sexual "risk-taking" assignments in the routine practice of sex therapy.

In contrast, given the strong societal emphasis on monogamy and long-term commitments in both heterosexual and homosexual relationships, it is hardly surprising that couple therapy and marital enhancement approaches are increasingly pivotal in the practice of sex therapy. We have commented extensively on the need for greater synthesis of couple and sex therapy interventions, particularly in the areas of male erectile disorder and HSD (Leiblum & Rosen, 1991; Rosen et al., 1994). Relationship dynamics are so often crucial to the genesis and maintenance of sexual difficulties, as power struggles, betrayals of trust, waning sexual chemistry, role conflicts, and intimacy problems are encountered. Similarly, relationship distress is among the most frequent sequelae of sexual dysfunction, as the strain of sexual incompatibility takes a major toll on the couple relationship. In this context, interpersonal and systemic approaches to treatment are likely to remain at the forefront of the field.

Finally, the clinical practice of sex therapy is being influenced increasingly by the changing health care climate in the United States, and the growing trend toward managed care and cost-containment measures in particular. Although limited coverage is still available in most plans for short-term treatment of sexual disorders, the limits and restrictions on reimbursement are real issues for the practicing clinician. As with all forms of individual or couple therapy, brief, symptom-focused treatment has become mandatory in many plans. Increased accountability and third-party monitoring of all client contacts is rapidly becoming the rule rather than the exception. On the other hand, less attention is being given to the intrinsic quality or appropriateness of treatment services. Clearly, these factors will have a major impact on the practice of sex therapy in the years to come.

REFERENCES

Althof, S. E., Levine, S. B., Corty, E., Risen, C., & Stern, E. (1994, March). *The role of clomipramine in the treatment of premature ejaculation.* Paper presented at the 19th annual meeting of the Society for Sex Therapy and Research, Atlanta.

Althof, S. E., & Turner, L. A. (1992). Self-injection therapy and external vacuum devices in the treatment of erectile dysfunction: Methods and outcome. In R. C. Rosen & S. R. Leiblum (Eds.), *Erectile disorders: Assessment and treatment* (pp. 283–312). New York: Guilford Press.

Althof, S. E., Turner, L. A., Levine, S. B., Risen, C., Kursh, E., Bodner, D., & Resnick, M. (1991). Long-term use of self-injection therapy of papaverine and phentolamine. *Journal of Sex and Marital Therapy, 17,* 101–112.

American Psychiatric Association. (1987). *Diagnostic and statistical manual of mental disorders* (3rd ed., rev.). Washington, DC: Author.

American Psychiatric Association. (1994). *Diagnostic and statistical manual of mental disorders* (4th ed.). Washington, DC: Author.

Assalian, P. (1988). Clomipramine in the treatment of premature ejaculation. *Journal of Sex Research, 24,* 213–215.

Assalian, P. (1994). Premature ejaculation: Is it really psychogenic? *Journal of Sex Education and Therapy, 20,* 1–4.

Bancroft, J. (1989). Man and his penis: A relationship under stress. *Journal of psychology and human sexuality, 2,* 7–32.

Barbach, L. (1975). *For yourself: The fulfillment of female sexuality.* New York: Doubleday.

Becker, J. (1994, June 26). *The new Victorianism.* Paper presented at the annual meeting of the International Academy of Sex Research, Edinburgh, Scotland.

Bitran, D., & Hull, E. M. (1987). Pharmacological analysis of male rate sexual behavior. *Neuroscience and Biobehavioral Review, 11,* 365–389.

Brindley, G. S. (1983). Cavernosal alpha-blockade: A new technique for investigating and treating erectile impotence. *British Journal of Psychiatry, 143,* 332–337.

Coleman, E. (1991). Compulsive sexual behavior: New concepts and treatment. *Journal of Psychology and Human Sexuality, 3,* 37–52.

Crowe, M. J., Gillan, P., & Golombok, S. (1981). Form and content in the conjoint treatment of sexual dysfunction: A controlled study. *Behaviour Research and Therapy, 19,* 47–51.

Donahey, K. M., & Carroll, R. A. (1993). Gender differences in factors associated with hypoactive sexual desire. *Journal of Sex and Marital Therapy, 19,* 25–40.

Everitt, B. J., & Bancroft, J. (1991). Of rats and men: The comparative approach to male sexuality. *Annual Review of Sex Research, 2,* 77–117.

Feldman, H. A., Goldstein, I., Hatzichristou, G., Krane, R. J., & McKinlay, J. B. (1994). Impotence and its medical and psychosocial correlates: Results of the Massachusetts Male Aging Study. *Journal of Urology, 151,* 54–61.

Hawton, K. (1992). Sex therapy research: Has it withered on the vine? *Annual Review of Sex Research, 3,* 49–72.

Hawton, K., Catalan, J., & Fagg, J. (1991). Low sexual desire: Sex therapy results and prognostic factors. *Behaviour Research and Therapy, 29,* 217–224.

Hawton, K., Catalan, J., & Fagg, J. (1992). Sex therapy for erectile dysfunction: Characteristics of couples, treatment outcome, and prognostic factors. *Archives of Sexual Behavior, 21,* 161–176.

Hawton, K., Catalan, J., Martin, P., & Fagg, J. (1986). Long-term outcome of sex therapy. *Behaviour Research and Therapy, 24,* 665–675.

Heiman, J. R., LoPiccolo, L., & LoPiccolo, J. (1976). *Becoming orgasmic: A sexual growth program for women.* Englewood Cliffs, NJ: Prentice Hall.

Heiman, J. R., LoPiccolo, L., & LoPiccolo, J. (1988). *Becoming orgasmic: A sexual and personal growth program for women* (rev. ed.). Englewood Cliffs, NJ: Prentice Hall.

Kaplan, H. S. (1977). Hypoactive sexual desire. *Journal of Sex and Marital Therapy, 3,* 3–9.

Kilmann, P. R., Boland J. P., Norton, S. C., & Caid, C. (1986). Perspectives on sex therapy outcome: A survey of AASECT providers. *Journal of Sex and Marital Therapy, 12,* 116–138.

Laumann, E. D., Gagnon, J. H., Michael, R. T., & Michaels, S. (1994). *The social organization of sexuality.* Chicago: University of Chicago Press.

Leiblum, S. R., & Pervin, L. A. (Eds.). (1980). *Principles and practice of sex therapy* (1st ed.). New York: Guilford Press.

Leiblum, S. R., Pervin, L. A., & Campbell, E. H. (1989). The treatment of vaginismus: Success and failure. In S. R. Leiblum & R. C. Rosen (Eds.), *Principles and practice of sex therapy* (2nd ed.): *Update for the 1990s* (pp. 113–140). New York: Guilford Press.

Leiblum, S. R., & Rosen, R. C. (Eds.). (1988). *Sexual desire disorders.* New York: Guilford Press.

Leiblum, S. R., & Rosen, R. C. (Eds.). (1989). *Principles and practice of sex therapy* (2nd ed.): *Update for the 1990s.* New York: Guilford Press.

Leiblum, S. R., & Rosen, R. (1991). Couples therapy for erectile disorders: Conceptual and clinical considerations. *Journal of Sex and Marital Therapy*, *17*, 2, 147–159.

Lief, H. (1977). Inhibited sexual desire. *Medical Aspects of Human Sexuality*, *7*, 94–95.

LoPiccolo, J. (1992). Postmodern sex therapy for erectile failure. In R. C. Rosen & S. R. Leiblum (Eds.), *Erectile disorders: Assessment and treatment* (pp. 171–197). New York: Guilford Press.

Lue, T., Hricak, M., & Tanagho, E. (1985). Vasculogenic impotence evaluation by high-resolution ultrasonograph and pulsed doppler spectrum analysis. *Radiology*, *155*, 777–781.

Masters, W. H., & Johnson, V. E. (1966). *Human sexual response*. Boston: Little, Brown.

Masters, W. H., & Johnson, V. E. (1970). *Human sexual inadequacy*. Boston: Little, Brown.

Michal, V. (1982). Arterial disease as a cause of impotence. *Clinics in Endocrinology and Metabolism*, *11*, 725–748.

Nathan, S. (1986). The epidemiology of the DSMIII psychosexual dysfunctions. *Journal of Sex and Marital Therapy*, *12*, 267–281.

Okami, P. (1992). Child perpetrators of sexual abuse: The emergence of a problematic deviant category. *Journal of Sex Research*, *29*, 1, 109–130.

Rosen, R. C. (1991). Alcohol and drug effects on sexual response: Human experimental and clinical studies. *Annual Review of Sex Research*, *2*, 119–179.

Rosen, R. C., & Ashton, A. (1993). Prosexual drugs: Empirical status of the "new aphrodisiacs." *Archives of Sexual Behavior*, *22*, 6.

Rosen, R. C., & Leiblum, S. R. (Eds.). (1992). *Erectile disorders: Assessment and treatment*, New York: Guilford Press.

Rosen, R. C., & Leiblum, S. R. (1995). Hypoactive sexual desire. *Psychiatric Clinics of North America*, *18*, 107–121.

Rosen, R. C., Leiblum, S. R., & Hall, K. S. (1987). *Etiological and predictive factors in sex therapy*. Paper presented at the annual meeting of the Society for Sex Therapy and Research, New Orleans.

Rosen, R. C., Leiblum, S. R., & Spector, I. (1994). Psychologically-based treatment for male erectile disorder: A cognitive-interpersonal model. *Journal of Sex and Marital Therapy*, *20*, 67–85.

Schover, L. R., & Leiblum, S. R. (1994). The stagnation of sex therapy. *Journal of Psychology and Human Sexuality*, *6*, 5–30.

Segraves, R., Saran, K., Segraves, K., & Maguire, E. (1993). Clomipramine versus placebo in the treatment of premature ejaculation: A pilot study. *Journal of Sex and Marital Therapy*, *3*, 198–200.

Tiefer, L. (1994). Three crises facing sexology. *Archives of Sexual Behavior*, *23*, 361–374.

Virag, R., Fryden, D., Legmans, M., & Virag, H. (1984). Intracavernous injection of paperverine as a diagnostic and therapeutic method in erectile failure. *Angiology*, *35*, 79–87.

Wagner, G., & Kaplan, H. S. (1993). *The new injection treatment for impotence: Medical and psychological aspects*. New York: Brunner/Mazel.

Wincze, J. P., & Carey, M. P. (1991). *Sexual dysfunction: A guide for assessment and treatment*. New York: Guilford Press.

Zilbergeld, B. (1978). *Male sexuality*. Boston: Little, Brown.

Zimmer, D. (1987). Does marital therapy enhance the effectiveness of treatment for sexual dysfunction? *Journal of Sex and Marital Therapy, 13,* 193–209.

PART I

Sexual Desire Disorders

Sexual desire disorders are among the most prevalent and challenging problems encountered in current sex therapy. Low sexual desire, in particular, occurs frequently in both men and women, older and younger individuals, and heterosexual and homosexual couples and may present as either the primary sexual complaint or secondary to another sexual dysfunction (e.g., male erectile disorder or female orgasmic dysfunction). Disagreement exists concerning the definition and diagnosis of hypoactive sexual desire (HSD), and recent research has implicated a wide variety of intrapsychic, interpersonal, and biological factors in the etiology of low desire. In the arena of treatment, there is a growing trend toward the use of cognitive-behavioral and systems–interactional approaches. Recently, pharmacological and hormonal interventions have also been explored. As we have noted, there is an unfortunate lack of treatment process or controlled outcome research in this important area (Rosen & Leiblum, 1995).

Given the frequency and significance of desire disorders in contemporary sex therapy, the first major section of the current volume is devoted entirely to this topic. The case studies presented offer an intriguing array of theoretical perspectives, clinical formulations, and treatment interventions. Certain commonalities are apparent, such as the prevalence of sexual abuse or early trauma as an etiological determinant. In Barry W. McCarthy's case (Chapter 8), for example, the low-desire husband shamefully reveals his early abuse at the hands of his mother's lover. Similarly, in Helen Singer Kaplan's case of the phobic virgin (Chapter 3), the patient was sexually abused at an early age by an elderly neighbor. Sexual relations occurred with a former therapist in the case presented by Arnold A. Lazarus (Chapter 4), and Cathryn G. Pridal and Joseph

LoPiccolo (Chapter 7) describe the shame and embarrassment associated with early sibling incest. While some therapists may overemphasize the role of early sexual abuse, according to McCarthy, it is striking how commonly such experiences are reported.

A history of depression is another frequent concomitant of low desire in both men and women (Donahey & Carroll, 1993; Schreiner-Engel & Schiavi, 1986). In fact, dysphoric mood is often present in both the identified patient and his/her sexual partner, as either the cause or the effect of reduced sexual intimacy in the relationship. Several cases in this volume illustrate the complex relationship between low desire and mood disorder. For example, the wife with inhibited desire in J. Gayle Beck's case (Chapter 2) is described as clinically depressed, as is the high-desire husband in the case by Pridal and LoPiccolo. Depression is a significant feature of Kaplan's description of the phobic virgin. Given the prevalence of mood disorders in these cases, it is not surprising that psychotropic medication is a frequent concomitant to therapy (Rosen & Leiblum, 1995). Psychotropic drugs are used adjunctively in the chapters by Stephen B. Levine (Chapter 5), Lazarus, Pridal and LoPiccolo, and Harold I. Lief (Chapter 6). A problem with the use of antidepressants, however, is that while affect and well-being may be improved, additional difficulties with sexual arousal and orgasm are frequently encountered (Rosen, 1991).

Several authors have noted the importance of intimacy or relationship difficulties in both sexual apathy and desire discrepancy problems. It is not uncommon in these cases for inadequate desire to serve as a mask or barrier for underlying relationship conflicts (Verhulst & Heiman, 1988). Similarly, individuals with inhibited or excessive desire are frequently handicapped by their inability to feel safe or secure in an intimate relationship and may use sex to avoid intimacy, or as a way of creating "pseudointimacy." This process is apparent in the cases presented in this volume by Bernard Apfelbaum (Chapter 1), Pridal and LoPiccolo, Beck, and Lazarus. Special intimacy concerns are apparent in lesbian or homosexual couples, as discussed by Margaret Nichols (Chapter 9).

Despite the variety of treatment interventions employed, certain common themes are evident. First, most therapists employ a flexible and individualistic approach to the scheduling and format of treatment sessions. Individual and couple therapy approaches are frequently combined, and most therapists make liberal use of bibliotherapy, couple communication training, and other psychoeducational interventions. Structured sex therapy assignments, such as sensate focus, are used less routinely nowadays, although Apfelbaum argues that these assignments are most useful in revealing the underlying resistances or "response anxiety" of the client. Finally, more traditional psychodynamic approaches are often employed, along with couple therapy and/or cognitive-behavioral interventions.

Overall, these chapters offer a fascinating and informative perspective on current treatment approaches to sexual desire disorders. Among the distinguished authors in this section are Kaplan and Lief, who independently identified HSD as a separate and discrete clinical entity. It is interesting to note how their clinical formulations and treatment interventions have evolved over the past 20 years. Psychodynamic and ego-analytical perspectives on low desire are provided by Levine and Apfelbaum, respectively, and the cognitive-behavioral and systems approaches are strongly represented in the chapters by Lazarus, Pridal and LoPiccolo, Beck, and McCarthy. The dynamics of sexual avoidance are illustrated in the case vignettes by Domeena C. Renshaw (Chapter 10), and the specific issues of low desire in the lesbian couple are clearly portrayed by Nichols. In short, these chapters provide a broad array of clinical perspectives on this common sexual complaint.

REFERENCES

Donahey, K. M., & Carroll, R. A. (1993). Gender differences in factors associated with hypoactive sexual desire. *Journal of Sex and Marital Therapy*, *19*, 25–40.

Rosen, R. C. (1991). Alcohol and drug effects on sexual response: Human experimental and clinical studies. *Annual Review of Sex Research*, *2*, 119–179.

Rosen, R. C., & Leiblum, S. R. (1995). Hypoactive sexual desire. *Psychiatric Clinics of North America*, *18*, 107–121.

Schreiner-Engel, P., & Schiavi, R. C. (1986). Lifetime psychopathology in individuals with low sexual desire. *Journal of Nervous and Mental Disease*, *174*, 646–651.

Verhulst, J., & Heiman, J. R. (1988). A systems perspective on sex sexual desire. In S. R. Leiblum & R. C. Rosen (Eds.), *Sexual desire disorders* (pp. 243–267). New York: Guilford Press.

I

Masters and Johnson Revisited: A Case of Desire Disparity

BERNARD APFELBAUM

INTRODUCTION

Although it has not been said outright, most authorities in the field think of Masters and Johnson's therapy as an exercise in futility. Their therapy is believed to rest largely on the effect of the sensate focus assignments, and it is thought that, as Witkin (1982) put it, "sensate focus is intended primarily to acquaint the couple with his (her) own and the partner's specific sensual likes and dislikes" (p. 112). When this simple intervention fails, as it usually does, the general view is that we must go beyond Masters and Johnson.

Most sex therapists say that they base their therapy on Masters and Johnson's work, but what is thought of as the MJI (Masters and Johnson Institute) approach has been assimilated to whatever model a sex therapist uses and may even then be considered an inadequate version of that model (Apfelbaum, 1985).

Witkin (1982) contends that the MJI assignments make it "relatively easy to avoid relating to the other [partner] in a spontaneous way" (p. 112). She recommends the "intimate shower," in which partners are forced to confront their resistances to intimacy.

Witkin here reflects the widespread objection to the Masters and Johnson assignments—that they block spontaneity. Ironically, this is precisely their objective. The fact that this is not generally known arises from Masters and Johnson's way of presenting their work. Outside of participation in their full-time training program or attendance at their training seminars there is no way to become familiar with many of the essentials of their model, a novel and perhaps questionable method of presentation in a scientific field. As a consequence, Masters and Johnson's contribution has been evaluated, even by their peers, on the basis of a reading of *Human Sexual Inadequacy* (1970), in which much of the presentation is limited to the assignments, and even the rationale for the assignments is given only the most limited coverage.

Not only has their model yet to be completely presented in published form, its deceptive simplicity has made it seem limited at best. This is a crucial misunderstanding. Masters and Johnson's therapy is a revolutionary departure, even from subsequently established approaches that are thought to be based on it and simply to go beyond it.

THE COMPULSIONS OF NORMAL SEXUALITY

Masters and Johnson's success rates launched the field of sex therapy as we now know it. Other therapists, expecting similar results from the sensate focus assignments alone, have popularized the explanation that given such a simple therapy, Masters and Johnson's patients must have had simple problems.

Kaplan (1979) revised Masters and Johnson's success rates from very high to very low, reporting a 10–15% success rate for Masters and Johnson's therapy as applied to cases of severe impotence and hypoactive sexual desire (HSD), hardly better than would be expected from waiting-list controls. This assessment was based not on data from the MJI (R. C. Kolodny, personal communication,September 1981) but on Kaplan's own and her staff's application of Masters and Johnson's therapy (M. A. Perelman, personal communication, March 1983). This is an instructive case in point because what Kaplan thought of as applying MJI therapy consisted simply of giving the sensate focus assignments, reflecting the belief that their assignments *are* the therapy.

Kaplan's data, apparently gathered informally from staff members' overall impressions, are what is to be expected from the application of the assignments alone. However, within the context of the Masters and Johnson approach, the sensate focus exercises cannot fail, or at least when they fail they also succeed—succeed, that is, in pinpointing performance anxiety and the compulsions it generates.

The complaint that Masters and Johnson's sensate focus assignments are too methodical, stifling spontaneity, epitomizes how elusive their insight has proved to be. The point of taking strict turns at being active and passive, and of not touching back when stroked, is that the compulsion to reciprocate is blocked. The pressure to reciprocate is one of the major compulsions of normal sexuality that Masters and Johnson (1970) identified ("rushing to return the favor"; p. 73). It is a much more subtle and pervasive example of performance pressure than is the fear of failure. Perhaps the profound effects of performance anxiety would be better grasped if it was called response anxiety (Apfelbaum, 1977b).

It might be easier to grasp the significance of the Masters and Johnson intervention if the pressure to respond is kept in mind. It might then also become clear that performance or response anxiety is, ultimately, bound by the compulsion to respond positively in sex. It is *this* pressure that pontentiates the pathogenic effect of anything other than an agreeable, encouraging, and good-natured response in sex. That is, this pressure makes it threatening not to have an upbeat, positive response to sex.

If we do not grasp this perspective, the sensate focus assignments can seem unnecessarily methodical, rule-bound, and restrictive. But it is significant that this kind of intervention can succeed *at all*. It was a startling discovery that, in the absence of instruction in erotic technique or any effort to create an erotic environment, and even by blocking spontaneity, symptoms of long standing can be reversed. The point is that the assignments block the way people spontaneously act in sex, which is compulsively driven, thereby making actual spontaneity possible.

What makes this revolutionary insight obscure is the fact that when sexual rituals are blocked, people typically experience the anxiety that has been ritually bound. They become all the more exposed to response anxiety and the fear of failure. The "failure" of the assignments makes it possible for the therapist to show patients their urgent need to respond positively, and therefore how threatened they are by anything that impairs that ability. The job of the therapist is to help patients deritualize their sexuality by including "turned-off" states of various kinds (Apfelbaum, 1984a, 1988, 1989).

INTENSIFYING PERFORMANCE PRESSURE

The downside of the sexual revolution has been a virtual epidemic of response anxiety. It is now as if being good in bed is what sex is all about. If the intensity of this pressure is not appreciated, the "failure" of the assignments can look like simple resistance. The fear of not being aroused then looks like a *resistance* to being aroused. As I pointed out in a review of *Disorders of Sexual Desire*:

Kaplan asserts that in all but the simplest cases Masters and Johnson's strategy of nondemand pleasuring and the avoidance of goal directedness is likely to fail because, underneath, the person "does not want to" perform. . . .

By declaring performance anxiety to be a cover for the wish to fail sexually and by insisting on successful performance and advocating working at sex, Kaplan has reversed all the essentials of Masters and Johnson's thinking. (Apfelbaum, 1981, p. 183)

Thus, when the presumed "Masters and Johnson therapy," meaning the assignments alone (plus giving information), does not work, a therapist is liable to conclude that the couple must be resisting or must have a dynamic investment in being symptomatic: a need to fail, to thwart the partner, to avoid intimacy, pleasure, or success. These are the classical *pre*-Masters and Johnson interpretations that non-sex therapists have applied to failures to fit the standard sexual script.

It is as if the assignments have been taken as a new sexual script, which is merely a variant of the standard one. If patients are unable to give up their original goal orientation to meet the new goal of not being goal oriented, the therapist appeals to the old psychodynamic paradigm. Bringing back the old paradigm has been thought of as "going beyond Masters and Johnson," thereby creating a new synthesis. Hence, Kaplan calls her approach "*psycho*sexual" or even the "new" sex therapy, and LoPiccolo calls his model "*post*modern."

The revival of these classical interpretations, albeit in a new guise, has justified reversing the Masters and Johnson strategy, that is, *intensifying* the pressure to perform. As in Kaplan's approach, the patient is aggressively confronted with the threat of failure (e.g., the loss of the relationship) and his/her presumed responsibility for it. As other exhortative therapies (rational–emotive therapy, Gestalt, est, Synanon) have demonstrated, authoritative reinforcement of self-blame can generate symptom relief. Also, performance anxiety typically does lead to performance rather than performance failure (Apfelbaum, 1977a, 1977b), and may even be seen as a primary motive for sex among normals if the Masters and Johnson breakthrough is properly understood.

My impression is that intensifying the pressure to perform is likely to require lengthy treatment and also is likely to be ineffective with desire problems. These expectations are borne out by Kaplan (1979; see also Apfelbaum, 1981).

The following case is an illustration of how easily other issues can obscure the causal role of response anxiety, the result being, in effect, a regression to more standard treatment modes and interventions, with the loss of the opportunity for a rapid, restorative, and ultimately *sexual* solution to the problem.

A CASE OF DESIRE DISPARITY

This case was noteworthy for its temptations to distract both the clinician and the patients themselves from the frontier of the problem: performance (response) anxiety.

First Hour

Jack, 48, had been a rapid ejaculator in his previous 6-year marriage. With Jane, 32, his present wife of 12 years, he had little difficulty with ejaculatory control. Unlike his first wife, Jane complied with his wish for light bondage and to have her wear lingerie. She had had no coital experience prior to Jack and had been apprehensive about her readiness to respond sexually. What worried her was the effect of sexual abuse at age 5 (she offered no further details of this experience), as well as her Catholic upbringing.

Jane was in concurrent once-weekly individual therapy and had been continuously for the previous 6 years. Her presenting complaint was rushes of fear that she sometimes experienced when Jack approached her sexually. She reported that she had been able to explore the feelings generated by the abuse but, as she put it, "I'm still not able to let go of the fear." Given her continuing distress, her therapist made the referral to couple sex therapy.

After the first 8 years of their sexual relationship, Jane refused to wear lingerie or agree to bondage. Since that time, Jack's earlier difficulty with ejaculatory control had not recurred but his desire waned and their frequency declined from three times a month to once a month or less. Jack also experienced a lowered level of excitement when they did have sex, both subjectively and as evidenced by intermittent erectile insufficiency.

Jack reported that although he now felt little interest in sex with his wife (or in general), from the beginning of the relationship he had felt dissatisfied, and that he typically felt he had to "beg" for sex.

At the end of the first session I explained that during the first 8 years Jack had been able to bypass Jane's apathy by using the fantasies (about her) that the bondage and lingerie could inspire. Being immersed in these fantasies made it possible for Jack to overlook his resentment at having to "beg" for sex and also to overlook both Jane's relative detachment and her apprehensiveness. This allowed Jack to enjoy sex more fully than ever before, and also relieved Jane of the worry that she would wreck their sexual relationship.

Jane acknowledged that it was only after she refused to go along with the lingerie and bondage ritual that she felt the rushes of fear. She added that it was only at her individual therapist's recommendation that she refused to engage in this behavior, although she could not now imagine resuming it.

I also said that Jack's complaint that he had to beg for sex was both an expression of feeling humiliated about feeling sexually unwanted and an implicit accusation of Jane, implying that she was withholding. Jane responded with relief that she felt Jack saw her as withholding. Jack freely admitted that he often did think Jane was punishing him. I said that it is almost universally true that the high-desire partner feels punished, and many therapists even believe that the low-desire partner has a motive to punish. Nevertheless, this impression is more apparent than real, and it looked as if rather than being withholding, Jane was trying too hard to suppress her fear and to be a good sport.

I told Jack and Jane that if they decided to continue, the approach to this problem would be to give them written stroking assignments and have them write reports on these assignments to be read aloud at the following session. Both the use of written instructions and the requirement of written reports are, as far as I know, unique to our center, reflecting our interest in discovering what the patient actually is responding to. Because the assignments are to be done three times, and as they take about 1 hour to do and a half hour to write up, I suggested that we allow 3 weeks to 1 month before the next visit, given their busy schedules.

This ended the first hour. In most cases, one session is sufficient to analyze the problem to this level. I think of this as a "functional" first hour, as contrasted with a focus on data gathering. Given this approach, there is no time for a diagnostic assessment, history taking, separate interviews with the partners, or other more leisurely carryovers from clinics and training centers.

My guiding assumption is that unpacking the problem is the "royal road" to the solution, and that it is easy to get sidetracked by irrelevancies, and thus to risk punching through the surface of the problem, and then get caught up in the common denominator of underlying psychopathology present in everyone.

Second Hour

When they returned in 3 weeks, Jack and Jane had not done the assignment, and both reported feeling guilty about and responsible for this. I explained that everyone feels that way about not doing assignments and nothing can be done about these feelings; they just seem to be a built-in reaction.

Nonetheless, their sexual frequency had gone up. They had attempted coital sex six times. Five had been initiated by Jane; the reason she gave was that she did not want to be seen as withholding. On four of these occasions Jack's excitement faded, as did his erection. He said that the problem for him was that "she chose the time and place."

Jane then said that she felt self-conscious about her small breasts, and that she had always felt that Jack found her physically unappealing. Jack agreed that he had teased her about her breasts and hips, arguing that he had no control over what turned him on, just as he had no control over his need for lingerie and bondage.

I agreed with Jack that he had no control over what excited him, and that his sexuality was just as automatic as it felt, but his having to fall back on automatic turn-ons was part of the problem. When one's focus turns to sexual marginalia, this means that more emotional, intimate, or spiritual turn-ons are lacking. My point was that body turn-ons are ways of bypassing the more personal side of sex. I could have added, although I did not in this case, that for most of us, sex *is* bypassing: a way of creating intimacy while also avoiding it.

Interrogating Jack made it possible to reconstruct his turn-on more specifically: It looked as if Jack had felt rejected by Jane's sexual apprehensiveness, and he had solved the problem, to the relief of both of them, by looking for a way to get turned on to Jane's body—that is, to bypass any more direct emotional connection with her. This made it especially frustrating to Jack when he had to notice aspects of Jane's body that did not appeal to him. He then solved *that* probem by having Jane wear lingerie, thereby creating an image of her as sexy and lustful. Bondage helped in that he could imagine that he was preventing Jane from punishing him and that he was overcoming her resistance to sex. Bondage also helped in that by pinning Jane's arms, Jack could think of her limited participation (limited reciprocation) as his doing rather than hers and so feel less rejected by it.

Jack's complaint that he had lost interest several times in the past 3 weeks because Jane chose the time and place may have been a reflection of feeling rushed by Jane's determination to prove she was not withholding but also may have reflected Jack's belief that it should nevertheless be exciting as Jane now was seemingly being forthcoming in just the way he had always wanted.

Jane's initiatives may have made it difficult for Jack to get his mind in gear in the way he needed to in order to sustain his excitement independently of her. It was as if Jane was interfering with the sexual relationship Jack was having with her.

Jane confirmed that although wearing lingerie was embarrassing (because she did not feel at all like a vamp), being pinned did relieve her of the pressure to be active and reciprocating.

I explained that that made good sense, and that the Masters and Johnson assignments employed a kind of bondage in that when in the passive role, partners were enjoined not to reciprocate. When this enforced passivity did not trigger anxieties, it could free people to more fully experience being caressed.

I also said that Jack and Jane were caught in a familiar circularity: Jack felt rejected by Jane's apprehensiveness and then had to bypass her in order to get turned on. Jane felt somewhat relieved by Jack's autonomous style but still felt sexually inadequate with him. This made her feel cold, as did Jack's jibes about her body and his "begging." The colder she felt, the more Jack had to turn *himself* on, using her only as a prop.

Jack acknowledged that this analysis seemed accurate. However, what he meant about Jane choosing the time and place was that she made sex into a power struggle. Jack explained that Jane's father had been a bully and a tyrant; consequently, Jane did not want to submit to Jack's sexual approaches. Jack thought this was why Jane seemed reluctant to do the assignments.

Jane said that her reluctance was a reaction to Jack's saying, "When are we going to do our little assignments?" "Little" to her meant that he trivialized the problem, possibly viewing it as a simple case of her being sexually uptight and needing special education.

I agreed that obviously they *were* in a power struggle—it could hardly be otherwise. They were each unwilling to be the one who had to *react* to the other's initiative. I pointed out that the pursuer is likely to pursue when in a state of readiness, although this might find the pursued in a state of unreadiness. I added that it would, of course, be easier if either one of them could say at such times that he/she was not ready or was not into it, but that in most cases it is not safe to say such things.

This was the end of the second hour. Already a number of seemingly primary pathogens have been identified: In addition to Jane's abuse experience and oppressive relationship with her father and Jack's paraphilias, there were Jack's hostile jibes, Jane's possible need to punish Jack and/or to resist sex, the power struggle, and their resistance to the assignments. From my perspective, these were secondary rather than primary causes.

These causes are generally seen as primary because they block the ability to respond positively in sex, and it is a given that responding positively is what sex *is*. In my view, following Masters and Johnson, this belief is the primary cause of sex problems.

In Jane's case the pressure to respond positively made her try to suppress or overcome her fear rather than to have it become part of her sexual relationship with Jack. Similarly, Jane felt it necessary to comply with Jack's sexual demands as much as she was able to; when she was unable to, she would withdraw rather than express her concerns.

A common response to this analysis is to argue that lovers are simply unable to tolerate negative feelings and therefore the task of sex therapy is to train people to bypass negative feelings. My answer is that lovers do indeed have this intolerance of negative feelings, and do in fact cope with such feelings by either spontaneous or deliberate bypassing (Apfelbaum & Apfelbaum, 1985). However, many patients are unable to bypass and therefore are screened out as too deeply disturbed to be candidates for sex therapy. Patients who are able but unwilling to bypass are likely to be thought of as resisting, as if they should be willing to make a sacrifice for the good of the relationship.

However, unless the primary cause (i.e., the pressure to respond positively) is the focus of therapy, the risk is that it will be reinforced by going directly to those issues that cause the patient to respond negatively. This focus is likely to precipitate a more intensive and lengthy therapy of the kind that Kaplan (1979) reports. Further, it is my experience that when patients are helped to play out their problems in sex, rather than to bypass them, many seemingly primary pathogens (power struggles, anger, sabotaging, and resistance of all kinds) disappear without having to be directly addressed.

As I see it, couple sex therapy makes possible more effective personality change than can be accomplished in psychotherapy, through deep self-disclosure and what Masters and Johnson call the exchange of vulnerabilties, in the intense intimacy that only sex can create—provided that the sexual relationship is such that vulnerabilities can be expressed and responded to ("counterbypassed") rather than bypassed (Apfelbaum, 1988).

Most couple problems are more effectively solved in the relationship than in therapy, and therefore the goal is to undo impasses and thus to make the *relationship* therapeutic.

Third Hour

Jack and Jane phoned for the third session 2 months later, explaining that they had been on a trip to Europe. Again they had not done the assignment but apparently felt less remiss about it, partly because they both felt that they had had relatively passionate sex three times during the vacation. When interviewing them about this occurrence, it appeared that in exotic locales, Jack found himself seeing Jane as sexy and attractive. She said that this effect may have been partly a consequence of her feeling less wary and distrustful.

However, several times during this period, when Jack attempted to embrace her, Jane felt the rush of fear. She had trouble particularizing it other than to describe a panic reaction, and also to make it clear that her focus was on trying to "let go" of the fear, as she had already indicated. Another part of this reaction pattern was feeling hopeless about ever being able to get over the fear.

Jane was so intent on disqualifying the fear that she had not even considered the obvious question: Was she aware of any differences between the times when she felt the fear and those when she did not? Jane was surprisingly quick to respond that she did not feel it in bed because they typically were not looking at one another, but when she saw Jack's face she was more likely to feel panic. I asked her to review what had been covered about that in her individual therapy and she said that this aspect had not come up.

After a struggle to find the right word, Jane guessed that what she reacted to in Jack's face was his looking "blank." When pressed to elaborate she reacted dismissively and impatiently. It was clear that she felt overextended and did not yet feel entitled to such experiences.

Feeling stung by Jane's characterization, despite its brevity, and as if to justify any way he appeared grim, Jack quickly interjected that Jane was "never" physically demonstrative. In the first session they had both said that it was not unusual for them to hug or to hold hands, although in sleep both kept to their own side of the bed. Now Jack added that when they did touch he "always" made the overtures, and that he might appear blank because he was always uneasy about the kind of reception he would get, especially as Jane always looked so icy and remote.

Jack delivered this defensive response in his seemingly unruffled, genial, and smiling way. His unperturbable bedside manner (he was a family physician) contrasted with her look of fragile hauteur, head tilted slightly back, as if narrowly scrutinizing (although actually coping with chronic anxiety and a low threshold for confusion).

I could have said, but did not, that people usually are shy about eye contact in sex since they may have the wrong expression, may look too serious or too rapacious or unresponsive, etc. Instead, I commented that Jack probably heard Jane to mean that he should not look blank, but he probably was doing the best he could not to look worried or anxious about getting rejected, just as he had done his best to make his sexual style rejection-proof (i.e., autonomous). I added that Jane had, after all, devoted years to trying to overcome her fear, and I did not think the solution was for Jack to look more animated.

Jane was unable in the time remaining in this third hour to discover more about the effect and meaning of Jack's facial expression, and I suggested that she take this up in her weekly individual therapy. I also commented that this sort of reaction is exactly what the assignments were designed to explore.

I said that the immediate cause of the problem was Jane's efforts to solve it, that is, to let go of the fear—to cope with it on her own. She needed to be able to bring the fear into their sexual relationship rather than to exclude it, but she needed words for that—she needed a repertoire of ways to express it. Jane had had a lot of practice at suppressing the fear and no practice at expressing it. I added that writing her reports on her experiences in the stroking assignments would help to build such a repertoire.

I pointed out that in most contexts, fear means that you are afraid of something and need reassurance about it; however, sex is like the theater: the last place one would express stage fright is on stage. Sex is easy for people who are able to have positive and encouraging responses, or at least who are able to conjure them up, but any less than positive responses are not only difficult to handle but also threatening because they can so easily be taken as a rejection by one's partner and can make one feel sexually inadequate. Consequently, it would be an accomplishment for Jane to develop the ability to broaden the scope of their sexual relationship. To confide her fears in Jack would have the effect of deepening their level of intimacy.

Fourth Hour

Three weeks later Jack and Jane presented their reports on the two (rather than the assigned three) times they had done the first stroking assignment. Jane said that she had not brought the problem up with her therapist because "we were on an entirely different track." I pointed out that as she could not even think of a way to work it into the conversation with her therapist, it clearly was going to feel counterinstinctual to bring it up in sex.

However, their notes on the first assignment (Appendix 1.1) were sufficiently revealing and unexpectedly graphic for this rather reserved and temporizing couple. First, Jane noted that once she made up her mind to do the assignment, she felt "a lot of resistance, which I thought might be a valuable clue." She meant a clue to her underlying sexual anxiety. At first she had gone along with their customary assumption that she was resistant to sex and that she should not be. But writing a report on her experience gave Jane permission to notice reactions that she had previously disqualified.

Thus, she went on to say that her resistance to the assignment might have been caused by Jack's being "embarrassingly critical" about her body. It also is true that reading the report aloud in the office atmosphere helps patients to own their experiences. The blockbuster in this first report was Jane's description of Jack's touch as "anonymous." Emboldened by her own critique, Jane ad-libbed that Jack's touch "lacked gentleness." She also reported feeling discouraged because Jack seemed to suffer being touched without much pleasure.

Here I took the opportunity to return to Jane's comment in the third hour about Jack's facial expression, the "blankness" that she had then treated as irrelevant. At this point, further questioning revealed that it could make Jack seem impersonal, distant, even sinister.

This dramatic turnaround is not unfamiliar when patients are required to write about their reactions and when there is a heavy emphasis on the actual experiences the patient is having rather than the experiences he/she is supposed to have. Even up to the point of reading what she herself had written, Jane felt that she had failed in the assignment. Only as she read her notes did it dawn on her that her reactions might have some validity. Relying on the implied permission of the assignments, as she read her own notes aloud she found herself making pointed complaints about *Jack's* coldness and suddenly felt vindicated. Jane was confronted with the ways she felt slighted and rebuffed by Jack.

Once a couple reaches a turning point of this kind, I feel that the job has been done, although it will take some time to develop its implications.

For his part, Jack had complaints about Jane, but this was familiar to both of them. He wrote that it disconcerted him that Jane's face was "like stone." He confirmed that he felt rather numb to her touch and that he felt she was just tolerating his touch.

In questioning them about their notes, I discovered that Jack found the assignments to be frustrating. His unresponsiveness to Jane's touch reflected his impatience with pleasuring—which can look like a resistance to pleasure. If that interpretive pitfall is avoided, it emerges as a resistance to vulnerability. Jack did not want to be dependent on Jane's desire to please him. As is true of many men, Jack's sexual style was as invulnerable as he could make it. Pronounced goal directedness is the linchpin of this sexual set.

I explained Jack's impatience on these grounds and further elaborated the rationale for the assignments, saying to Jack that his urge to get to penetration and orgasm reflected a degree of tension and drivenness that limited his level of excitement. Becoming more relaxed might expose him to worries about keeping up his level of arousal and being dependent on Jane's mental state, but it also had the potential to free him to become more aroused than had heretofore been possible.

Making Jack temporarily the identified patient had the predictable effect of further emboldening Jane, as became apparent in the next session.

Fifth Hour

They were to repeat the first assignment twice. The second time Jack initiated, and Jane felt somewhat more relaxed. They each reported feeling a certain degree of unaccustomed warmth. Jane commented that the thorough stroking required by the instructions made her feel more accepted by Jack, although she thought this must be an illusion. Jack disagreed, saying that not having to think about getting turned on made it easier to pay attention to Jane and even to enjoy her body.

They were to return for the sixth hour in 3 weeks, having done the second assignment three times, but for reasons that became apparent in the next session, they canceled and did not return for 4 months.

Sixth Hour

When they did return, they reported that they had done the second assignment soon after the last visit. Apparently hoping to speed things up, they had skipped to the third part of this assignment (Appendix 1.2), which concludes with the active partner doing some extended genital stimulation, manually, using a teasing touch, with a lubricant, Albolene. Jane wrote that it felt as if Jack was doing a pelvic, and she could barely contain her anger.

She found that her tension and anger were growing, although her individual therapist continued to direct these feelings back to their early source. This led to some significant breakthroughs in her relationship to her father but left her with no good way of organizing these feelings in her relationship to her husband.

Although Jane apparently at no time considered dropping out of therapy, she nevertheless coped with her anger by withdrawal, and it was at least 2 months before she could bring herself to do another assignment. She avoided sexual contact entirely, although Jack made some overtures. The significant event occurred at the beginning of the next time they did the assignment. Jane told Jack that she felt tense and angry and was not sure she could go ahead with it. She was braced for what she called a "counterattack" from Jack but it never came. To her astonishment, Jack seemed to become tender and attentive.

Jack reported that when Jane told him she felt tense and angry, it was easy for him to see that she was in acute distress. This seemed to bring out all his caretaking ways. Jack also noticed that Jane's face seemed relaxed for the first time in the assignments, and to *his* astonishment he felt a surge of erotic feeling.

Although they had been advised not to use the assignment as foreplay (i.e., when it was being done for the purpose of reporting on it), this time they went on to penetration on Jack's initiative, and they both described feeling an unfamiliar degree of warmth and intimacy. This was their only coital experience during this 4-month period.

The second time they did this assignment was marked by Jane's feeling that Jack was more responsive to her touch and that he liked, apparently for the first time, how she touched his penis.

At this point it appeared that the assignments had served their purpose, and I wanted to turn the couple's attention to a detailed look at what happens to them in a spontaneous sexual encounter, especially at the beginning. They were to write about it as they would an assignment. This time we agreed to allow 2 weeks, and they returned on the date planned.

Seventh Hour

Jack and Jane had forgotten exactly what they were supposed to do and, as it happened, came up with a better agenda than the one I suggested. Rather than concentrating on one encounter, they did a diaristic account of the 2 weeks. Unexpectedly, they had some kind of sexual contact every day, usually at bedtime. Apparently they had coital sex about half of these times, with orgasm by one or the other two or three times.

Their daily frequency during this 2-week period was generated by Jane's wish to work on overcoming her fear as well as by Jack, who apparently was, not surprisingly, practicing looking more animated, although with no apparent effect on Jane.

The climactic event in this series happened on the third day. Jane felt the panic as Jack approached to embrace her. She called a writing break, as she had practiced doing in the second assignment. Her diary entry indicated that this move took her out of the narrowed-down state that was induced by her panic and the pressure to bypass her panic.

I have sometimes suggested to patients that consciousness tends to narrow in physically intimate encounters. By breaking and avoiding touch, they can invite "staircase wit," that is, the thoughts and feelings that only surface after separating.

Jane's instinct was to meditate on the experience before writing and this induced a reverie in which she flashed back to the abuse experience and especially to the face of her abuser. She was reluctant to elaborate and I did not press her because yielding to the pressure to disclose or relive an abuse experience risks revictimization, much as a rape trial can be worse than the rape.

Jane also recognized that in sex, and in the absence of Jack's otherwise omnipresent geniality, what she now described as Jack's grim, almost resentful expression not only was terrifying but also immobilized her. This triggered a regression to the traumatic incident, which, in short, took the prototypical form of flatness and depersonalization.

Jane found that as a result of this exercise, she felt more relieved about the childhood experience than about her present distress. Previously she had felt complicit in the abuse because she interpreted her immobilization as cooperation, which had the expectable effect of intensifying her guilt. When she saw how Jack could provoke the same reaction, she understood that this paralysis was a reaction to being abused as a child by a seemingly loving adult. She now realized that what had seemed like complying with the abuse actually was a reaction to it.

However, with Jack she again thought that she needed to be able to "let go" of the fear because it now seemed even more obviously to be a reenactment. She felt the panic to a greater or lesser degree several other times during this period and handled it by ending the encounter with a writing break.

I said that in recognizing a repetition, there is always the risk of disqualifying it as a distortion of the present in terms of the past. Thus, it is common to think of the abuse victim as having to learn to discriminate between the present partner and the abuser. I suggested that this approach is not only laborious and stressful but can be misleading. What can be missed is the way that although past trauma distorts present reality, it also makes the victim especially sensitive to the ways that the present partner actually does resemble the abuser. If Jane had not had this sensitivity, she might have been better able to accommodate to Jack's sexual style, much as his ex-wife apparently had, which would then have left Jack with the sexual inhibitions that had been identified in the assignments.

A less "damaged" partner would have been able to overlook (i.e., bypass) Jack's drivenness. In our discussion of Jack's notes, we found a deeper meaning of his complaint that Jane chooses the time and place. Jack really did need to be the initiator and the active partner. Enforced passivity had "failed" for him. He had no way to enjoy being passively pleasured. He was too vulnerable to slights. This was one reason for his soothing geniality. He avoided making demands and much preferred doing favors to asking for them. At bottom he felt that Jane would have *no reason* to caress him.

Given this rationale, I argued that they had not yet had a chance to develop their sexual relationship, and that like most people they felt compelled to bypass any anxiety or insecurity, with the result that, notoriously, sex becomes vulnerable to depression, worrying, and catastrophizing. Ideally, sex would be an opportunity for relief from such feelings and for a profound kind of reassurance, but this ideal is seldom realized because the compulsions of normal sexuality defend against the exchange of vulnerabilities.

Jack's drivenness had defined their sexual relationship, with the effect that little erotic feeling, and much less passion, was generated in either of them. I suggested that rather than bypassing his fear of rejection, Jack needed to express it to Jane; similarly, Jane needed to give up the futile effort to bypass her fear and needed to turn to Jack for reassurance.

The assignment was for them to escalate from writing breaks to talk breaks, in which they both tried to put their fears into words. I also gave him instructions for a third stroking assignment in which the emphasis is on each locating and attempting to relieve the other's tensions as they are physically expressed (Appendix 1.3).

Eighth Hour

At the eighth session, 1 month later, Jack and Jane again reported daily encounters, but it now appeared that my reframing in the last session had critically altered their sexual set. Jane said that Jack looked entirely different (ironically, given the standard advice, it was Jack, not Jane, who learned to differentiate himself from the abuser). Her panic did not reappear and Jack said he felt a great weight had been lifted from his shoulders. They both reported moments of erotic feeling, which looked like the beginnings of passion. At a 6-month follow-up, they both checked "very satisfactory" regarding their level of sexual enjoyment and reported a frequency of three to four times weekly. My own rating of their progress per session would place them in the top 20% of my case load.

Commentary

Although this case illustrated defining features of the Masters and Johnson breakthrough in general, and of my ego-analytic application in particular (Apfelbaum 1984b, 1988; Apfelbaum & Apfelbaum, 1985), I should identify the aspects of the treatment that were specific to this one couple. They were in a withdrawal–withdrawal pattern that would have worked against more intensive or more lengthy therapy. They were always on the verge of withdrawing from therapy and from the assignments, as well as from each other. Had they been expected to meet on a weekly schedule, or to do the assignments more regularly, I believe they would not have continued. Ideally, the therapy would have been more extensive, with more closely spaced visits. Although a daily schedule is probably the most effective, only certain couples have the motivation and the mental set that makes it possible. Ultimately, the patient sets the pace.

Although termination was, of course, left open, such brief therapy (8 hours spaced over 10 months) must be limited in scope and clearly risks relapses. However, my key objective is to reverse an adversarial pattern and thus to make the sexual relationship itself therapeutic.

AN EVOLUTIONARY PERSPECTIVE

Clearly, this couple confirmed Witkin's (1982) observation that the assignments make it "easy to avoid relating . . . in a spontaneous way" (p. 112). However, the assignments did bring out the spontaneous ways this couple avoided relating. The assignments succeeded in their diagnostic function. As Masters and Johnson (1985) put it:

> The judicious use of sensate focus exercises has multiple clinical applications. For example sensate focus exercises are now intitially used to identify and evaluate levels of inhibited sexual desire and/or states of sexual aversion. Thus, sensate focus techniques are employed both as diagnostic and as therapeutic modalities. (p. 7)

Sensate focus exercises in the context of Masters and Johnson's therapy are an elegant diagnostic and exploratory device.

The subtle insight that has been the basis of Masters and Johnson's therapy is that Jane's fear is a liability because we expect her to perform. We all too easily agree with her that her fear has no place in sex. In effect, we do not notice her fear of her fear, that is, her belief that her fear will ruin sex. We are even farther from realizing that because her fear is triggered in sex, it is in sex that her fear should be allayed.

All sex therapists recognize how common it is for people to feel the compulsion to fit the standard sexual script. However, the expectations that create the standard script have been narrowly construed as the "foreplay" mental set and the preoccupation with erections and orgasm. If we recognize that the expectation of a positive response is the crux of the standard script, we are in a position to vastly broaden our conception of sex and of our sexual potential rather than to fit people to a compulsively restricted version of sex.

Given what is still the dominant view of sex, we find a variety of pathogens (e.g., a restrictive sexual upbringing, depression, distractibility, grudges, pleasure anxiety, a negative body image, Oedipal guilt, fear of failure, and fears of being used, rejected, unloved, or abandoned), all of which are seen as pathogenic simply because they interfere with one's ability to respond positively. The point is that in sex as we construe it at this time in our psychological evolution, these reactions have no place. This is what potentiates them, that is, makes them appear to be primary pathogens—which makes it appear to be the task of therapy to modify these pathogens *rather than the task of sex itself*.

To put this another way, modifying Jane's fear in order for her to fit her own and everyone else's expectations would be a laborious and stressful process. The ego-analytic alternative is to change her way of relating and responding to the fear, a much more easily reached objective, and one that may give us a glimpse of future developments in the evolution of our sexuality.

APPENDIX 1.1. BSTG STROKING ASSIGNMENT

The purpose of this assignment is to set up a simple standardized situation to collect impressions about what goes on between you when you are touching one another: what you experience and what you imagine that your partner experiences. We are interested in the discomforts that arise, because tensions and insecurities are easier to relieve when they can be brought out in the assignment and then discussed in the office.

Read over these instructions at least once before you do the assignment, and also have this sheet at hand to refer to when doing it.

The idea is to do a structured stroking assignment, meaning that you will be taking clear turns and will be following a methodical procedure. One partner gets stroked for half the time and the other for the other half. There will be enough time to see what it is like to touch and to be touched, to collect clear impressions of what each experience is like with your partner.

You will be doing a light fingertip stroke all over your partner's body. Ideally, the one being stroked will say what feels good and where it feels good, and how the touch could be improved, but don't expect to be able to do this right away.

This assignment is done without clothes, using a bed. There should be at least enough light to see what you are doing, and the assignment should not be done unless the room is comfortably warm, since any chill blocks other sensations. Don't try to create a special mood with wine or music, since the idea is to get a kind of baseline impression.

To make your strokes glide smoothly, rub a small amount of baby powder between the hands (be careful to avoid breathing it) and renew it periodically. Cornstarch can be used as a substitute.

Stroking movements should blend into one another in a slow continuous motion without losing contact with your partner's body. The idea is to do a teasing touch, especially in sensitive areas: lips, ears, anus, breasts, genitals. These should be included without special attention, although patterns of goose bumps should be attended to further since, if the room is not cold, this is a sign of successful stroking. If you hit areas of ticklishness use a heavier touch and then progress to a lighter one.

First you do both backs, then both fronts. Each turn should last 10–15 minutes. It is important to keep things simple and, as much as possible, to not vary the assignment in any way. All other sexual activity should be avoided on the day the assignment is done.

Backs: The passive partner lies face down on the bed. Preferably the active partner sits on the edge, but some people will need back support, leaning on an arm, pillow, or against a wall or headboard. If possible, avoid lying down on your side and try to use both hands.

Begin with the back above the waist, using a light fingertip stroke. Spend a few minutes covering this area, lightly dragging your fingers in long sweeping motions or in slow circular ones. Then move up to the neck and shoulder area, and along the sides of the arms. At the buttocks add a kneading motion, spreading and moving the muscles. Then go down the backs of the legs and back up the outside and down the inside of the legs. Feet can be done with the flat of the hand or gently kneaded.

Fronts: The partner whose back was done first now lies facing upward with eyes generally closed. The active one then does the chest and stomach area, then neck, head and face, arms, and down over the pubic area and the hips to the legs.

Notes: Since the purpose of this assignment is to collect impressions and experiences, try to notice what you are thinking and feeling and what, if anything, is said. Write down as much of this as you can. *Notes are essential* even though you may think you will remember what went on. Make a point of having pads or paper available for this. Write your notes as soon as possible after the assignment is done, and include as much detail as you can.

What your notes should cover: Label the four parts: active and passive backs; active and passive fronts. Your reports should cover both what you felt, physically and emotionally, and also what thoughts you were having, in each of the four parts, as well as your impressions of what was going on in your partner. Be sure to include the date, as well as who initiated the assignment and how you felt about doing it.

Feel free to talk over your experiences doing the assignment, but we recommend that you do not read each other's notes, because that may inhibit you in writing them.

APPENDIX 1.2. BSTG STROKING ASSIGNMENT (2)

Our purpose now is to focus on genital stimulation without intercourse or orgasm. Continue to avoid any other sexual activity on the days the assignment is done. Be sure to do your reports, the more detailed the better, following the format described at the end of the instructions for the previous assignment.

Note breaks: Interrupt the assignment for two ten-minute periods any time during a session and jot down notes to use in your reports. Either partner may initiate these breaks.

Talk breaks: Talking about what you are thinking and feeling during an assignment session is optional, although the active partner will need to know how the stroking is going. However, if things do not feel right to one of you— if there is some vague discomfort or something that needs to be said that cannot be said in the stroking situation— stop altogether and separate, preferably sitting at some distance from one another. Then take turns talking, with one of you saying what is on your mind for a few minutes, and then the other. Then resume the session. If things still do not feel right, try another talk break or else discontinue the session and write it up.

First session: Repeat the previous assignment, but this time limit the stroking to 5–10 minutes per side. After finishing the front, and without changing roles, spend another 5–10 minutes focusing on sensitive areas, using the same light teasing touch. Trace around the ears, lips, breasts, genitals, insides of upper thighs.

Erections and lubrication may appear in this assignment, and if so, the idea is to accept them as signs of pleasure, continuing stroking at the same pace and avoiding the compulsion to push for more intense sexual responses. Of course, resisting the pressure to accelerate at such times may be frustrating to both partners. If so, be sure to include this in your reports.

Second session: As in the first session, again do 5–10 minutes of stroking, backs and then fronts, and as part of doing the fronts, cover the sensitive areas, working up to the genitals, with the active partner sitting at the side of the passive partner facing the feet.

Now when doing the male genitals try to get more information about your partner's preferences. Explore the whole genital area as well as the penis, asking how it feels. If erections appear, practice sustaining them for periods of several minutes, avoiding vigorous or heavy stroking and orgasm—then allow erections to subside by stroking other areas or, if necessary, by stopping all stimulation.

In doing the female genitals, once again the idea is to get more information about your partner's preferences. Explore the whole vaginal area as well as the clitoris, asking how it feels and varying the speed and pressure. If lubrication occurs this can be used to reduce friction, but there should be an opportunity to practice stroking while the area is dry. This means using feather-light strokes and also moving the surface skin over the underlying areas, for example, sliding the clitoral hood or moving the outer vaginal lips. You will need to do a lot of checking. Again, the idea is to sustain excitement, to let it subside, and then to resume genital stimulation.

Third session: This assignment is a repeat of the previous one, with the addition of a lubricant, Albolene ("Liquifying Cleanser," in older jars called Albolene "Cream"; scented or unscented), not other hand creams or vaseline.

For men, small amounts of Albolene should be used only after some degree of erection has occurred, but for women Albolene should be used at the beginning of genital stroking.

Whether or not arousal occurs, Albolene should be used to practice the different kinds of stroking made possible by the use of a lubricant. Again practice sustaining excitement and letting it subside.

APPENDIX 1.3. BSTG STROKING ASSIGNMENT (3)

This assignment extends the method of taking turns up to, and possibly including, orgasm for one or both partners. The idea in this assignment is to make orgasm enough of a possibility so that staying relaxed is more difficult and tensions can be noticed that may have been missed in the simpler assignments. Again use note breaks and, if necessary, talk breaks. When one of you feels uncomfortable or has something that needs to be said, say "Let's take a break," and then either try to say what you are experiencing or ask your partner to interview you about it (the interviewer should take notes on what is said).

Follow the same progression of strokes that you have by now worked out, but we now want to see if you can locate deeper levels of tension. This means doing some deeper strokes, without attempting a thorough massage. On the back: Try kneading the neck and upper back, moving the shoulders. With the fist of your hand move the muscles on either side of the spine (avoid pressing the spine). Using both hands, push up folds of skin. Also use a broad pinching motion with each hand. The pelvis can be lifted slighty and rotated and the thigh muscles pinched and kneaded. Try pressing on both sides of the lower back while your partner exhales, as in the old method of artificial respiration. Do this for five exhales.

On the front: Try smoothing out the forehead and cupping the eyes, using a mild pressure for a 60-second count. Kneading the scalp is good for those who don't mind having their hair mussed or pulled. Using the same artificial respiration procedure, press gently but firmly on the center of the chest, using both hands, one on top of the other. The passive partner should make a low noise as the breath is being forced out. The active partner should try to make the noise come out louder by pressing a little harder.

At this point check for signs of body tension: Lift each forearm, bend it at the elbow, and let it drop. Do the same with the lower legs. If the limbs don't fall freely or if there are other signs of tension, either work on areas that still seem tense or take a talk break.

If a fairly relaxed state has been reached, go on to genital caressing. Use Albolene in the same way that you did in the last assignment. However, this time you should keep your left hand free of it. Limit Albolene to just the penis and the vulva (the vaginal area).

Here is where the active partner has to keep on his/her toes to watch for signs of tension in the passive partner. Many people automatically get tense as they become aroused. Note any pelvic tension in your partner and mention it. Help your partner to avoid thrusting motions and also to avoid tightening the vaginal muscles and the muscles at the base of the penis.

As the passive partner becomes more aroused, look for obvious signs of tension like muscle tightness and shallow breathing. Often just mentioning what you have noticed is sufficient to relieve the tension. One effective procedure is to suggest that the passive partner take a very deep breath, holding it for a few seconds and letting it out, then doing this one or two more times. Another useful procedure is to stroke another part of the body with the left hand, or just to rest that hand elsewhere while doing genital stroking. Resting the left hand on the forehead can be especially effective.

If tension continues, either call a talk break or go back to overall body stroking for a time, or both. Don't return to genital caressing in this session unless your partner is relaxed.

Try to avoid the temptation to accelerate your strokes when and if your partner comes close to orgasm. For those who reach an orgasm easily, be especially sure not to trigger an orgasm too abruptly. Of course, you will need to follow your partner's instructions about how to do the genital stroking. Avoid orgasm altogether if it requires any special effort to achieve it. Simply move up to whatever level of arousal it is possible to reach without straining by either partner.

REFERENCES

Apfelbaum, B. (1977a). Sexual functioning reconsidered. In R. Gemme & C. C. Wheeler (Eds.), *Progress in sexology* (pp. 93-100). New York: Plenum Press.

Apfelbaum, B. (1977b). On the etiology of sexual dysfunction. *Journal of Sex and Marital Therapy 3*, 50–62.

Apfelbaum, B. (1981). Review of H. S. Kaplan, *Disorders of sexual desire* and other new concepts and techniques in sex therapy. *Journal of Sex Research 17*, 182–189.

Apfelbaum, B. (1984a). The ego-analytic approach to individual body-work sex therapy: Five case examples. *Journal of Sex Research 20*, 44–70.

Apfelbaum, B. (1984b). Ego-analytic sex therapy: The problem of performance-anxiety anxiety. In R. T. Segraves & E. J. Haeberle (Eds.), *Emerging* dimensions of sexology: Selected papers from the proceedings of the Sixth World Congress of Sexology (pp. 127–132). New York: Praeger.

Apfelbaum, B. (1985). Masters and Johnson's contribution: A response to "Reflections on sex therapy," an interview with Harold Lief and Arnold Lazarus. Journal of Sex Education and Therapy 11, 5–11.

Apfelbaum, B. (1988). An ego-analytic perspective on desire disorders. In S. R. Leiblum & R. C. Rosen (Eds.), Sexual desire disorders (pp. 75–104). New York: Guilford Press.

Apfelbaum, B. (1989). Retarded ejaculation: A much-misunderstood syndrome. In S. R. Leiblum & R. C. Rosen (Eds.), Principles and practice of sex therapy (2nd ed.): Update for the 1990s (pp. 168–206). New York: Guilford Press.

Apfelbaum, B., & Apfelbaum, C. (1985). The ego-analytic approach to sexual apathy. In D. C. Goldberg (Ed.), Contemporary marriage handbook (pp. 439–481). Homewood, IL: Dorsey Press.

Kaplan, H. S. (1979). Disorders of sexual desire. New York: Brunner/Mazel.

Masters, W. H., & Johnson, V. E. (1970). Human sexual inadequacy. Boston: Little, Brown.

Masters, W. H., & Johnson, V. E. (1985, October). Sex therapy on its 25th: Why it survives. Unpublished address to the annual meeting of the Society for Sex Therapy and Research, Minneapolis.

Witkin, M. H. (1982). Showering together: A way to improve marital-sexual communication. Medical Aspects of Human Sexuality 16, 111–112.

2

What's Love Got to Do with It?: The Interplay between Low and Excessive Desire Disorders

J. GAYLE BECK

INTRODUCTION

Typically, sexual dysfunctions are defined and conceptualized with reference to a dyadic relationship. Nowhere is this more clear-cut than in cases in which low desire is present in one partner while excessive desire is reported by the other. Although the following case may not be typical, it illustrates the importance of careful assessment and specific intervention strategies. In addition, this case portrays an interesting functional interrelationship of two markedly different sexual problems.

This case falls within the broad category of sexual desire disorders. Historically, early descriptions of desire disorders focused almost exclusively on low or hypoactive sexual desire problems, with emphasis on unconscious emotional conflicts (Kaplan, 1979) or biological influences such as low androgen levels (Bancroft, 1983) as etiological factors. Although considerably more is known about low-desire disorders relative to hyperactive sexual desire disorders (e.g., Leiblum & Rosen, 1988),[1]

[1]It should be noted that consensus does not exist regarding whether hyperactive sexual desire should be categorized as a *sexual* disorder. In particular, some authors feel that hyperactive sexual motivation may reflect a variety of nonsexual

it is clear that both disorders involve disturbance of sexual *drive*. In the case of excessive (or hyperactive) sexual desire, the primary disturbance appears to be an incessant, intrusive level of sexual drive, which may motivate a high frequency of sexual behavior (Levine, 1988). Although hyperactive desire disorder is not distinguished from the paraphilias, mania-induced hypersexuality, or character disorders within the fourth edition of the *Diagnostic and Statistical Manual of Mental Disorders* (DSM-IV; American Psychiatric Association, 1994), it is important to note that this sexual disturbance involves an unusually high level of sexual motivation rather than images of paraphiliac object choices or mania-induced hypersexuality.

In contrast, low sexual desire disorder is characterized by a persistent or recurrent absence of sexual fantasies and little motivation for sexual activity. Within DSM-IV, this disorder is termed "hypoactive sexual desire disorder" (HSDD). In diagnosing HSDD, clinicians typically do not rely on the patient's frequency of contacts with a sexual partner, as this may reflect traditional prescriptions concerning initiation and acquiescence with sexual requests rather than a patient's level of sexual motivation per se (Beck, 1992). It is not unusual for both males and females with HSDD to report fewer sexual fantasies and less sexual daydreaming relative to sexually functional samples. Interestingly, one study on HSDD suggests that men with this disorder masturbate more frequently than do normal samples, while there were no differences in the frequency of masturbation between women with HSDD and female controls (Nutter & Condron, 1983, 1985). Although considerably more information is needed in order to understand both forms of sexual desire disorders, it is clear that HSDD and excessive levels of sexual desire often share common features, including complex interpersonal dynamics within the sexual relationship and the possible presence of comorbid disorders such as affective or anxiety disorders (e.g., Schreiner-Engel & Schiavi, 1986).

To date, there are no data regarding the prevalence of hyperactive sexual desire disorders. And the scant data regarding the prevalence of HSDD indicate that a marked increase in its presentation may have occurred in sex therapy practices over the past decade (Spector & Carey, 1990). Despite this, the clinician typically is faced with a number of

---

needs and drives, such as emotional compensation for actual or perceived failures (e.g., Levine, 1988). Alternatively, other authors (e.g., Carnes, 1983) have conceptualized excessive sexual desire as an addictive disorder. Given the relative lack of information concerning hyperactive sexual desire problems, it is difficult at present to resolve this issue.

questions in clinical management. One such issue is the extent to which marital factors need to be addressed in addition to sexual problems. As illustrated in this case, it is always necessary to assess the couple's pattern of relating, as well as specific aspects of sexual functioning. Sometimes, complete disclosure of relevant information may not occur at the outset of treatment for a variety of reasons. Thus, versatility and flexibility are required when the presenting complaint is HSDD.

Moreover, the clinician may feel hampered by a relative lack of valid and reliable measures to use in pretreatment assessment and case formulation of patients with HSDD. Although it is ideal to employ measures with adequate psychometric properties, often this is impossible in the case of desire phase disorders. Thus, the clinician may be forced to construct measures that are individualized to specific patients, such as daily self-monitoring and other forms of idiographic assessment. These types of measures are sensitive to gradual therapeutic change, are more precise, and assess behavior at a molecular level relative to available standardized questionnaires (e.g., Barlow, Hayes, & Nelson, 1988). In addition, self-monitoring devices are ideal for repeated administration during the course of treatment. Typically, standardized assessment batteries are mixed with individualized measures, to assess change at both molecular and molar levels. In the case presented here, the batteries involved administration of several self-report inventories before and after treatment, while self-monitoring was used to assess daily change during the course of treatment. In some respects, inclusion of self-monitoring was central in the formulation of this case.

Another point that deserves comment is the interplay between low sexual desire and excessive sexual desire in this couple. Although this combination of problems is rare, the interaction of marital and sexual issues is highlighted most clearly through this synergy. Given the complexity of this couple's problems, the formulated treatment goals and interventions include a variety of strategies, ranging from traditional sex therapy approaches to cognitive-behavioral interventions, Gestalt techniques, and interventions designed for use with individuals with deviant patterns of sexual arousal. This eclecticism followed guidelines provided by Friedman and Hogan (1985); specifically, these guidelines emphasize the importance of utilizing a multidimensional approach to treatment, including interventions designed to target affective responses, foster development of insight, focus on dyadic functioning, and include behavioral homework. As noted below, this case also included a combination of individual and couple sessions.

This case falls within the broad category of disorders of sexual desire. In considering this rather complex couple, it is important for the reader to remember that in any case, unexpected surprises are possible and when they do occur, one needs to revise the treatment plan accordingly.

CASE EXAMPLE[2]

Judy and Richard had been together for 15 years at the time of initial contact. Judy presented as a poised, attractive 40-year-old who was employed as a senior partner in a large law firm. Despite the fact that he was 43, Richard appeared younger than his wife and was noticeably more concerned with his looks. He was employed as a junior vice president for a major company. The couple did not have children, having decided that their careers would preclude a family.

Both Judy and Richard had obtained graduate degrees (a J.D. and a Ph.D., respectively) and described themselves as hard working and achievement oriented. Several years prior to seeking treatment, they had purchased their "dream house" in an affluent section of town. Despite the effort involved in acquiring this house, neither spent much time at home. Judy's job required extensive international travel and Richard reported a wide variety of hobbies, such as sky diving, which filled his time.

Judy and Richard met one another during graduate school. Despite a stormy relationship, the couple maintained close contact when Richard relocated to another city to take a job. When Judy completed law school 1 year later, she joined Richard in a city "where I knew no one, didn't have a job, and had no means to support myself emotionally or financially." After cohabiting for 1 year, the couple married, only to legally divorce 1 month later because of the tax benefits. At the point of initial contact, neither found this arrangement unusual.

Presenting Complaint

The chief complaint was infrequent sexual contact stemming from Judy's apparent lack of sexual interest. The problem was long standing, although there were discrepancies in identifying when the problem began. Judy stated that the problem had begun 5 years ago, while Richard noticed a change 2 years prior to seeking professional help. Their frequency of sexual contact averaged once every 2 months, with Judy refusing Richard's overtures on other occasions because she was not "in the mood." Judy described their sexual interactions as mechanical and emotionally unsatisfying, although she experienced adequate lubrication, subjective arousal, and orgasm. Richard was distressed solely by the infrequency of sexual contact, stating that he enjoyed intercourse and wished that it would occur more often. Neither reported problems with pain during or after intercourse or inadequate arousal. Judy masturbated once per week; Richard stated that he did not masturbate.

[2]This case was previously presented in a different form in Beck (1993).

History

Judy was the eldest daughter of a large family. She described her mother as stern, strong willed, and loving. Her parents divorced when she was 12, owing to her father's alcoholism. Judy described her childhood as a quest for her father's approval; in her memory, nothing was ever adequate by his standards. Judy excelled in math and science courses throughout prep school, as this earned high praise from her father. After her parents' divorce, Judy remained in contact with her father while living with her mother and five sisters. During college, she recalled that her father did not approve of her steady boyfriend. By the time that she was in law school, her father's drinking had progressed to the point that he was involuntarily hospitalized, which Judy organized and financed using a family trust fund. Her father died shortly after Judy married Richard; the family felt that his death was a release from years of trouble caused by alcoholism.

Judy's sexual history was unremarkable. Her first sexual relationship occurred in college with a steady boyfriend. She described this relationship as "terrific" and stated that they have remained friends. She experienced no difficulties with sexual desire, arousal, or orgasm at this time. She met Richard at a party when she was in law school and found him charming, funny, and elusive. Judy and Richard characterized the relationship as difficult from the outset, with Judy pursuing Richard while he withdrew, often dating other women in the interim. When Judy would withdraw from the relationship, Richard would court her and seek to reestablish intimacy. This pattern continued for 2 years, prior to Richard's relocating to start his first job.

Richard was an only child; his mother died of cancer when he was 8 and he was sent to a military school shortly afterward. Two years following his mother's death, his father married a woman who had two daughters and who did not welcome Richard in "her" house. Subsequently, visits at home were shortened and many school holidays were spent with friends' families or alone in the dorm. Richard confided that between the ages of 14 and 18, he had a sexual relationship with one of his stepsisters on those rare occasions when he went home. This was his first sexual experience. Although none of the other family members ever discovered the relationship, Richard recalled considerable apprehension surrounding these contacts. During college, Richard dated many women and derived a sense of self-esteem from being pursued by them. He was an above-average student but never put full effort into his studies. After college, he worked for 2 years before entering a Ph.D. program. He dated many women during this interval but would end a relationship once sexual contact was initiated. Given his high level of sexual activity, he did not masturbate, although he fantasized almost constantly about women. Upon entering a Ph.D. program, Richard became more serious about his career. He excelled in his classes and enjoyed a reputation as one of the brightest students in the program.

Richard described the beginning of his relationship with Judy as "pleasant." Although he was not looking for a steady girlfriend, Judy was interesting, pretty, and highly intelligent. He recalls feeling pressured by her for emotional closeness and, at times, would distance himself. Their sexual relationship followed the course of this emotional tango, with problems arising whenever the tension of prolonged emotional intimacy became too great for Richard. At these points, he would date other women. When he would attempt to reestablish contact with Judy, she would lose her interest in sex, which frustrated him. This pattern was repeated no fewer than six times during the 2 years they dated. Despite recounting their history together, neither Judy nor Richard saw the parallel with their current situation.

Three years prior to entering therapy, Richard confided to Judy that he had been involved in an extramarital affair. He revealed this information because he felt burdened by guilt and wished to reconcile with Judy. After several sessions of pastoral counseling, Judy and Richard reported an interval of closeness and marital satisfaction, including sexual satisfaction. This was their only previous mental health contact.

Assessment

Prior to the selection of an assessment battery, I interviewed both Richard and Judy individually. Case formulation indicated that the presenting problem was maintained by an amalgamation of individual and dyadic factors. Given their history of ambivalent attachment to one another, disturbed communication, and somewhat discrepant accounts of the problem onset, the aim of these individual interviews was to determine each partner's perspective on the problem and to develop treatment goals.

During her interview, Judy indicated that she had never felt that Richard wanted or approved of her. Much like her childhood experience with her father, Judy continually felt pressured to prove herself to Richard in order to be accepted and loved by him. She reported considerable depression, with disturbed sleep, apathy, and feelings of sadness, and indicated that she rarely gained Richard's approval. She was angry at Richard for his past affair but felt that this was not the reason for her current sexual apathy. Judy believed that if she could feel Richard's commitment to her on a consistent basis, her sex drive would be normal. The extent to which Judy minimized the importance of the affair was notable in this discussion. Judy could not acknowledge that there was a problem with intimacy between them or the destruction of trust that Richard's transgression caused for her. Her sexual fantasies revolved around romantic themes, often including Richard. Judy tearfully acknowledged that she was afraid that therapy would reveal that Richard did not want to be her partner, and she worried that therapy would lead to separation.

During his interview, Richard was guarded and inappropriately cheerful. He stated that he did not understand his wife's sexual apathy and that he tried to meet her needs. Although he acknowledged that this was a problem that involved both of them, he appeared to hold his wife completely responsible for their infrequent sexual contact. When I asked about his sexual history, including his incestual relationship with his stepsister, his high level of sexual activity with many different women preceding marriage, and his past affair, he indicated that he had a strong sex drive but otherwise perceived these activities as part of normal male development. This was difficult for me to believe given Richard's level of education and sophistication. However, when pushed by my statement that incest was not usually considered normal, Richard expressed remorse and confessed that he found forbidden and illicit sexual contact extremely arousing. He reported sexual fantasies involving anonymous partners (e.g., sex with a flight attendant on an airplane) but denied acting on these fantasies. Richard felt alone in his marriage and, like his wife, feared that separation was a realistic, albeit undesired possibility.

Following these individual interviews, Richard and Judy completed a questionnaire battery selected to assess both individual and dyadic factors. This included the Dyadic Adjustment Scale, Derogatis Sexual Functioning Inventory (DSFI; an omnibus instrument that assesses 10 areas of responding, including sexual fantasies, satisfaction, and attitudes, and includes the Brief Symptom Index [BSI] as a measure of general psychological status), Beck Depression Inventory (BDI), and Sexual Arousability Inventory (SAI). Table 2.1 lists relevant pretreatment scores and the interpretation of these values relative to available norms. As the table illustrates, both Richard and Judy reported extreme marital unhappiness, particularly around issues of affection, leisure time, and sex. On the DSFI, Judy reported average levels of sexual drive (her ideal frequency of sexual contact was one to two times per week) and typical sexual fantasies (e.g., fantasies involving oral–genital sex and intercourse). Judy scored in the clinical range on the BDI and reported distress from depressive and anxiety symptoms. In contrast, Richard's scores on the BDI and BSI were within the normal range. On the DSFI, he reported a high level of sexual drive, indicating that ideally he would prefer to have sexual contact

TABLE 2.1. Questionnaire Assessment Battery: Pretreatment Scores and Norms

	Richard	Judy	Norm for nondistressed individuals
Dyadic Adjustment Scale[a]	71	63	115
Derogatis Sexual Functioning Inventory[b]			
Information	70	61	50
Experience	70	49	50
Drive	81	52	50
Attitude	48	53	50
Symptoms (BSI)	See text		
Affects	Not administered		
Gender role	56	53	50
Fantasy	See text		
Beck Depression Inventory[c]	5	18	0–10
Sexual Arousal Inventory[d]	90	83	80–91

[a]Spanier (1976); [b]Derogatis (1979); [c]Beck, Ward, Mendelson, Mock, and Erbaugh (1961); [d]Hoon and Chambless (1986).

several times per day. On the fantasy subscale, he endorsed items describing sex with multiple partners, having a forbidden lover, and watching others perform sexually as arousing images, in addition to fantasies involving sex with his spouse. Both Richard and Judy reported adequate levels of arousal to a wide variety of sexual activities on the SAI.

After completing the questionnaire battery, I asked Judy and Richard to maintain daily self-monitoring records of their sexual urges, fantasies, and activities. Included were ratings of subjective desire, feelings of sexual arousal, genital response, and sexual activity. I instructed both individuals to maintain private records in order to reduce bias. I asked Richard to record the complete range of sexual fantasies, including fantasies involving illicit or anonymous sexual contact.

Formulation and Selection of Treatment

Based on results of the pretreatment assessment, I outlined several treatment goals, derived from both interview and self-report sources. A major theme was identified concerning Richard's poor tolerance for emotional closeness. He tended to interpret Judy's requests for intimacy as sexual overtures, although typically Judy was seeking support and comfort. When rebuffed, he would withdraw, which would lead to Judy's pursuit and eventual anger at him. Judy appeared to lack the communication skills for direct expression of her emotional needs. Rather, she would mask her needs by attempting to excel (at work, hobbies, etc.) in order to win Richard's approval and love. When they were not forthcoming, Judy would withdraw, which was perceived by Richard as a preoccupation with her work. In addition, Richard appeared to live much of his sexual life alone, fantasizing about taboo images. These fantasies were quite arousing, although he denied acting on them. However, I felt that the presence of these fantasies distracted Richard from engaging emotionally with his wife. Thus, I outlined four treatment goals:

1. To alter Richard and Judy's pattern of sexual initiation and interaction. Preceding treatment, this consisted of Richard pressuring Judy for intercourse; if she consented, sexual activity included minimal involvement on Judy's part and was oriented around intercourse.

2. To stop the emotional pursuit between Judy and Richard. In particular, the issue of emotional intimacy appeared unresolved, with Judy seeking closeness and approval and Richard distancing himself when this became overwhelming.

3. To strengthen marital communication so that this couple could express emotional needs and desires directly and honestly. In particular, both individuals desired the development of negotiation skills.

4. To monitor Richard's use of taboo sexual fantasies as a distraction from interaction with Judy. Although he denied masturbation involving these fantasies, Richard's nearly constant sexual fantasies detracted from attention to his wife.

The intervention strategies selected to address these goals included exercises derived from the Gestalt tradition designed to heighten sensory awareness in order to teach both Richard and Judy to differentiate sensual versus sexual feelings. Other strategies included communication skill enhancement (including negotiation skills), exploration of differences regarding emotional closeness via cognitive restructuring and role plays, and behavioral homework designed to expand the couple's sexual repertoire. I selected these interventions following guidelines provided by Friedman and Hogan (1985). I instructed both individuals to continue self-monitoring throughout the course of treatment.

Course of Treatment

The course of treatment with this couple was divided into several phases. In the first phase, sensory awareness was heightened through body awareness exercises, including sensate focus exercises. The purpose of these exercises was to teach Richard and Judy to attend to bodily cues of emotion, to recognize and label feelings, and to verbally share these emotions with each other. Both positive and negative feelings were emphasized, as neither Judy nor Richard attended to or articulated emotions well. Given the long-standing pattern of distancing and pursuit that was noted, these exercises also were intended to help the couple learn to respond verbally to each other instead of resorting to their entrenched interaction pattern. Although I placed a ban on intercourse, I included nongenital sensate focus exercises in order to increase sensual contact and to differentiate sensual touch from sexual activity. Because communication is an intrinsic part of sensate focus, the inclusion of this exercise set the stage for later communication training.

The first treatment phase was greeted enthusiastically by Judy, who reported enjoying the opportunity to express herself emotionally to Richard. In contrast, Richard stated that he found the awareness exercises "odd" and was not quite sure what to say. Although he did not avoid participating in these exercises, Judy clearly took the initiative. She reported feeling closer to Richard following each exercise but indicated that Richard had not reciprocated in emotional expression. Judy expressed anger at this imbalance and said that she felt as if Richard was blaming the problem on her. Although Richard enjoyed sensate contact, he expressed frustration with the ban on intercourse and requested removal of this restriction. Despite my restatement that it was necessary to avoid repetition of their dysfunctional sexual and communication patterns, Richard continued to push for intercourse. A review of his self-report records indicated an increase in taboo sexual fantasies during the 3-week interval that they practiced awareness exercises. It appeared that Richard was responding to these exercises with an increase in sexual desire but was avoiding emotional contact with Judy.

This development prompted an individual session with Richard to further explore the issue of taboo fantasies. During this session, Richard revealed that he had a long-standing masturbatory pattern, involving fantasies of sex with strangers. He admitted to masturbating one to two times per day using these fantasies and was quite ashamed of this. In Richard's opinion, this pattern was deviant and he had attempted repeatedly to stop. He said that he had acted on these fantasies only twice, in situations in which he thought he would not be discovered (e.g., at conferences). His wife was uninformed of the nature and frequency of his masturbatory activities and of his prior sexual contact with strangers. Richard was understandably apprehensive about her reaction and had not disclosed this information at the outset of treatment because he believed that if sex with Judy were to occur more frequently, his masturbatory pattern would be easier to control.

This new information necessitated a revised treatment formulation.

In many respects, Richard's masturbatory pattern resembled that seen in sexual deviants, with a high daily frequency of fantasies and infrequent performance of the behavior. A major difference, however, was the nature of the behavior; fortunately, in this case it did not involve illegal sexual contact (as seen, for example, in cases of voyeurism). However, given Richard's preoccupation with these taboo fantasies and the extent to which they superseded sexual and emotional contact with Judy, it was necessary to decrease his masturbatory urges with a separate treatment component. The goal was to reduce Richard's arousal to taboo fantasies. Based on the available literature on sexual deviation, a combination of masturbatory satiation and covert sensitization procedures was selected and described to Richard. Although Richard consented to these procedures, he was reluctant to inform Judy of the true nature of his arousal pattern. In-session role playing with Richard helped him to face Judy with this information, which he did during the next conjoint session.

Session 5 involved Richard's revelation of his masturbatory pattern to Judy and discussion of this pattern as it related to the couple's ongoing marital distress. Judy was distraught to hear of Richard's sexual contact with strangers, particularly given concerns about AIDS (acquired immune deficiency syndrome). Moreover, this information confirmed her belief that Richard did not want to be her partner and she expressed ambivalence about her ability to remain in therapy. With discussion, however, she agreed to stay in treatment for a 3-month trial to strengthen their communication skills, as this would be helpful irrespective of whether they remained together. Individual treatment with Richard was scheduled during this interval. Judy also requested that Richard undergo AIDS testing. The ban on intercourse remained in place, but the couple was encouraged to continue with the experiential and sensory awareness exercises.

The second phase of treatment involved eight sessions of structured communication training with Richard and Judy, scheduled over a 3-month interval. Emphasis was placed on understanding how specific irrational beliefs impeded clear communication. For example, Judy's belief that Richard was not interested in her needs and desires was explored as follows:

JUDY: It just seems that everytime I express my feelings, he either changes the topic or walks away. It's hard enough to share my feelings but when that happens (*tearfully*) I feel like giving up—I think he doesn't care about me.

RICHARD: That's not true. I don't walk away from you. I just don't know what to say sometimes.

THERAPIST: This is a good example of a situation when active listening skills are called for, Richard. See if you can paraphrase the feelings that Judy is expressing right now, instead of defending yourself.

RICHARD: Well Judy is saying that I don't listen to her—that I just leave the room.

THERAPIST: And is she saying anything else?

RICHARD: I guess she's saying that I don't love her.

JUDY: (*Sobbing*) Exactly.

THERAPIST: Judy, how would you like Richard to respond at those times?

JUDY: I just want him to listen to me—not to give advice or leave me alone or talk about something else.

THERAPIST: Let's try practicing this, to make sure that both of you know how to communicate with each other at these times.

Communication training included the techniques of reverse role playing, active listening (as illustrated above), problem solving, and anger management. Richard and Judy both noted a significant decrease in marital conflict during this interval. During the sixth session of this phase, Judy expressed renewed interest in maintaining the relationship, although her level of spontaneous sexual interest did not increase appreciably.

Simultaneous with these conjoint sessions, Richard was seen individually on a weekly basis for 3 months. These meetings involved covert sensitization scenes, which paired auditory fantasies of taboo sexual activities with aversive outcomes. Appendix 2.1 provides an abbreviated example of a typical covert sensitization scene. This procedure was implemented in a two-room chamber with intercom communication in order to maintain privacy during the sessions. Richard practiced masturbatory satiation as homework during this interval. This technique asks the patient first to masturbate using desired sexual fantasies (in this case, fantasies of consensual sexual contact with Judy). Following ejaculation, Richard was asked to masturbate for an additional 15 minutes using undesired, taboo fantasies in order to associate deviant fantasies with the period when arousal and interest were at their lowest. Richard was asked to perform satiation homework daily and was instructed to state his fantasies aloud and to audiotape each practice occasion. This permitted me to assess his compliance with the satiation homework and to ensure that he was following instructions accurately. Richard reported that the taboo fantasies gradually became less arousing during this interval and occurred less frequently. In the final 3 weeks of this phase, Richard began to experience spontaneous fantasies involving Judy for the first time in years.

The third phase of treatment involved several techniques designed to address the issue of emotional intimacy and to expand this couple's sexual repertoire to include greater flexibility in initiation and sexual interaction. Ten conjoint sessions spaced over a 4-month interval were involved in this phase. Treatment discussions focused on the implications of intimacy (e.g., what it would mean if they became closer to one another and how this change would impact their current priorities for time management). In this context, Richard expressed fears that he would be overwhelmed by Judy if emotional intimacy were to last for too long. Exploration of these issues revealed that Richard feared that he would lose his independence and would end up "like my father—smothered and controlled by my stepmother." Cognitive restructuring techniques were employed to change self-statements such as this one and to help Richard perceive Judy's requests for emotional closeness as an affirmation of love and commitment. Judy was taught to identify pursuit behaviors and to replace them with verbal requests for support and intimacy in order to interrupt their distance–pursuit pattern. The couple was given the assignment to date one another at least weekly, alternating responsibility for arranging the date and inviting one another out.

In this phase of treatment, sensate focus exercises were used as the starting point for enhancing this couple's sexual repertoire. Given that Richard and Judy had been practicing sensate focus for 3 months, their communication of sexual likes and dislikes was well practiced. In order to expand their range of sexual behaviors, I asked them to read and discuss together several popular sex manuals (e.g., *The Joy of Sex*, Comfort, 1972). These readings generated a collection of sexual behaviors that both found appealing and wanted to explore. Although the ban on intercourse was still in place, Richard and Judy were instructed to experiment with genital pleasuring, incorporating new activities, with emphasis on communication. Responsibility for initiating these sexual contacts alternated between Judy and Richard. Judy reported an increase in sexual desire shortly after this phase began, which helped her to accommodate this treatment strategy. They reported mutually satisfying sexual interactions within 1 month, at which point the ban on intercouse was lifted.

Figure 2.1 illustrates the changes in sexual desire reported by Judy and Richard during the course of treatment. These ratings were derived from self-monitoring records, which were maintained throughout the 8 months of treatment.

Termination

The final three treatment sessions were devoted to preparing for termination. This involved fading my influence by loosening the structure of treatment in order to develop the couple's ability to handle relationship issues independently. During one of these sessions, Richard asked Judy for forgiveness for neglecting her and for his past trangressions with other women. Judy stated that her forgiveness was expressed by her actions, by the fact that she was committed to remain with Richard and to work through the barriers that had separated them emotionally. The couple

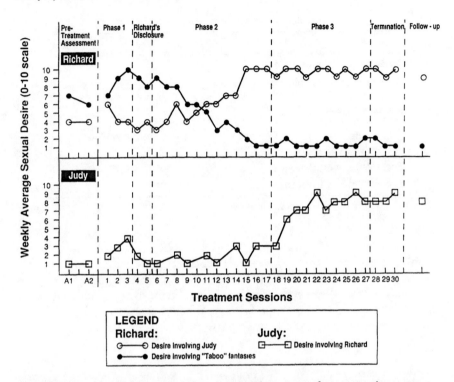

FIGURE 2.1. Self-reported sexual desire during the course of treatment (average ratings of strength of subjective sexual desire and urges for sexual contact on a 1–10 scale, where 1 = none and 10 = maximum). Phase 1 included sensory awareness training; Phase 2 involved dyadic communication training and individual sessions with Richard using covert sensitization and masturbatory satiation; Phase 3 addressed emotional intimacy and expansion of sexual repertoire.

decided to continue their regular dates and to schedule "talk times" in order to maintain their level of communication. Judy also informed Richard that she had requested a reduction in her job-related travel, as she felt that this disrupted the continuity of their marriage. While this reduction was not scheduled to occur for several months, Richard expressed relief and appreciation.

Prior to the final session, the couple completed the battery of self-report questionnaires for posttreatment assessment. These scores are shown in Table 2.2. Both Richard and Judy reported significant increases in marital and sexual satisfaction. Judy no longer experienced significant depression and reported adequate levels of sexual interest. Although Richard's level of sexual interest remained higher, I attributed this to a desire discrepancy (Zilbergeld & Ellison, 1980) rather than a dysfunc-

TABLE 2.2. Posttreatment Questionnaire Scores

	Richard	Judy
Dydadic Adjustment Scale	120	110
Derogatis Sexual Functioning Inventory[a]		
Information	75	73
Experience	70	65
Drive	81	59
Attitude	54	56
Gender role	55	54
Beck Depression Inventory	5	8
Sexual Arousal Inventory	90	95

[a]Other subscales not administered.

tion or a problem area. The couple reported satisfaction with the frequency and variety of their sexual contacts and indicated that they planned to continue their "sex education" reading. Richard reported that occasionally he would have a taboo fantasy. When this occurred, he was careful to mentally switch the fantasy partner to his wife.

Follow-Up

A follow-up meeting was scheduled 3 months after termination. This meeting was scheduled to provide a booster session and was designed to assess this couple's maintenance of treatment gains. When Richard and Judy arrived for this session, they announced their decision to get married legally and Judy proudly displayed her engagement ring. Although the regularity of their dates and talk times had been somewhat inconsistent, both partners were content with their level of marital communication. They did not report any recent instances of the distancer–pursuer pattern that had characterized their relationship before treatment.

During the follow-up interval, sexual interactions had continued at about the same frequency as noted posttreatment and both partners were satisfied with the quality of their sexual contact. Richard revealed that he had experienced a burst of taboo fantasies during an interval of work-related stress. He had handled this by returning to daily masturbatory satiation exercises for a 3-week period, during which the frequency and intensity of these images were reduced. Although it is unusual for a patient to reinstate this aversive procedure voluntarily, Richard was unusually motivated. His long struggle with these intense urges seemed unpleasant enough to motivate him, particularly because of the extreme marital problems that had resulted when these fantasies were present. Richard's commitment to Judy was noticeably stronger and his willingness to be legally married to her (in spite of the loss of tax benefits) stood as firm evidence to Judy that he indeed wanted to be with her. Judy reported experiencing sexual desire three to four times per week, which is about average for women in light of available data (Beck, Bozman, & Qualtrough, 1991). Overall, the couple was confident with their ability to handle sexual and relationship issues as they arose.

COMMENTARY AND DISCUSSION

Although this case is hardly a "prototypical" example, there is considerable uncertainty regarding the modal characteristics of sexually disordered patients. The use of daily self-monitoring proved critical in the successful resolution of this couple's sexual problems because it permitted reformulation of the case after Richard disclosed his arousal pattern. In addition, a variety of therapeutic techniques, including strategies designed to heighten sensory awareness and to expose long-standing relationship patterns, was important for the resolution of this case. Moreover, inclusion of strategies borrowed from the treatment of sexual paraphilias was necessary to reduce excessive sexual interest, as observed by Levine (1988) and others. These strategies were integrated with procedures designed to address the sexual and marital problems that reduced sexual desire in the other partner.

Fortunately, neither partner was resistant to change. From the outset, both were quite motivated and were frightened about completely destroying their relationship. Both Richard and Judy were likable and highly verbal, although they lacked sophistication about the extent to which their own behavioral patterns affected the quality of their marriage. Although Richard initially withheld important information from me, this is not unusual in cases in which atypical arousal patterns are present. Once Richard revealed his secret to me, he and Judy reached an important turning point. Although there was some concern that Judy might end the relationship on learning the true nature of her husband's sexual arousal pattern, her consent to remain in therapy was a major step in her commitment to Richard. After this point, treatment proceeded well and with the full cooperation of both partners.

At present, there are no normative data regarding the average length of treatment for sexual desire disorders, nor is it known whether therapeutic complications (such as resistance or sabotage efforts) are common. Clearly, as this case suggests, much remains to be learned about the clinical spectrum of sexual desire disorders.

APPENDIX 2.1. AN EXAMPLE OF A TYPICAL (ABBREVIATED) COVERT SENSITIZATION SCENE USED WITH RICHARD TO DECREASE AROUSAL TO TABOO FANTASIES

You're in a restaurant in New Orleans, where you've been attending a conference. It's been a rough week and you're feeling relaxed and happy to be away from it all. You notice one of the waitresses—she's about 5'3" and shapely, with beautiful red hair. You begin to watch her as she moves around the tables near to you—her movements are sexy and you can't help but stare at her large breasts. She can tell that you're watching her—she looks back and smiles every time she passes you. You start to think about how you can talk to her when all of a sudden, she's standing next to you. She says, "I'm sure glad that this place isn't crowded—it makes everything so much easier and I get a chance to know the customers—is everything alright?" You can feel yourself getting aroused and hope that she doesn't notice the bulge in your pants. You start to talk to her, asking her about herself—does she like her job? how long has she been working here? All you can think about is how much you'd like to undress her, to fondle those large firm breasts—you can almost hear her moan with pleasure as you talk to her, fantasizing about having sex with her. She excuses herself and moves away to serve another customer. You decide to ask her to go out for a drink, thinking how much you'd like to get her into bed tonight. As you are paying your check, she comes by you and you grab her hand, asking her if she'd like to go for a drink later. She smiles, teasingly, and says, "Sure, I'm finished here now." You wait outside for her—when she comes out, she's wearing a tight pair of slacks that reveal an incredible body. She walks you to her car and says, "I know just the place where we can go." Driving to the bar, all you can think of is her naked body—ripe, full breasts, her great legs. You walk into the bar with your arm around her, she is giggling and teasing you. As you sit in the dark bar, you start to fondle her, slowly touching her body over her clothes—her firm breasts, her legs, her pussy. She is responsive and begins to kiss you, slow, passionate kisses. Although the bar is dark, you notice some people standing several feet away, watching you. You look up and it's your boss, your wife, and your best friend. They are watching in horror as you fondle this woman and seduce her. They have seen everything and know what a sickie you are, how you just can't stop thinking about seducing every woman you see, how you can't think of anything else. You've been caught red-handed and everyone is glaring at you. You start to mumble an excuse but you feel sick and embarrassed, you can feel your dinner churning in your stomach. Your wife removes her wedding ring and throws it at you as she walks away. Your boss says, "Richard, we don't respect this type of behavior from one of our executives." You are so humiliated as you sit there, halfway undressed by this strange women, embarrassed in front of the people you care about most. You know that you're sick and disgusting to these people, that you've lost their trust and respect. They know that you're a chronic womanizer and you feel like you're going to throw up. But suddenly, you get away. It was only a dream. You wake up and you can relax, your stomach doesn't hurt and you're glad that you're away from womanizing, free from seducing strange women. You relax again.

REFERENCES

American Psychiatric Association. (1994). *Diagnostic and statistical manual of mental disorders* (4th ed.) Washington, DC: Author.

Bancroft, J. (1983). *Human sexuality and its problems.* London: Churchill, Livingstone.

Barlow, D. H., Hayes, S. C., & Nelson, R. O. (1988). *The scientist–practitioner.* New York: Pergamon Press.

Beck, A. T., Ward, C. H., Mendelsohn, M., Mock, J., & Erbaugh, J. (1961). An inventory for measuring depression. *Archives of General Psychiatry, 4,* 561–571.

Beck, J. G. (1992). Behavioral approaches to sexual dysfunction. In S. M. Turner, K. S. Calhoun, & H. E. Adams (Eds.), *Handbook of clinical behavior therapy* (2nd ed., pp. 155–173). New York: Wiley.

Beck, J. G. (1993). Low sexual desire disorder. In C. G. Last & M. Hersen (Eds.), *Adult behavior therapy casebook* (pp. 217–234). New York: Plenum Press.

Beck, J. G., Bozman, A. W., & Qualtrough, T. (1991). The experience of sexual desire: Psychological correlates in a college sample. *Journal of Sex Research, 28,* 443–456.

Carnes, P. (1983). *Out of the shadows: Understanding sexual addiction.* Minneapolis: Comp-Care.

Comfort, A. (1972). *The joy of sex.* New York: Crown.

Derogatis, L. R. (1979). *Sexual Functioning Inventory* (rev. ed.). Baltimore: Clinical Psychometrics Research.

Friedman, J. M., & Hogan, D. R. (1985). Sexual dysfunction: Low sexual desire. In D. H. Barlow (Ed.), *Clinical handbook of psychological disorders* (1st ed., pp. 417–461). New York: Guilford Press.

Hoon, E. F., & Chambless, D. (1986). Sexual Arousability Inventory (SAI) and Sexual Arousability Inventory—Expanded (SAI-E). In C. M. Davis & W. L. Yarber (Eds.), *Sexuality-related measures: A compendium* (pp. 21–24). Syracuse: Graphic Publishing.

Kaplan, H. S. (1979). *Disorders of sexual desire.* New York: Brunner/Mazel.

Leiblum, S. R., & Rosen, R. C. (Eds.). (1988). *Sexual desire disorders.* New York: Guilford Press.

Levine, S. B. (1988). Intrapsychic and individual aspects of sexual desire. In S. R. Leiblum & R. C. Rosen (Eds.), *Sexual desire disorders* (pp. 21–44). New York: Guilford Press.

Nutter, D. E., & Condron, M. K. (1983). Sexual fantasy and activity patterns of females with inhibited sexual desire versus normal controls. *Journal of Sex and Marital Therapy, 9,* 276–282.

Nutter, D. E., & Condron, M. K. (1985). Sexual fantasy and activity patterns of males with inhibited sexual desire and males with erectile dysfunction versus normal controls. *Journal of Sex and Marital Therapy, 11*, 91–108.

Schreiner-Engel, P., & Schiavi, R. C. (1986). Lifetime psychopathology in individuals with low sexual desire. *Journal of Nervous and Mental Disease, 174*, 646–651.

Spanier, G. B. (1976). Measuring dyadic adjustment: New scales for assessing the quality of marriage and similar dyads. *Journal of Marriage and the Family, 38*, 15–28.

Spector, I. P., & Carey, M. P. (1990). Incidence and prevalence of the sexual dysfunctions: A critical review of the empirical literature. *Archives of Sexual Behavior, 19*, 389–408.

Zilbergeld, B., & Ellison, C. R. (1980). Desire discrepancies and arousal problems in sex therapy. In S. R. Leiblum & L. A. Pervin (Eds.), *Principles and practice of sex therapy* (1st ed., pp. 65–101). New York: Guilford Press.

3

Sexual Aversion Disorder:
The Case of the Phobic Virgin,
or an Abused Child Grows Up

HELEN SINGER KAPLAN

INTRODUCTION

Sexual aversion disorder is one of the two clinical variants of disorders of sexual desire (American Psychiatric Association, 1987, 1994). Sexual desire disorders do not involve the impairment of genital function. The essential clinical feature of these syndromes is a pathological deficit in sexual motivation. In other words, these patients have no desire for sex or for sex with their partners but may well be capable of physiologically normal erections and orgasms.

Disorders of sexual desire are highly prevalent. On average, about 30% of patients who are currently seeking help at sexual disorder clinics have complaints relating to deficient sexual motivation or desire.[1]

Masters and Johnson, who invented modern sex therapy in the 1960s, originally focused exclusively on the functions and dysfunctions of the genitalia, and they did not include sexual desire or disorders of sexual desire in their studies of human sexual inadequacy (Masters &

[1]According to Leiblum and Rosen (1988), the prevalence of disorders of sexual desire reported by different U.S. and European sex therapy programs range between 1% and 63%.

Johnson, 1964, 1970; Masters, Johnson, & Kolodny, 1994). Their treatment approach, which was highly successful, was devised for genital-phase dysfunctions such as psychogenic impotence, premature ejaculation, retarded ejaculation, anorgasmia, and vaginismus. As originally conceived, however, the standard sex therapy format, which centers around the sensate focus exercises, is not particularly effective for patients with sexual desire disorders and may actually aggravate the severity of these symptoms.

In fact, it was by studying our treatment failures in the early 1970s that I became aware that one group of our nonresponders had become sexually dysfunctional simply because they had tried to make love without feeling desire. It was then I first realized that sexual desire disorders (SDDs) constitute a separate clinical entity, and that these patients require a new and different treatment approach.

CLINICAL FEATURES

The primary symptom of sexual aversion disorder is a fear, phobia, or intense aversion to genital contact with a partner, or to some specific nongenital aspect of sex, such as kissing or breast touching, along with a compelling urge to avoid the feared or repulsive sexual activity. If "trapped" in an unavoidable sexual situation, sexaphobic patients, especially those with concomitant anxiety disorders, may experience genuine, terrifying panic attacks.

It is important to distinguish sexual aversion disorders, which are characterized by an active phobic avoidance of sex, from hypoactive sexual desire (HSD), which involves a "quiet" loss of sexual desire in the absence of a phobic component. While hyposexual or "sexually anorexic" patients have no appetite for erotic interchange with their partners, unlike the sexaphobics, they are not actively repelled or afraid.

THE PSYCHODYNAMICALLY ORIENTED APPROACH
TO THE TREATMENT OF SEXUAL AVERSION DISORDERS

The psychodynamically oriented sex therapy approach to disorders of sexual desire is based on the same integrated sex therapy model that was originally developed for the treatment of the genital phase dysfunctions (Kaplan, 1974, 1979, 1986), and it employs the same basic format. However, the specific interventions used are different in order to accommodate the specific and unique therapeutic requirements of these sexually anxious patients.

More specifically, therapeutic behavioral "homework assignments," which the patient or couple conducts in the privacy of their homes, are used to modify the *immediate causes* of the patient's sexual symptoms, in this case the malignant link between sex and fear, while psychodynamically informed therapy, conducted in the therapist's office, is used to explore the patient's deeper emotional and sexual conflicts and, most important, to manage the resistances that almost invariably arise to the rapid modification of sexual symptoms.

The Behavioral Aspects of Treatment

Each type of psychosexual dysfunction is the product of a unique set of immediate or currently operating causes that impair the genital reflexes or sexual motivation in specific ways. These different causes respond to different types of therapeutic interventions, and therefore different specific behavioral protocols have been devised for each of the psychosexual disorders listed in the revised third and fourth editions of the *Diagnostic and Statistical Manual of Mental Disorders* (American Psychiatric Association, 1987, 1994; Kaplan, 1974, 1975, 1979, 1986).

Thus, for example, "quiet" HSD is often seen in patients who unwittingly downregulate their sexual desires by evoking negative thoughts and feelings while avoiding effective sexual stimulation (Kaplan, 1995). It follows that the treatment approach for HSD emphasizes the use of cognitive interventions to modify these immediate or currently operating antisexual behaviors and thought processes, while therapeutic libido-enhancing behavioral assignments are used to counteract these patients' tendency to screen out and avoid erotic input (Kaplan, 1995).

By contrast, the thrust of the treatment approach for sexual aversions is quite different and focuses on eliminating the patient's pathological sexual fears with techniques derived from learning theory.

Extinguishing the Sexaphobic Response

Once again, the immediate cause of sexual phobias, sexual panic, and sexual aversion is the malignant link between fear/aversion and sex. This destructive association must be modified in order for the patient to improve. The behavioral interventions that are used for this purpose center around the systematic, gradual *in vivo* exposure of the patient to partner-related genital stimulation or to that specific aspect of sex that triggers his/her phobic avoidance.

The therapeutic *in vivo* desensitization assignments are structured so that the patient will be exposed to the feared or repellent sexual situation gradually and progressively under calm, emotionally safe, and supportive circumstances, until the phobic response to sex is extinguished, and he/she is free to experience normal sexual pleasure.

More specifically, the sexaphobic patient is instructed to attempt to remain physically in the presence of a small, manageable piece of the feared and previously avoided sexual situation, which might, for different patients, entail kissing, body caressing, genital touching, looking at the partner's nude body, just holding hands, etc., until his/her negative feelings have abated. After the patient becomes entirely comfortable with that level of exposure, the partner and patient advance to the next step.[2]

THE CASE OF GRETA B

Greta B, an Austrian immigrant, was a 39-year-old single woman and virgin who requested treatment for her sexual aversion and avoidance of relationships with men.

The patient had a severe, lifelong aversion to sex and was particularly repelled by the idea of kissing.

Greta B was a virgin. She had not had intercourse, nor had she ever engaged in any sort of physical intimacy with a partner, not even holding hands. The very thought of meeting a man who might make sexual advances filled her with dread, and she had avoided any and all potentially romantic situations on that account. Thus Greta had never dated or danced with a man, nor had she ever engaged in flirtatious banter. Declining social invitations that involved the presence of men, Greta generally spent evenings and weekends alone. Apart from her job as a bilingual secretary for the Roman Catholic Diocese, and her volunteer work at an old-age home, which she found gratifying, Greta led a lonely and pleasureless life.

The patient's aversion to and phobic avoidance of sex was limited to contact with a partner. Greta had no difficulty fantasizing and masturbating to orgasm when she was by herself.

---

[2]*In vivo* desensitization should be distinguished from systematic desensitization, a technique developed by Joseph Wolpe which uses imagery but no direct physical exposure to the phobic stimulus (Wolpe, 1958). In the experience of our group (see below), systematic desensitization is not effective for treating sexual disorders.

This patient also had a history of a disabling panic disorder with agoraphobic features for which she had been treated the previous year at another facility. She had responded well to a course of imipramine, 150 mg per day, and cognitive therapy. When Greta became my patient, she was still on a maintenance dose of 75 mg of imipramine and she was functioning well in all spheres: She worked, she traveled without any difficulty, she was able to enjoy some holidays with her women friends, and she had experienced no further panic attacks since the end of her treatment. However, there had been absolutely no corresponding improvement in her sexual symptoms, which were as severe as ever.

Greta realized that her fear of sex was destroying her life, and she was now determined to seek help to overcome this problem.

History and Etiology

The central core and immediate cause of Greta's sexual problem was her intense aversion to kissing, which could be traced directly to the sexual abuse she had endured as a child. Between the ages of 6 and 10, Greta was repeatedly molested by an elderly neighbor who lived down the hall. The man would wait for her when she came home from school and drag her into his apartment, where he would hold her tightly while he pressed his "stinking" mouth on her lips. At the same time, he forced the child to stimulate his penis and would not let her go until he ejaculated. A shy, lonely little girl, raised by her widowed mother—a reclusive woman who was probably also a agoraphobic—Greta told no one of her ordeals and suffered in silence. These repeated traumatic experiences had forged a link between feelings of disgust and aversion with kissing and sex.

A second tier of immediate causes of this patient's sexual problem, which would also have to be modified in therapy, was Greta's unattractive, antiseductive appearance, which presumably served to protect her from unwelcome sexual approaches. This defense had originated in Greta's attempts as a little girl to become "sexually invisible" and unappealing in the vain hope that she could slip by her tormentor unnoticed.

Persons who are afraid of sex often adopt a countersexual persona and assume a cloak of sexual invisibility or unattractiveness in their efforts to avoid sexual relationships, and like Greta, these individuals often remain single and celibate. However, the absence of a partner complicates the outlook for sexaphobic patients because the usual course of treatment for this disorder involves a systematic program of *in vivo* desensitization assignments, which are designed to expose the phobic patient gradually to the sight, sound, touch, feel, smell, and taste of the lover's body and genitalia. Therefore, the availability of a cooperative, an attractive, and, above all, a trustworthy partner is considered an invaluable asset if not an essential condition for treating sexaphobic and/ or sexually aversive patients.

The unavailability of a sexual partner presents an even greater handicap for women patients than it does for men because hired sexual partners, such as sexual surrogates, masseuses, and prostitutes, can effectively substitute for intimate partners for the purpose of conducting the therapeutic desensitization exercises. But whereas it is quite acceptable and customary for men to pay for sex, single sexaphobic women tend to object to this and must therefore first solve the considerable problem of *attracting* a sexual partner to work with, before they can be treated.

The risk of contracting AIDS from casual sexual partners is now diminishing this gender difference, as men are also becoming wary of sex with strangers. For this reason, increasingly, the objective of the first phase of treatment for single, dysfunctional patients is to support their quest for appropriate sexual partners.

Treatment

The challenge posed by trying to cure a lifelong, severe sexual aversion and avoidance and phobic social anxiety in an obese, unattractive woman of 39, who had no sexual experience, who had never dated, and who had no partner or any imminent prospects of finding one, was considerable.

Transference

As a first step, I became Greta's "good mother." A strong positive transference is an important ingredient in the success of this brief treatment method. An amiable transferential state boosts the therapeutic process by virtue of patients wanting to please, and this also allows them to identify with the therapist and to adopt his/her more liberal and permissive sexual attitudes. A positive transference is especially important with sexually dysfunctional patients who, like Greta, have experienced inadequate or destructive parenting and/or poor gender-appropriate role models during the critical phases of their psychosexual development.

Greta was "ready" for a good mother, and a firm therapeutic alliance was rapidly established on that basis. Thereafter, I gave Greta "grooming" and "appearance" homework. More specifically, I advised her to have a cosmetic "makeover" consultation at a department store, and I suggested that she clean and mend her clothes. I then asked her to wear her prettiest colored blouse to our next session. Greta was eager to win my approval, and I let her know that she did, when she came in looking much better the following week.

Because Greta had no partner with whom she could conduct the therapeutic exposure assignments, I first tried to reduce her sexual anxiety with *covert desensitization*. Toward that end I asked her to watch kissing scenes on television and to practice visualizing couples kissing, but this had little effect.

I also used a cognitive maneuver in an attempt to "detour around" her repugnance of kissing by pointing out that it was perfectly possible for her to make love to a man without necessarily allowing him to kiss her.

At the same time, in every session we worked on uncovering and working through Greta's traumatic childhood experiences. We reviewed the sexually abusive incidents she had endured in great detail and talked at length about how she had felt at the time. I made a special effort to clarify the destructive impact these events had on her psychosexual development and on her present problems. After a few sessions of this Greta seemed to become a little bored by the topic, which suggested to me that she was beginning to come to terms with her painful memories.

Greta was making progress. In addition to her growing insight into the consequences of her traumatic childhood experiences, she also became visibly more attractive and cheerful. However, she continued to avoid social contact with men.

Treatment was at an impasse. It was apparent to me that no further meaningful progress could be made unless somehow, actual partner-related therapeutic experiences could be arranged.

Greta had a lovely feminine speaking voice, which was seasoned with her charming Viennese accent, and I decided to use this asset as a starting point for helping her overcome her social anxiety and avoidance.

I asked the patient to place an advertisement in the personals column of a local magazine. I pointed out that she could expect to receive many letters from men who would want to meet her. In the attempt to forestall her anticipated objections, I reassured Greta that her contacts with men would be entirely under her own control, as the letters would be addressed to an anonymous box number provided by the magazine. She could choose to call only those men whose letters appealed to her.

But Greta resisted this assignment. She claimed that only crazy men would answer personal ads and, besides, she maintained that she could not afford it.

Resistance

At this point I confronted the patient with her resistance. I told her that I thought her objections to placing the ad were merely rationalizations and excuses for continuing her avoidance of men and sex. At the same time, I balanced this relentless stripping away of her old defenses with my understanding and support. Thus I was very warm and empathic with the difficulty of her situation, and I expressed my view sympathetically, that her intense fears and avoidance of meeting men were entirely understandable under the circumstances and that no one could fault her for this.

I also "joined the patient's resistance" by lowering my fee to compensate for the cost of placing the advertisement. Finally, with deep misgivings, Greta agreed to place the ad.

We then proceeded to compose the ad together. This turned out to be an excellent therapeutic opportunity to begin to modify the negative image Greta was projecting, which was one of the more effective defenses against sex in her considerable armamentarium.

In her initial draft of the ad, Greta described herself as fat and unattractive, while mentioning none of her positive qualities. The patient had no insight that this was an expression of her fear and avoidance of sex and practically guaranteed that no sane man would answer her ad.

With my steadfast support of the positives, and my unrelenting vetoes of the negatives that Greta kept trying to slip into the text of the advertisement, she eventually composed an appealing yet entirely honest description of herself, to which she received over 100 replies.

Greta was astonished and thrilled when she saw how many men wanted to meet her. However, she was also terrified of and very resistant to the idea of contacting them.

I then *reduced* the assignment. I suggested that Greta pick out the 25 most promising letters and call only three of these men each week. I tried to further decrease her anxiety by limiting the purpose of the phone calls so that these would be less threatening. I told Greta that the calls were only *exercises* meant for learning and practicing how to conduct a pleasant appropriate social conversation with a man, but they were *not* to be the occasion for arranging dates.

We also rehearsed the phone calls. I advised Greta to start the conversations by telling each man that she liked his letter, and that she just wanted to chat and get to know him a little. For the time being, she was specifically asked *not* to arrange to meet any of the men. In case a conversation became unpleasant, the patient was instructed to hang up the phone at once.

But despite the slow, careful pace of the desensitization program, and despite my continuing support amplified by our strong therapeutic alliance, all my attempts to bypass Greta's resistances with cognitive and behavioral tactics failed and the patient remained paralyzed by her intense anticipatory anxiety.

MANAGING RESISTANCES IN PSYCHODYNAMICALLY ORIENTED SEX THERAPY

Greta's resistance was typical and expected. In virtually every case, patients and couples with sexual disorders resist the process and/or the outcome of sex therapy.

Resistant patients miss their appointments, "misunderstand" the therapist's instructions, start fights with their lovers, attack the therapist, get into accidents, get pregnant, get ill, run out of money, or, as in Greta's case, fail to comply with their assignments.

Resistance may be mobilized by the *process* of sex therapy, or by its *outcome*, that is, by the rapid improvement of sexual functioning which typically occurs with this method. But Greta was not ambivalent about a positive outcome. She was ready to enjoy a normal sex life, and as far as she was concerned the sooner the better. However, the *process* entailed in reducing her sexual anxiety and her phobic avoidance of men was overwhelmingly difficult for this patient and she resisted her assignments tenaciously.

It should be noted that when treating sexually dysfunctional couples conjointly, resistances may be mobilized in the sexaphobic individual, as well as in the sexually asymptomatic partner, whose anxiety is often raised by his/her spouse's rapid improvement and increasing desire, while in many cases both partners take turns sabotaging treatment.

A key to a successful outcome in conjoint psychosexual therapy is the therapist's ability to overcome the partner's resistances and to enlist his/her unqualified cooperation. This is often an awesome task, and the only advantage of treating Greta as a single person was that I did not have to concern myself with partner resistance.

Bypassing the Deeper Causes

When treatment fails to progress as expected because a patient (and/or the partner) is resisting, I proceed on the assumption or theory that these obstacles are manifestations of the patient's underlying unconscious intrapsychic conflicts about love and sex, and/or deeper ambivalences toward the partner, which originated in early childhood. Presumably, these are the same deeper issues that gave rise to the patient's desire disorder in the first place.

However, initially we do not try to interpret this material. Our first-line strategy for dealing with the resistances to the behavioral therapeutic sexual exercises is to attempt to "detour around" or "bypass" these with a systematic, sequential program of gradually intensifying behavioral and cognitive interventions. These progress from the simple *repetition* of the assignment *to reduction* of the intensity of the exercise to *cognitive reframing* of the problem in less threatening terms to active *confrontation*.

In many cases, the patient's resistances are mild, and such brief cognitive-behavioral therapeutic maneuvers, which may be characterized as "superficial" from a psychodynamic perspective, succeed in bypassing or bridging the deeper sources of the patient's sexual symptoms, deficits, and resistances to experiencing normal sexual feelings for his/her partners. There are many cases in our files where patients' sexual functioning and desire improved to normal levels purely in response to such behavioral and cognitive interventions, while they gained virtually no insight into the presumed unconscious roots of their sexual symptoms and/or destructive interactions with their partners.

However, we have seen an equal number of cases in which the patient and/or the couple were impervious to the *in vivo* exposures, repetitions, reductions, medications, restructuring, support, permission, and confrontation.

When this happens and a sexaphobic patient shows no improvement in response to the behavioral, cognitive, and pharmacological interventions, in sharp contrast to therapists who do not believe in unconscious motivation or insight therapy, *we do not give up on the case*. Instead, we shift into our second-line psychodynamic mode wherein the goal then changes from *bypassing* the deeper unconscious causes of the patient's sexual symptoms to *insight* and resolution.

Many patients who were initially unresponsive to exclusively behavioral and cognitive interventions, who would surely have ended up as treatment failures, have been salvaged by the addition to our treatment regimen of our second-line, psychologically "invasive," insight-promoting psychodynamically oriented interventions.

One might ask why insight-promoting methods should be deferred until it is clear that the patient is truly resistant to the cognitive-behavioral approach—why not start with psychodynamically oriented interventions in the first place? A simple and partial answer is that this is frequently unnecessary. For although there is little doubt in anyone's mind that the vicissitudes of early life play a significant role in shaping adult destiny and psychopathology, it does not necessarily follow that each patient's childhood needs to be explored intensively, or that everyone must attain insight into the deeper and unconscious causes of their sexual symptoms in order for their functioning to improve.

When it became clear that Greta's therapy was not moving forward despite my most artful "bypass" maneuvers, I shifted to a more "invasive," "insight-fostering" strategy. More specifically, I now attempted to fortify the behavioral program with psychodynamic explorations of the childhood roots and the deeper causes of Greta's sexual fears and of her resistances.

But Greta would have none of this. For example, during one week I gave Greta three assignments, but she did only two. She successfully carried out a masturbation–fantasy exercise with a vibrator, and she attended her first session of Overeaters Anonymous. However, Greta resisted her third and most important assignment, she failed to place any of the three prescribed calls to men who had answered her ad.

Dream work is often very useful in facilitating a patient's insight into the deeper meaning of his/her resistances, and in many of my cases the well-timed interpretation of a patient's dream has catalyzed a genuine therapeutic breakthrough. Therefore, in an effort to illuminate the unconscious psychic infrastructure of Greta's tenacious resistance, I asked her whether she had had any dreams that week.

Greta told me that she had dreamt that she had three umbrellas. She had given two away to a friend but kept one of the umbrellas for herself, "in case it rained."

I tried to interest the patient in considering the notion that this dream might be a metaphor for her inner conflicts about therapy and her resistance to giving up her defensive avoidance of men. I suggested that the umbrellas might symbolize her defenses, which she was being asked to give up in therapy. I proposed the idea that by doing two of the assignments she had given up two of her protective defenses or "umbrellas" against sex, namely, she had allowed herself to experience erotic feelings by fantasizing and masturbating and she was beginning to work on improving her appearance by trying to overcome her obesity. But, I said, the dream suggests that she was not yet ready to give up her "last umbrella," her ultimate defense against being hurt sexually again by a man, namely, her avoidance of contact with potential sexual partners.

Greta was totally unimpressed by my clever interpretation and she dismissed my efforts as comparable to "Gypsy tea-leaf readings."

I continued to see the patient for a total of 14 sessions. Although it seemed that Greta had obtained no insight into her deeper conflicts, on an experiential level she had made slow but significant progress: Despite having lost no weight, her appearance had improved, she had become quite skilled and much more confident in her phone conversations with men, and the wounds caused by the trauma of her unfortunate childhood sexual experiences seemed to be healing. But Greta still had not had a single date with a man or even a face-to-face conversation.

The clinic closed for the summer and I saw her once again 2 months later in the fall. I was alarmed when Greta began the session by telling me that she had been "picked up by a policeman."

I feared that perhaps therapy had somehow unleashed an unsuspected latent psychopathic or self-destructive tendency in this patient, and that she had gotten herself into trouble. But Greta quickly reassured me that what she had meant was that a *cute* policeman had picked her up in the *park* and they were now having a pleasant sexual relationship, although she admitted that she still did not care much for the kissing part.

From the beginning, I understood some of the deeper underlying pathogenic issues that possibly contributed to the origin and maintenance of this patient's sexual symptoms. For example, I believe that the death of her father when she was very young could have made her particularly vulnerable to sexual assault by a "father" figure, while the emotional neglect by her mother might have predisposed the patient to becoming insufficiently assertive and self-protective with men. However, although these insights shaped my behavioral interventions, these issues never came up as such in treatment. Thus, for example, my understanding of this patient's dynamics motivated my exceptionally protective "maternal" behavior toward her, as well as my emphasis, while we role-played the phone calls, on modeling appropriate assertiveness with men. But we never discussed the impact of Greta's relationship with her parents on her sexual problems.

SEXUAL TRAUMA AND ABUSE

As noted earlier, it is a basic principle of psychodynamically oriented sex therapy that we begin treatment by attempting to modify the patient's sexual symptoms directly with behavioral-cognitive methods, while the underlying or historic issues are explored later, and only if the patient resists the initial bypass tactics. But there is an exception which was illustrated in this case. I do not consider it appropriate or effective to attempt to circumvent the deeper causes of a patient's sexual symptom when this involves sexual trauma such as sexual child abuse or adult rape. *Patients with posttraumatic sexual stress syndromes*, such as Greta B, do not let down their defenses against sexual feelings easily, and they tend to resist sex therapy until they have worked through the original traumatic injury. For patients with a history of sexual trauma, it feels better, and it makes more sense from the standpoint of treatment, first to attempt to "detoxify" the traumatic memory by helping them to uncover this fully, and to explore the subsequent impact on their psychosexual development prior to giving any assignments that might expose the patient to a sexual situation reminiscent of the original, damaging trauma.

SEXUAL PANIC STATES

We have found a very high concordance between anxiety disorders and sexual aversions and phobias in our patient population.[3]

The treatment of patients who are highly anxious presents special difficulties irrespective of whether the patients meet the criteria for panic disorder, because in extremely anxious individuals the association between fear and sex is particularly intense, tenacious, and difficult to extinguish, and the treatment format for sexaphobic patients, especially those with concomitant anxiety disorders, must be carefully adjusted and fine-tuned to accommodate to their high anxiety levels.

It is not possible to achieve such requisite flexibility with traditional sex therapy methods. For example, sex therapists frequently assign the sensate focus (SF) exercises in an attempt to relax their patients. But severely sexaphobic individuals tend to panic in response to SF exercises. The lengthy exposures to nudity, physical contact, and forced intimacy that are entailed in the SF exercises tend to overwhelm phobic patients and to mobilize their resistances. Because this procedure often backfires with these patients, I consider the SF exercises contraindicated for patients with sexual desire disorders, except in carefully selected cases.

Most patients with sexual panic states require a much slower pace of desensitization with very small increments of exposure to the previously avoided sexual situation, and in some cases, it may be necessary to repeat each tiny step as many as 20 to 30 times before their anxiety abates.[4]

---

[3]More than 25% of the 373 patients with sexual anxiety states (sexual aversions and the phobia of sex) who were seen at the Human Sexuality Program of the New York Hospital–Cornell Medical Center and at our private practice group between 1976 and 1986 met the DSM-III criteria for panic disorder, while another 25% of these patients showed atypical symptoms and signs of anxiety disorders (Kaplan, 1986). These results have yet to be replicated by other investigators.

[4]The behavioral literature reports some successes with "flooding" the patient with intense anxiety for the treatment of (nonsexual) phobias. However, in our experience, exposing the patient to the phobically avoided sexual situation while he/she is in a state of panic is not useful and may aggravate these conditions.

The Concept of an
"Optimal Therapeutic Anxiety Level"

The sexual exercises prescribed for sexaphobic patients should be individualized and controlled so that the patient's anxiety remains within a "therapeutic range" during the duration of the therapeutic exercise.

According to learning theory, the experience of a certain amount of anxiety is necessary for the success of the process of desensitization. If an assignment evokes absolutely no anxiety or fear in a patient, obviously, no extinction can take place. However, excessively high anxiety levels are equally countertherapeutic; for if the patient has a panic attack while she is engaging in a therapeutic homework assignment with her partner, her sexual fears will not be extinguished but may become reinforced and more severe.

For example, the first homework assignment I gave to one of my patients, a woman who was referred to our program by a Masters and Johnson type of clinic because she had a panic attack in response to the SF exercises, was to look briefly at her husband's genitalia (which she had not done in the 4 years of their marriage). Only when she was finally comfortable with looking was she asked to touch his penis, and initially this was only for 10 seconds.[5]

With regard to the case described herein, had Greta continued to sit home alone, she would not have experienced any sexual anxiety but neither would she have improved. On the other hand, had I asked her to attend a singles event, which is a common assignment for sexaphobics without partners, chances are that she would have been flooded with intense anxiety and remained frozen in a fearful state to the point where no extinction could occur. I used the phone-call tactic because this gave me better control over the patient's anxiety, and I was able to maintain this anxiety at moderate levels, which were conducive to exposure therapy.

PHARMACOLOGICAL CONTROL OF ANXIETY

It is often difficult or even impossible to control the intense fears of patients who have underlying anxiety disorders and to keep this within a therapeutically useful range. Even the most painstakingly slow and well-conceived therapeutic exposure assignments may evoke intense uncontrollable anticipatory anxiety and counterproductive panic attacks in

---

[5]This case, which was described in a previous publication (Kaplan, Fyer, & Novick, 1982), was brought to a successful conclusion in 20 sessions.

these patients. Moreover, even if these anxious patients do not actually experience overt panic attacks, they tend to *remain* suspended in an intensely anxious state during their desensitization assignments, and as extinction can only occur if the patient's fears *diminish while he/she is in the presence of the phobic situation*, these overanxious patients often do not calm down sufficiently for deconditioning to take place, no matter how small the exposures are.

In many such cases the adjunctive use of antianxiety and/or panic-blocking drugs, such as alprazolam or trazodone, can resolve this therapeutic dilemma by bringing the patient's anxiety down to manageable levels.

As was seen in Greta's case, drugs alone do not cure sexaphobic patients. But in good responders, the adjunctive use of panic-blocking or antianxiety medications can reduce anxiety sufficiently during the *in vivo* exposures to facilitate the permanent extinction of the sexaphobic responses in patients who would otherwise be too anxious to cooperate with or benefit from sex therapy.

It is, of course, impossible to determine what role, if any, the drugs Greta was taking played in the successful outcome of her treatment. It is clear that medication is not always necessary for patients with sexual panic states because we have been able to cure a number of sexaphobic patients with concomitant anxiety disorders who, for various reasons, were not medicated, and perhaps this patient would have been among those. However, I believe it would have been extremely difficult, if not impossible, and at the very least much more stressful, for the patient if she had to undergo treatment in an unmedicated state, unprotected against her panics.

REFERENCES

American Psychiatric Association. (1987). *Diagnostic and statistical manual of mental disorders* (3rd ed., rev.). Washington, DC: Author.

American Psychiatric Association. (1994). *Diagnostic and statistical manual of mental disorders* (4th ed.). Washington, DC: Author.

Kaplan, H. S. (1974). *The new sex therapy*. New York: Brunner/Mazel.

Kaplan, H. S. (1975). *The illustrated manual of sex therapy*. New York: Quadrangle Books.

Kaplan, H. S. (1979). *Disorders of sexual desire*. New York: Brunner/Mazel.

Kaplan, H. S. (1986). *Sexual aversions, sexual phobias, and panic disorders*. New York: Brunner/Mazel.

Kaplan, H. S. (1995). *The sexual desire disorders: Dysfunctional regulation of sexual motivation*. New York: Brunner/Mazel.

Kaplan, H. S., Fyer, A. J., & Novick, A. (1982, Spring). The treatment of sexual phobias: The combined use of anti-panic medication and sex therapy. *Journal of Sex and Marital Therapy, 8* (1), 3–28.

Leiblum, S. R., & Rosen, R. C. (Eds.). (1988). *Sexual desire disorders.* New York: Guilford Press.

Masters, W. H., Johnson, V. E. (1964). *Human sexual response.* Boston: Little, Brown.

Masters, W. H., & Johnson, V. E. (1970). *Human sexual inadequacy.* Boston: Little, Brown.

Masters, W. H., Johnson, V. E., & Kolodny, R. C. (1994). *Heterosexuality.* New York: HarperCollins.

Wolpe, J. (1958). *Psychotherapy by reciprocal inhibition.* Stanford: Stanford University Press.

4

Adjusting the Carburetor: Pivotal Clinical Interventions in Marital and Sex Therapy

ARNOLD A. LAZARUS

INTRODUCTION

Many drivers have experienced car problems that seem to indicate an extreme mechanical disorder. The vehicle may stall, sputter, jerk, shudder, and backfire, and the hapless owner might feel resigned to bear the expense of a complete overhaul. How comforting to learn from an honest mechanic that little more than an adjustment of the carburetor (and perhaps some spark plugs and an oil change) will be needed. The following case exemplifies this analogy in the clinical/psychotherapeutic arena.

An experienced social worker referred Mrs. Z to me after treating her for a year with only minor improvements. Concurrently, Mr. and Mrs. Z also underwent an unsuccessful course of marital counseling with a family–marital therapist for over a year. Previously, Mrs. Z consulted several therapists, one of whom diagnosed her as suffering from a borderline personality disorder. The marital therapist described Mrs. Z as aggressive and resistant, and characterized her husband, Mr. Z, as equally defiant and oppositional. It was easy to see why these professionals had characterized Mr. and Mrs. Z in this way. She was demanding, somewhat histrionic, argumentative, accusatory, and often self-defeating.

When I met with Mr. Z, he was combative, defensive, and angry. His major complaint was that, at his wife's insistence, there had been no sex for the past 4 years (of a 20-year marriage). They were on the verge of divorce, and Mr. Z stated that the only reason he had not yet consulted attorneys was because of financial constraints.

My first impression was that this couple needed extensive intervention, a veritable "engine replacement," and that prognosis was guarded at best. And yet as therapy proceeded, a few pivotal issues came to the fore—rather simple and obvious concerns that called for little more than didactic instruction and a small touch of clinical artistry. The end result was remarkably gratifying.

Before presenting the case, some additional orienting remarks may be in order. In my experience, it is rare to find harmonious marriages wherein all goes well except for some specific sexual problem. Typically, there is an inextricable link between the couple's interpersonal ambience and what goes wrong in the bedroom. Thus, the need to integrate marital and sexual interventions is fairly standard. With Mr. and Mrs. Z, sexual accord necessitated very precise relationship corrections and attitude adjustments before their chronic sexual impasse could be addressed.

As will be seen, the use of bibliotherapy (i.e., recommending or prescribing particular self-help books) was a focal element that not only expedited the therapy but strongly reinforced the psychoeducational approach that was employed. Most clients seem to resonate to the notion that if a picture is worth a thousand words, certain selected books can be worth, not a thousand sessions, but give or take a dozen or two. It is often helpful to stress that counseling and therapy need to be viewed as education rather than healing, as growth rather than treatment. When clients realize that overcoming emotional and sexual problems is an educational process, the concept of *self-education* is easily understood. They become more inclined to *do* something constructive and to take responsibility for effecting change. As the old adage states, they are not merely handed fish to eat but are equipped to do their own fishing.

When dealing with volatile and hypersensitive individuals, therapists have to be extremely wary to avoid "pushing their clients' buttons." Perhaps the most obvious pitfall into which many clinicians fall is the observation–interpretation trap. As Wile (1981) underscored, too many therapists make accusatory interpretations (e.g., referring to "dependency needs" or implying that someone is "infantile and demanding"). Distressed couples "are already feeling discouraged and self-critical about their situation. Being told that they are dependent, competitive, greedy, and so on would increase their alarm and defensiveness" (Wile, 1981, p. 98). As will be seen, Mr. Z's previous marital therapist fell into this unfortunate trap, thereby negating his ability to be of therapeutic assistance.

INITIAL SESSIONS WITH MRS. Z

Mrs. Z, a 50-year-old commercial artist, appeared tense and guarded. The first session was largely devoted to obtaining background information and building rapport. She was asked to take home and complete the Multimodal Life History Inventory (Lazarus & Lazarus, 1991). It presented a verbal portrait of Mrs. Z as emotionally isolated, distant from her husband, at odds with her adult son and daughter, having no "love life," being "stuck," lacking in self-esteem, feeling unable to help herself, and consequently experiencing a profound sense of depression and demoralization.

Two initial interventions revealed the extent of the client's suspiciousness and hypersensitivity. First, Mrs. Z misperceived the suggestion to consult a biologically oriented psychiatrist to determine whether antidepressant medication was indicated as an attempt to reject her by referring her elsewhere. Nevertheless, it was not difficult to reassure her that the intent was not to dismiss her but simply to enlist the help of another professional (two heads are better than one). "I'd like to avoid drugs, if possible," she said.

The other incident stemmed from a fantasy question that was posed to Mrs. Z. After she expressed how little she could offer, how boring and dull her company tended to be, she was asked to imagine that arrangements had been made for her to spend the day with a most intelligent and attractive man. "Would this hypothetical stranger confirm the self-denigrating comments you have just made about yourself? Would he come away from the experience agreeing that you are dull and boring?" On the face of it, this exercise proved successful. Mrs. Z stated that under such circumstances, she would exert a tremendous effort to be pleasant and engaging and that the man would probably tap into her sense of humor and appreciate some of her profundities, and he would emerge after a day in her company feeling that it had been enjoyable and worthwhile. This led to the affirmation of a healthy "inner core" that was submerged by "external baggage."

However, when Mrs. Z arrived for her next appointment she mentioned that the foregoing exercise had occasioned a great deal of anxiety in her. She wondered whether I was making a sexual overture or pass at her and she had discussed this with the social worker who made the initial referral. The social worker advised her to raise the matter in her next session with me. Her grounds for suspicion were examined and the appropriate reassurances were provided, at which point she alleged that about 10 years ago she had consulted a psychiatrist who had seduced her. She said that they had been lovers for several months until she decided to call a halt to it. This, in turn, occasioned the opportunity to delve into her sexuality and to examine what had gone wrong in the marriage. The major issues seemed to revolve around steadily increasing mutual resentments that she and her husband were harboring, his lack of bodily hygiene, and some myths she held regarding sexual activity after having had a hysterectomy.

The next five sessions followed a routine format. Mrs. Z was eager to share and review significant aspects of her life history; her anger and her insecurities were examined, her entitlements were explored, and emphasis was placed on developing an effective interpersonal style (e.g., assertive vs. aggressive communications). An avid reader, she asked for bibliotherapy and initially I gave her a copy of *I Can If I Want To* (Lazarus & Fay, 1992); subsequently she read *Marital Myths* (Lazarus, 1987) and *PQR: Prescription for a Quality Relationship* (Fay, 1994). These books specifically address a variety of adaptive interpersonal styles and refute several specific illusions. It was evident that Mrs. Z took the trouble to read each one thoroughly and intelligently and was endeavoring to transfer what she had gleaned from her readings to her daily living. She asked for more books and I loaned her several by Albert Ellis and his associates on rational–emotive therapy.

One of the first major cognitive-behavioral shifts occurred at this juncture (during the eighth session). Mrs. Z often expressed frustration and rage at the fact that many of her needs were not being met, especially by her husband. The following brief dialogue led to some immediate and profound changes:

MRS. Z: I need a vacation desperately, but my husband is too cheap to consider going to some decent place. When I am on vacation I need to have luxurious accommodations and lots of comforts or I end up being miserable. So I have the option of going to France and staying with my relatives which only obligates me to them—and that's the last thing I need, or we can spend some money and have a nice time visiting Italy and Holland which I've wanted to do for years. But I really need to get away.

THERAPIST: This seems like a good opportunity to examine the way in which you confuse *want* with *need*. I notice that you do this in many areas of your life, and I think you have now read enough on the subject to appreciate the difference and apply it to your life. Do you know what I'm referring to?

MRS. Z: That I need to have what I want to get?

THERAPIST: Well, let's talk about some of your *needs*. Perhaps everyone's greatest need is for oxygen. If someone shuts off your air supply, you'd soon grow desperate, and if it were not rapidly restored, you'd be dead. That's a real need! And you sure need water or liquid. Without it, you'd also die. And ditto to food or sustenance. But you don't need love and respect from your children—you wish for it, desire it and want it, but you can live with or without it. And you don't need Mr. Z to help you around the house. You would prefer it, you would like it, you want it and you'd probably appreciate it. But I repeat, it is not a basic need. And you don't need a vacation. You very much want one. As long as you define your wants as needs, you will feel desperate if they are not met or fulfilled. If you are deprived of a luxury vacation and you equate this with the deprivation of oxygen, food, or water, you'll feel downcast, sad, angry, anxious and depressed. But if you can say, "I don't need it, I can take it or leave it, I can live with or without it, but if possible I'd like to have it," you will avoid a sense of desperation and manage to approach the matter calmly and rationally, and thereby most probably end up getting what you want.

This simple intervention had a significant calming effect on Mrs. Z who succeeded in differentiating between her needs and desires and thereafter reported that she had started viewing the world quite differently. "I can't fully explain it," she said, "but by realizing that, as Ellis would say, it is not a dire necessity for me to have everything I want, that all my wishes don't have to be granted, I am approaching everyone and everything very differently." At this point I emphasized that, with her permission, I would like to meet her husband with a view to determining how to upgrade their marriage. She fully accepted the precept that without involving them as a couple, their marital and sexual impasse would probably not be resolved. However, she was uncertain whether Mr. Z would agree to meet with me because his previous experiences with mental health professionals had turned him against "all shrinks." She recommended that I call him rather than have her serve as my messenger. I complied and the reluctant Mr. Z agreed to meet with me.

MEETING MR. Z

Mr. Z's opening remark set the tone of our first meeting. "I've lost a wife and I've lost a friend, and I don't think there's a damn thing you can do about it." This 55-year-old mechanical engineer, was overweight, was casually attired, talked very loudly, and described himself as "fiercely competitive." He appeared to be extremely insecure and therefore the first line of therapeutic intervention seemed to call for unbridled positive reinforcement. "Your wife tells me that you are extremely intelligent. She called you a 'self-made man,' and stated that you are very popular socially and that you have always been committed to family values. I believe you also have several patents to your credit." Mr. Z appeared to calm down in response to this initial emollient, but he replied, "Look, I don't give a shit. If I could afford it I'd get a divorce." "That makes perfect sense if all the love is dead," I replied, "but I believe that Mrs. Z still has plenty of love left for you." He then railed on about his wife's unfair treatment, her withdrawal, obvious resentment, incessant criticisms, litany of complaints, and disapproval.

According to Mr. Z, the marital therapist made two "fatal blunders." First, he had called Mr. Z "a games player," which the client heard as derogatory and pejorative. Second, Mr. Z took exception to the fact that the therapist labeled him "hostile." He stated: "That's no help to me, and besides, I think I have every reason to feel that way . . . I wonder if Dr. X would feel hostile if he never got laid."

At the end of this initial interview, Mr. Z agreed to attend four conjoint sessions. He was asked to complete the Multimodal Life History Inventory but stated outright that he was not about to fill in a 15-page questionnaire. Consequently, he was given the Expanded Structural Profile (C. N. Lazarus, 1993; see Appendix 4.1), which he agreed to complete. Subsequently, Mrs. Z also filled one in, which brought to light several additional clues for helping this couple. For example, it proved useful to point out some specific similarities and differences (e.g., he was more of an "action person," whereas she was decidedly a "people person") and to discuss ways and means of developing a "live and let live" philosophy that would take cognizance of their respective preferences. The profile also showed the extent to which Mr. and Mrs. Z both craved human touch and sexual intimacy.

Mr. Z inquired why I had not recommended something for him to read, given the fact that I had plied Mrs. Z with several books. I had just completed the first draft of my book *Don't Believe It for a Minute!* (Lazarus, Lazarus, & Fay, 1993) and loaned him a copy because it addressed several toxic ideas to which he seemed to subscribe.

CONJOINT MEETINGS WITH MR. AND MRS. Z

"First, you need to become friends and reestablish trust," they were told. Nevertheless, during the first two meetings, Mr. and Mrs. Z were both extremely accusatory, blamed each other for a myriad of problems, expressed innumerable resentments, and dwelled on negative incidents that sometimes went back over 20 years. Attempts to interrupt this combative spiral were unsuccessful. "I told you it's hopeless," Mr. Z retorted.

Mrs. Z called 2 days later to say that Mr. Z refused to return for therapy, whereupon I called him and explained that both he and Mrs. Z needed to appreciate that neither one was to blame for anything that had gone wrong with their relationship, but that misunderstandings and untoward circumstances had ripped them apart and kept them apart. Mr. Z finally agreed to attend the third conjoint session. The emphasis here was on *total nonblaming*. A turning point came when Mrs. Z turned to her husband and said, "I can see now that it was not your fault that we drifted apart. I played a definite role in it. . . . If I had done some things differently, you would have responded differently." After warning her to avoid needless self-blame, the treatment focus shifted to the development of a noncritical, noninterfering, mutually supportive *modus vivendi*. Mr. Z acknowledged that he too had "played some of my cards badly," and they came away from this session pinpointing specific misunderstandings, faulty perceptions, and miscommunications (rather than willful intent or spiteful retaliation) that had undermined their relationship. They were asked to "try on for size" a totally noncritical and nonblaming lifestyle for the next 2 weeks (i.e., before the fourth conjoint session).

At the fourth conjoint meeting, although the couple reported that peace and harmony had reigned in their home, Mr. Z stated that "nothing else had changed." He went on to express his profound dissatisfaction at the absence of sex and emphasized that he was unwilling to live a life of celibacy. They were instructed in the nonerotic tactile exercises that Masters and Johnson (1970) called sensate focus sessions and encouraged to implement them.

BREAKING THE SEXUAL IMPASSE

Mr. and Mrs. Z dismissed sensate focus training as "artificial, unnatural, contrived, and above all, adolescent." Mr. Z emphatically stated that he had made up his mind years ago never to endure any further sexual rejection. Mrs. Z explained that her husband had always responded very negatively whenever she had declined his sexual advances. "After my hysterectomy, he showed no sensitivity for what I was going through and took my refusals as a personal assault." The nonblaming philosophy was reiterated and the couple was encouraged to find nonpejorative explanations for their sexual plight. The best that they could come up with was that each had developed the same stubborn posture: "I'll teach you a lesson by withdrawing from you sexually." The following dialogue ensued:

Mr. Z: I'm telling you, I won't put myself on the line again. I was rejected a hundred times too many. She has to make the sexual advances if we are ever to get together again.

Mrs. Z: What kind of an agreement is that? Why do I have to take all of the responsibility?

Therapist: Perhaps because men have egos that are more fragile than women's.

Mrs. Z: That's rubbish. I don't accept that. It would be a one-way street.

Mr. Z: Do you know how many times I have approached you in the past and how many times you have said "no"?

Mrs. Z: I haven't kept score.

Therapist: This is a very sensitive issue. (*turning to Mr. Z*) Tell me, do you intend to give her a taste of her own medicine? If she agrees to make the overtures, do you look forward to saying "no"?

Mr. Z: That's not the way I work. (*turning to his wife*) You know that.

Mrs. Z: I don't know anything anymore.

Therapist: (*To Mrs. Z*) Are you willing to take the initiative?

Mrs. Z: I'm not sure how to go about it.

Therapist: (*Joking*) How about simply saying, "Let's screw!"

Mrs. Z: That's not my style.

Therapist: How about, "Honey, would you like to meet me in the bedroom?"

Mrs. Z: (*Seriously*) I guess I could say that.

Mr. Z: We have separate bedrooms, you know.

Therapist: How about if she says, "Honey, would you like to meet me in my bedroom?"

Mrs. Z: I still don't see why the entire onus rests on me.

Therapist: Right or wrong that's his script. He's pointed to a path through the jungle. In my opinion, if you need to be the sexual initiator, so be it. Later, we can find a quid-pro-quo item that he can use for balance. Oh, by the way, it's fully acceptable for you to ask him to shower, splash on some after-shave and brush his teeth before coming to the bedroom.

At the end of the session, as the couple was about to leave, I assumed the stance of a priest and offered a prayer and a benediction. The couple were extremely amused and Mr. Z said, with affection, "You're a character." I said: "Well, I've done all I can do. I can't force you to make love. So it's now in the hands of God."

Between the third and fourth conjoint meeting, I had an individual session with Mrs. Z during which I inquired whether she had any anticipatory concerns about her own sexual response if and when they resumed sexual relations. "I was afraid that I might be dry," she said, "but since

I am on estrogen I don't worry anymore." I then stated that it was likely that Mr. Z, given all the emotions that were involved, might experience potency problems. An explicit discussion of sexual technique followed that candidly and graphically included the hows and whys of applying lubricants, implementing tactile stimulation, performing fellatio, and, above all, exuding a nondemanding ambience. "I've been reading up on the subject," Mrs. Z assured me, "and I know what I have to do."

A month later, I met with Mrs. Z. "It's like a miracle," she said. "We made love about five or six times. . . . Sex is very important to him. He's a totally different person. . . . I've never seen him so mellow." There had indeed been some initial potency problems as anticipated, but these were shortlived. "I've become quite a bombshell in the bedroom!" Mrs. Z declared.

DISCUSSION

As in many cases of sexual disturbance, Mr. and Mrs. Z presented with a considerable amount of psychic debris that had to be cleared away before a path toward coital intimacy could be established. A seemingly intricate impasse responded to simple rapport building followed first by the important distinction between "necessities" and "preferences" and then by the implementation of a nonpejorative and nonblaming *modus vivendi*. Of course, the treatment trajectory has few obstacles when the clients are both reasonably cooperative and genuinely motivated to make specific changes.

A major factor in this case was the way in which Mrs. Z resonated to the tenets of "rational thinking." By replacing categorical imperatives with specific preferences, Mrs. Z was in a position to respond very differently to frustration and was able to educate Mr. Z to do likewise.

The importance of cognitive and interpersonal interventions in sex therapy can hardly be overstated. As mentioned in the introduction, it is rare to come across clients who are sexually incompatible or disturbed but have no significant cognitive and interpersonal deficits and excesses. Rather, the norm points to the prevalence of predominant errors of omission and commission, based largely on degrees of misinformation and missing information in behavioral, cognitive, and interpersonal modalities (Lazarus, 1989, 1992). In clients who are less responsive to "carburetor adjustment" than Mr. and Mrs. Z were, it is usually necessary to devote far more time and effort to the correction of faulty behaviors, cognitive distortions, and interpersonal disquietude. Sexual problems that rest on (or coexist with) extreme anxiety and insecurity, abject misery, hidden agendas, accumulated resentments, malignant misperceptions, and pernicious demands are not apt to respond to didactic rehearsals and specific readings. Such clients, and particularly those with clear-cut psychopathology, call for more heroic and robust methods, including prescribed medications.

Returning to the case in question, it seemed worth exploring the effects (or lack thereof) of Mrs. Z's sexual exploitation by a previous therapist. She insisted, however, that this was "in the past and mostly forgotten" and was obviously reluctant to examine it. When I reminded her that a certain level of suspiciousness that seemed to stem from this liaison had almost derailed our own therapy, she dismissed it as irrelevant. I decided not to pursue the subject.

At the time of this writing, Mrs. Z was contacted (10 months after the final session) and stated, "I'm enjoying my new self and so is my husband." I asked: "And does he have a new self?" She answered: "You bet. He's a completely different person."

APPENDIX 4.1. EXPANDED STRUCTURAL PROFILE

NAME _____ DATE _____

THE SEVEN DIMENSIONS OF PERSONALITY

(1) DOING . . . ACTION =	BEHAVIOR	B
(2) FEELINGS . . . MOOD . . . EMOTIONS =	AFFECT	A
(3) SENSING (sight, sound, touch, etc.) =	SENSATION	S
(4) IMAGINING . . . FANTASY . . . VISUALIZING =	IMAGERY	I
(5) THINKING . . . INTERPRETING . . . "SELF-TALK" =	COGNITION	C
(6) SOCIAL . . . RELATING =	INTERPERSONAL	I.
(7) BIOLOGICAL . . . PHYSICAL . . . HEALTH =	DRUGS	D.

Behavior
Affect
Sensation
Imagery
Cognition
I.nterpersonal Relationships
D.rugs/Biological Factors

B   A   S   I   C   I.   D.

Reprinted with permission from Clifford N. Lazarus, Ph.D., Comprehensive Psychological Services, 330 N. Harison St., Princeton, NJ 08540.

(1) Behavior

Behaviors are our actions, reactions, and conduct. Behavior is how we *act* in various situations or under certain conditions. Examples of behaviors include: sleeping, eating, playing tennis, crying, walking, yelling watching television, reading, riding a bicycle, etc. Thus, just about anything we *do* can be considered a behavior.

Some people may be described as "doers"—they are action oriented, they like to keep busy, get things done, take on various projects. On the scale below, circle the number that best reflects how much of a doer you are.

	very little		moderately		very much	
1	2	3	4	5	6	7

In the space below, try to make a note of at least one specific behavior that you would like to do *less* of, and also one specific behavior you would like to do *more* of.

I would like to do less (or stop):

I would like to do more (or start):

(2) Affect

Affect is the psychological term for *feelings*, *moods*, and *emotions*. Some affects are positive (such as joy) while others can be characterized as negative (such as depression). Other examples of affects include: happiness, annoyance, contentment, anxiety, jealousy, anger, excitement, guilt, and shame.

Some people are very emotional and may or may not openly express it. How emotional are you? How deeply do you feel things? How passionate are you?

	very little		moderately		very much	
1	2	3	4	5	6	7

In the space below, try to make a note of at least one emotion you would like to feel less of, and at least one emotion you would like to experience more often.

I would like to feel less:

I would like to experience more:

(3) Sensation

Sensation refers to the five basic human senses of *sight, sound, smell, touch, and taste.* In addition, the sensation dimension involves elements of sensuality and sexuality. Sometimes sensory experience is pleasant (for example, the smell of a fresh rose, sexual intimacy, or the taste of apple pie) while at other times sensations can be unpleasant (for example, the pain of a stiff neck, a tension headache, or the smell of rotten eggs).

Some people attach a lot of value to sensory experiences, such as sex, art, food, music, and other "sensory pleasures." Some people often focus on their sensations and pay much attention to pleasant and/or unpleasant inner experiences (such as inner calm and relaxation, or minor aches, pains, and discomforts). How "tuned into" your sensations are you?

        very little   moderately   very much
        1   2   3   4   5   6   7

Below, make a note of some sensations you would like to experience less of and more of.

I would like to experience less:

I would like to experience more:

(4) Imagery

Imagery refers to peoples ability to form *mental pictures* or representations of actual or imagined things, events, and situations. When we fantasize, daydream, or just see pictures in our "mind's eye" we are engaging in mental imagery.

How much fantasy or daydreaming do you engage in? How much and how clearly do you "think in pictures" or see things projected onto the screen of your imagination? (This is separate from thinking or planning.) How much are you into imagery?

        very little   moderately   very much
        1   2   3   4   5   6   7

Make a note below of at least one thing, event, or situation you would like to imagine less of and at least one thing you would like to imagine more.

I would like to imagine less:

I would like to imagine more:

(5) Cognition

Cognition is thinking or the mental faculty or process by which information is obtained. Reasoning, knowledge, and thought are all aspects of cognition. Often, people's thinking takes the form of private "self-talk." Self-talk is the tendency we all have to silently talk to ourselves and to tell ourselves things in the privacy of our own thoughts. Sometimes, our self-talk or cognitions make us feel good about ourselves. For example, when we tell ourselves things like: "That was a really good job I did," or "I'm really an okay person," we tend to feel good. At other times, however, our cognitions can make us feel unhappy with ourselves. For instance, when we tell ourselves things like: "I'll never be able to get the hang of this," or "I must really be a worthless person," we tend to react with unpleasant feelings.

Some people may be described as "thinkers" or "planners"—they are very analytical, reflective, and tend to think things through. How much do you "talk to yourself"? How much of a thinker or a planner are you?

	very little		moderately		very much	
1	2	3	4	5	6	7

Below, try to make a note of some cognitions you would like to have less of and some thoughts you would like to have more often.

I would like to think less:

I would like to think more:

(6) Interpersonal Relationships

Most of us live in richly social environments in which we are constantly interacting with other people across a variety of situations. Not surprisingly, some of our personal interactions are pleasant (for example, making love, or playing a friendly game of cards) while other are not so pleasant (for example, fighting and arguing).

This is your self-rating as a social being. How important are other people to you? How important are close friendships to you, the desire for intimacy, the tendency to gravitate toward people? The opposite of this is being a "loner." How much of a "people person" are you?

	very little		moderately		very much	
1	2	3	4	5	6	7

Below, try to note some interpersonal or social activities you would like to decrease and others you would like to increase.

I would like to decrease:

I would like to increase:

(7) Drugs/Biological/Health Factors

When you come right down to it, we are basically biological, biochemical creatures governed by the activities of our body and brain chemistry. Many of the things we do (that is, many of our behaviors) impact on our biology and hence influence how we think, act, and feel. Included in this aspect of human personality are such things as our general eating and exercise habits, how much alcohol we drink, whether or not we smoke or take drugs, whether or not we should lose some weight or get more regular sleep, etc.

Are you healthy and health conscious? Do you avoid bad habits like smoking, too much alcohol or caffeine, overeating, etc.? Do you exercise regularly, get enough sleep, limit junk food, and generally take care of your body?

very little		moderately		very much	
1	2	3	4	5	6	7

Below, note some things concerning biological factors that you would like to decrease and some things relating to biology you would like to increase.

I would like to decrease:

I would like to increase:

Comments or Additional Information

REFERENCES

Fay, A. (1994). *PQR: Prescription for a quality relationship*. San Luis Obispo, CA: Impact.

Lazarus, A. A. (1987). *Marital myths*. San Luis Obispo, CA: Impact.

Lazarus, A. A. (1989). *The practice of multimodal therapy*. Baltimore: Johns Hopkins University Press.

Lazarus, A. A. (1992). Multimodal therapy: Technical eclecticism with minimal integration. In J. C. Norcross & M. R. Goldfried (Eds.), *Handbook of psychotherapy integration*. New York: Basic Books.

Lazarus, A. A. & Fay, A. (1992). *I can if I want to*. New York: Morrow.

Lazarus, A. A. & Lazarus, C. N. (1991). *Multimodal Life History Inventory*. Champaign, IL: Research Press.

Lazarus, A. A., Lazarus, C. N., & Fay, A. (1993). *Don't believe it for a minute!* San Luis Obispo, CA: Impact.

Lazarus, C. N. (1993). *Expanded Structural Profile.* Princeton, NJ: Comprehensive Psychological Services.

Masters, W. M., & Johnson, V. E. (1970). *Human sexual inadequacy.* Boston: Little, Brown.

Wile, D. B. (1981). *Couples therapy: A nontraditional approach.* New York: Wiley.

5

The Vagaries of Sexual Desire

STEPHEN B. LEVINE

INTRODUCTION

Four important questions about sexual desire have periodically been addressed by clinicians, researchers, and writers from the humanities: What is the nature of sexual desire? How is desire to be measured? What are the sources of its deficiencies and excesses? How is the line between normal and abnormal sexual desire to be drawn? The first three of these questions have been addressed with a new directness during the last 15 years by a number of clinicians who specialize in sexual problems (Leiblum & Rosen, 1988). Prior to Kaplan's (1977) formulation, desire was discussed in terms of the instinct, "libido," a concept dating from early 20th-century psychoanalytic assumptions about how minds operated. Today, when biological assumptions are in vogue for explaining mental phenomena, the concept of libido has fallen further out of fashion. "Libido," "sex drive," and "sexual desire" are now often used synonymously to connote a neurotransmitter-based organizer of sexual behavior. The observations that this organizer can be inhibited by serotonergic and other pharmacological compounds and by many organic disease states and can be stimulated by some dopamine agonists is of great heuristic interest. Understanding desire as consisting of the mind's integration of testosterone-dependent biogenic drives, psychologically based motivations, and socially based expectations (Levine, 1987) appears to be complex beyond either a psychoanalytic or a biological model, however.

Definitive answers to these four questions have not yet been widely agreed on. The delineations of the sexual dysfunction labeled either "hypoactive" or "inhibited" sexual desire have failed to produce a clear-cut biological finding of great power to explain the absence of sexual interest in a chosen partner in the vast majority of cases. The failure of research has an important implication for clinicians.

The vicissitudes of sexual desire still belong to the province of clinicians. The scientific power of clinical work is well understood: Psychotherapies can generate but not prove hypotheses. Clinicians' work depends on their ability to synthesize the complex interaction of numerous factors in their patients' lives. Their interaction is typically beyond the capacity of scientific methods to separate for statistically valid, replicable ascertainment.

Unfortunately, there are numerous clinical perspectives from which to view any sexual desire problem. These are usually stated as the behavioral, psychodynamic, and systems theory mental health ideologies. But, another important problem—viewpoint—makes clinical work exasperating to the scientist. Clinical data reflect the viewpoint of the patient, the spouse, the couple working together, the therapist or, usually, unknown admixtures of each. I summarize this complexity to myself by assuming that every case presentation simultaneously reflects the sensibilities of the patient and the presenter and that it is invariably not clear which is which at times.

CASE PRESENTATION

Here is a story of evolving sexual desire in a couple. The story unfolded over a period of several years during which the sexual desire of both partners dramatically changed. The facts of the story derive from the husband's viewpoint. Its telling, however, derives from my memory and is influenced by my purposes: (1) to give readers a sense of familiarity with their own clinical experiences, (2) to suggest how the study of people's struggles can illuminate the complex origin of significant desire problems, (3) to suggest that the basic tactic of therapy is to help people to listen to themselves so that they can discover the meaning of the vagaries of their sexual desire, and (4) to caution that effective therapy in any branch of medicine rests on an understanding of pathogenesis, and that therapists must not get carried away with techniques for problems whose causes cannot be quickly understood.

The Initial Presentation

A middle-age college-educated businessman sought individual therapy saying that he was emotionally exhausted, depressed, periodically impotent, and no longer able to participate in his marriage of 21 years. Sex was a central part of the problem and the cause of his abiding resentment of his wife. For 2 months, ever since he decided he was going to leave home, his sleep and concentration at work had been interrupted by guilt. He knew that their sexual relationship was a complex by-product of her inhibitions, their unsatisfactory nonsexual interactions, and his own difficult-to-pinpoint psychological patterns. Because their past individual and couple therapy (with me and others) led to no lasting changes, he felt their marriage was hopeless. He wanted help with leaving the marriage.

"My life is filled with paradox." He had a passionate commitment to maintaining an intact family, and now he passionately wanted to leave it. He felt faithful to his wife, yet there had been insignificant exceptions. He felt that he modeled prudence in his interactions yet his children showed no signs of acquiring it. He continued to ask for sexual experiences several times per month even though he disapproved of how they were conducted and hated himself for bothering. And most acutely disturbing, although he wanted nothing to do with his wife—wanted to be rid of this "asexual" creature, in fact—he was gripped by episodes of jealousy imagining she was already having an affair.

For most of their sexual experiences over two decades, his wife pulled her nightgown up to her waist and disdainfully allowed penetration while she endured his "animalistic" need. As he spoke of being made to feel like a rapist, he cried. Her only orgasms had been stimulated by a vibrator and only during the last decade. His wife repeatedly told him that he caused their abject sexual experiences by ignoring her, preferring the company of his friends to her, never expressing affection, and sharing little of what he was thinking with her. "You, my dear husband, have a major intimacy problem!"

He discussed his situation in individual therapy for months before he moved out of his home, leaving a 16-year-old daughter—often sarcastically called his princess — and his wife. Their 20-year-old daughter —"a psychopath in training"—was away at college. These discussions enabled him to sleep, concentrate, and feel his mood was normal once again. By the time he left home, he was euphoric. His desire eager.

The Background

Twenty-one years ago, he and his thin, attractive girlfriend had an immediately and intensely sexual courtship. After 1 week of almost constantly being in each other's presence, they moved in together. The obstacle to their continued pleasure that emerged during the following months was the growing discomfort between his mother and his girl-friend. By the wedding, neither woman was comfortable near the other. He felt forced to choose between them. For months his wife did not stop criticizing him for paying his family's wedding expenses without discussing it with her. "I could afford it, they could not, and she disapproved." Within weeks of their marriage, two persistent patterns began: a disdainful, dutiful caring for his "primitive" sexual needs; his wife's polite cold avoidance of his mother. Each overwhelmed him.

"I was too young to appreciate what all her confusing family relationships meant in terms of her past and her future." His wife came from a divorced family in which her mother left her two children in the care of a grandmother when she went off with one of her several surreptitious lovers ("Her mother was some kind of slut!"). His wife has had a lifelong loving devotion to her brother and grandmother—which he admired— an intense disdainful tolerance of her mother—which he understood—and a warm but limited relationship with her father's second wife from which he benefited in terms of family life. The members of her family easily interacted with him and apparently were quite fond of him for his sociability, friendship, and generosity.

"Life was not so great in my family either." His family unit was broken by his father's sudden death at age 7. Severe financial problems left the family in immediate jeopardy; his mother went to work and eventually began an affair with a married man. Their poverty became an organizing principle in his life: He vowed never to want for money and had directed his life toward that goal since childhood. His mother's lover, who did not divorce, was a source of disgrace to the patient. He became the source of rage when the patient overheard the man pressuring his mother to find more time away from her children. When the man left his family and moved to a new city, his mother, sister, and he joined him. The patient soon discovered that the man was pressuring her to send him and his sister to live with relatives. The preteen patient was enraged that his mother even considered his outrageous demands. Several years later, his mother refused to care for her mother when she was incapacitated with dementia. She abruptly "shipped" her to a nursing home rather than deal with her. Thus, his disdain for his mother stemmed from both her relationship with this man and her treatment of his grandmother; it continued after his mother was abandoned by the man.

Both the patient and his wife intended to fix their history of family chaos with their own new intact family. Her singular ambition was to be a mother and to provide the stable environment that she never had. This was profoundly attractive to him; her academic failure during her semester of college was not important. Despite their identical familial ambitions, after several months he felt the marriage was a colossal mistake and began thinking of leaving. His mental drama was interrupted by the discovery of their first pregnancy. "I just could not suggest an abortion; she was so happy. I just hoped it would get better. The whole situation was too much for me. What a mistake! I should have ended it then and there!"

The patient became financially successful prior to marriage. With time, he dressed expensively, drove expensive cars, and was generous with time and money to a number of charities. He prided himself on his fund of knowledge of many subjects and had an impeccable reputation for honesty in business. He moved easily in many circles, had a keen analytical mind, and gravitated to the big picture—movements in society, state of medicine, real estate woes, international markets, activities in the fine arts. He loved moving in powerful circles, involving himself with the accomplished in many fields. He had a large circle of friends—men, women, and couples. He loved to hear about the problems of others and often was sought out for advice. He was socially active, frequently out most nights of the week after coming home earlier than most fathers from work. He indulged himself in material things but worried about the materialistic preoccupations of his wife and children, who seemed obsessed with clothes and goods. "I have been staying in this marriage for years for the sake of the children, enduring my unhappiness, only to realize that they have turned out to be self-centered, self-indulgent people without any positive regard for their father, empathy for others, and without a clue as to how the rest of the world actually lives." The final straw that moved him to seriously consider leaving the home was his perception that his "princess" regarded him only as a money source. While blaming himself and his wife for this, he always maintained that his wife was a wonderful mother who faithfully devoted her life to care for the needs of both of their children. Although deeply disappointed in his girls, he kept their difficulties in perspective: Neither had drug problems and many of his friends' children had worse problems.

The Departure from the Marriage

During the first 2 months of therapy, the angry noncommunication with his wife led to her informing him during "another" argument that she would be relieved if he left. He was waiting for these words. He had located an apartment and so he decided to rent and have it decorated. As was his pattern in all things, he planned an orderly departure to the apartment when it was completely finished. He personally devised a separation agreement. As he contemplated leaving, however, he was fearful that he would not be able to find women to date and that he would not be sexually adequate.

Thinner than he had been in 20 years, regimented into a healthy diet and regular exercise, encouraged by confidant–friends who were sure he was about to have a good time, he moved out feeling that his life was beginning and vowing that he would never go back to such a sick, emotionally abject life—*never*! He had not had any sexual desire for his wife in months and had no further sexual contact after a few humiliating repetitions of their "if you must" pattern.

The Next 6 Months

He discovered that his fears of people's lack of interest in him were ridiculous. For 6 weeks, he was busy almost every night having intimate conversations with either eligible women or his friends. He was reassured that he had no intimacy problem; "I just didn't like my wife well enough." He then settled into an almost exclusive relationship with a 40-year-old divorcee with several children. He was impotent for 3 weeks but otherwise was having wonderful sexual experiences. His desire was not a problem. His erection just faded at intromission. He discovered the joys of providing pleasure to his partner. He was astounded that she found his body nice. Despite the fact that he loved the devotion she had to her children, it gradually became clear to him that he wanted her to be alone with him much more and free to travel, and he did not want to be a stepfather even to one teenager. She came to represent the problem with a large segment of eligible women—they had children whose needs came first. As he dated others, he analyzed the implications of every conversation so he could ascertain whether the relationship had a future. He realized what he did and did not want. He wanted someone who was good at something, someone he respected for her accomplishments. When he realized that a woman was not suited for him, he left the relationship—disappointing several.

In the meantime, people were frequently spontaneously telling him how surprised they were that he stayed with his wife so many years. They characterized her as the most publicly demeaning, negative person they had ever seen. Friends described their discomfort being with them as a couple because of her attitudes toward him. Numerous people said that they tolerated the relationship as a couple to be with him and that he was one of the nicest people they had ever met. These experiences enhanced his self-esteem and confidence but led him to feel that he was a fool for having stayed so long. He repeatedly asked me why he had stayed for over two decades, fearful that we were missing something in our explanations—children, values, intact family, hope through therapy, wish not to hurt, etc.

He met an accomplished professional woman, ambitious, attractive, mid-30s, who was eager and excited about him. For 2 months he was involved with this "superwoman" in a long-distance relationship. Their meetings were sexually exciting, psychologically intimate, but often ended abruptly because of her work deadlines. An evening with her and her "off-the-wall" daughter ended his participation in the relationship because he perceived that she was inattentive to her starving-for-affection child. Memories of their affair, however, preoccupied him for several months. She became to him the generic accomplished woman trying to have it all. "No thanks, I want there to be real room for me in a woman's life."

The Family

Three important processes were simultaneously occurring. His wife was moving from angry to depressed; from glad-you-are-out-of-here to we-should-try-to-reconcile. His princess was taking an emotional nose-dive—grades dropping, cutting school, her fine academic record sullied, automobile accidents, raging at him and her mother, and cutting more psychotherapy sessions than she attended. His wife and daughter were so effectively preoccupied with his every social move that he discovered he had few actual social privacies.

He was surprised at the depth of his wife's despair and was taken aback by her competitiveness with the women he dated. I would never go back with her—*never*! When they attended a funeral together, she cried that she missed him and his body and asked if they could date. He considered it for several weeks and agreed. Within a month, he was repeatedly uttering this sentence to his confidants and enjoying its irony: "Now I have a girlfriend and a mistress who happens to be my wife!"

His wife's sexual behaviors changed dramatically. She was now endlessly interested in sex, came to his apartment for that purpose, had sex downstairs in their home when he came over to get the mail, and so forth. She wanted to do everything—even oral sex. She told him she wanted to be his sexual slave. For the first time in decades she lubricated without an artificial lubricant. Even when she developed lumbar disk symptoms from the intense exercise program she started herself on to lose weight, she wanted sex. He was enjoying this; not as love or reconciliation but as making up for 20 plus years. This was power; the tables were turned. He was watching the taming of the shrew in his house and he did not do anything but allow her to get a glimpse of what life might be like without him.

HUSBAND: Is it the Prozac she is taking?
DOCTOR: No, it is just that she is attempting to reclaim her husband.

Within several months of their dating, she intensified her requests that he move back and stop his relationships with others. He was enjoying her social transformation—weight loss, social pleasantness, and no longer demeaning in public or private. He kept repeating, "A leopard does not change its spots; but this one is." But he valued his independence and was slowly informing her that he did not think it would work—he was too preoccupied with their past while he was enjoying their present. "I don't think I can get over it." But the fact that his daughter looked like she was a tragedy waiting to happen made him more cautious about ending the apparent growing reconciliation. "There is no more than a ten percent chance that I will reconcile."

His wife decided to have her disk fixed surgically. She developed a rare postoperative complication that prolonged her rehabilitation. He was faced with the need to care for her at home until he at least learned whether she was going to recover. He surrendered and did the "moral" thing. Because his princess was coming home after a summer away and would need supervision, he agreed to be faithful during his wife's rehabilitation. This highly conflicted decision was accompanied by a brief sexual experience with a daring sadomasochistic woman he viewed only as a sexual plaything—a curiosity—something to which he felt entitled. His wife made steady progress physically; within 3 months she was almost pain free. She continued to be sexually active throughout this period. He joked with her that he was renewing his commitment to her 1 week at a time and would revoke it as soon as she proved nasty again. "There is no more than a thirty percent chance that I will reconcile."

As they became socially reintegrated as a couple, his friends could not get over the transformation that had occurred to her. She was warm to people she previously treated abruptly, was openly affectionate to her husband, and seemed to have lost her fault finding with others. She could not admit to her husband that she ever had any serious role in their troubles, feeling instead that his therapy enabled him to be kinder and to talk and that she had only been reacting to his rejection of her from the early weeks of their marriage.

He felt that hers was an overly simple view, but he was interested in her perspective. Her main one was that he hated his mother and transferred the hatred from her to his wife early after the marriage. He thought that it surely must have some explanatory merit. He had emotionally abandoned his mother to a modest economic life, and he could still feel the moral outrage over her behavior during his painful early years. He also felt angry that his mother did not maintain any interest in his girls over the years, even though he recognized that his wife posed a serious obstacle. While he found his wife's ideas useful, he continued to feel that their tragic relationship was not all explained by transference but, "One can never be certain about psychological matters."

Settling In

With his wife recovered, he began a faithful life with her. His resentment for what he endured for over 20 years continued. The thrill of the taming of the shrew passed after several months. He often thought of his many exciting times as a separated man without regret. He learned that he wanted his life to go the way he wanted his life to go. He was not interested in many compromises. He wanted to be with a woman he could respect.

"I have a history with my wife!" He did not speak of loving her and, if love is comfort, contentment, and pleasure in a wife's being, he did not love her. He tried to be kind and considerate to her. Her complaints, delivered with more restraint, resurfaced: "You are not affectionate!" "You are not intimate!" "You push me away." "I need more from you!" These were justified in his view.

They began to have sex twice a month. "I can take it or leave it." It offered him little joy. Morning sex when he transiently felt horny was convenient. He did not fantasize about his wife or their past sexual experiences. Although he frequently recited her many positive points to himself, he returned to his lack of respect for her lack of interest in the world and her comfort without education. He regained his weight and felt slothful again. He traveled with his wife to several exciting places but found no pleasure in her company and no interest in the things she wanted to do.

He began thinking again about leaving her and decided to wait either for her to realize that they could not be happy together and end their marriage or for his princess to further stabilize. He was not involved with another woman but strongly suspected that his ability to stay home in fidelity would probably quickly disappear if he were to meet an accomplished person with no or grown children who found him good enough as he was.

His life was still gripped by paradox. He did not want a marriage of compromise but he reestablished it for the sake of his enduring values. He wanted the sexual excitement he had when he was out of the house, but he slipped into a pattern of infrequent, unsatisfying, and unmotivated sex. He wanted sexual passion but ran from it.

DISCUSSION

Can the vicissitudes of this man's sexual desire be understood biologically? Not very well. He periodically made mention of feeling "horny" and that it was the relief of this bodily feeling that led him to have the demeaning sexual experiences with his wife. I had the impression that this every-2-weeks-or-so phenomenon was the expression of an ordinary drive endowment because it found consistent expression in periods of despair, liberation, social dilemma, and resignation.

Can the fluctuations in this man's sexual desire be understood in terms of the motivational component of sexual desire? Yes, his willingness to bring his body to the sexual experience in a series of new relationships was motivated by his need to explore his attractiveness to others, to enjoy the sensual experiences that he missed during his adulthood, to get to know women and their psychology more completely, to further understand his wife's inhibitions, and to put his past and future marriage into better perspective. After his separation, he was willing to bring his body to his wife to enjoy the "taming of the shrew," to explore his capacity to feel lovingly attached, and to regulate his sexual tensions.

Can the vagaries of his desire and sexual behavior be understood in terms of the social, conscience, or wish component of sexual desire? Not as crisply, but he and his middle-age friends of both sexes expected that he would be extremely sexually active upon leaving his marriage. "Take your time. . . . Don't rush into things. . . . Experience a lot of women to help you clarify what you really want. . . ." were examples of the often-repeated advice given to him by "people who had been there." He was kept from exploitative sexual behavior by three traits: his ability to listen intently to and comprehend the personal strivings of the women he dated, his aspiration to be a civilized man, and his wish to keep his reputation for integrity. In the battle with his conscience, however, he did give into one entitled episode of acting out sexually when his wife's illness forced him to "do the moral thing" and be at home. On their first meeting, the woman he found irresistible revealed herself as loving sadomasochism.

If sexual desire reflects the mind's capacity to integrate the biological, psychological, and social organizers of sexual behavior, his desire can be understood by understanding what was on his nonsexual mind during this 2-year period. He created new rules for his participation in marriage in a shift of power. His wife preferred to think that he was unable to love and be truly intimate. He temporarily answered this important query with, "I am unable to love and be intimate with her; I do not respect her enough." But, in more disquieting moments, he wondered whether his wife was correct. "Can I deeply love anyone?"

I do not believe that sophisticated therapies fix things as much as they enable people to realize the complex dimensions of their lives. It helps them to own their paradoxes and find solutions to them that are acceptable to themselves and those they value. The study of sexual desire, whether within the so-called normal range or that which qualifies for a diagnosis in the *Diagnostic and Statistical Manual of Mental Disorders* (American Psychiatric Association, 1994), introduces the therapist to irony, paradox, complexity, hypocrisy, conflict—all those very things that writers in the humanities have known about as long as recorded time (Updike, 1993). With tact, compassion, timing, and supportive humor, it is the responsibility of the therapist to assist the patient in the quest to see how his/her life fits into this essential human trap.

ADDENDUM

The editors have asked me to expand this contribution. I have decided to respond to their thoughtful questions in a separate section rather than significantly changing the original submission. They have asked me to elaborate on the four questions about desire posed in the introduction. What is the nature of sexual desire? Sexual desire is the psychobiological force that tends to produce sexual behavior. It precedes and accompanies sexual arousal, often being mediated by visualizations that vary from vague and fleeting images to well-formed fantasies called scenarios or scripts. I suspect that desire is the earliest form of the emotion called sexual arousal. Desire is simultaneously a cognitive and an emotional (psychic) process and a bodily (somatic) process. Knowledge of this psychosomatic physiology is limited. The manifestations of desire evolve during the life cycle. Age is the best known correlate of its evolution. Age effects its changes through the influences of biology, personality maturation, and changing life demands. Other more subtle influences on desire—such as moral sensibilities, sexual identity, personality structure, and education—are probably also involved.

How is desire to be measured? Sexual desire's complexity makes its measurement for research and clinical purposes arbitrary, imprecise, and relatively unreliable. Even when a person presents with easy-to-diagnose inhibited sexual desire—that is, describes a deficiency of sexual fantasies, spontaneous genital tingling, or tumescence; is motivated to avoid sexual behavior in all forms; and finds no arousal in response to esthetically pleasing persons, movies, readings, or pictures—future conversations often yield contradictory evidence. And when desire is judged to be excessive, the frequency of sexual behaviors, the time after orgasm when the person feels the need for another, and the capacity to concentrate can be clinically estimated. However, clinicians do not actually know whether the person has too much drive, motive, arousal, or frustration. In physiological terms, five questions illuminate the problem:

1. Is this a defect in neurohumoral transmission?
2. Is this a failure of the satiety mechanism?
3. Is this the product of overuse of erotization defenses against current despair?
4. Is this the product of overuse of erotization defenses against the emergence of memories of past physical and sexual abuse?
5. Is this the product of the couple's failure to understand each other's need for physical intimacies?

So we measure desire, sexual interest, frequency of orgasmic attainment, or some parameters and assign it a semiquantitative form—absent, low, ordinary, excessive.

The sources of desire's deficiencies are addressed in this volume through the case history method. Hypotheses about the sources of desire's excesses can be deduced from the list of five questions above. The line between normal and abnormal desire is not usually arbitrarily drawn by researchers or clinicians; rather, professionals allow the help seeking public to declare their desire problematic.

The editors have also asked me to elaborate my model of desire and to reference it. I have repeatedly offered the notion that desire possesses an elegance (Levine, 1989)—it appears to be a simple, unitary phenomenon, but it is deceptive and complex. Its unity is the result of the mind's synthesis of three shaping influences on our sexual behaviors. There is a testosterone-receptor-dependent physiological process that creates fantasy, early genital arousal, and heightened awareness of esthetically attractive people. This I call drive; I believe drive to be hardwired into each nervous system. Its purpose is ultimately reproductive—to ensure propagation of the species.

There is the deeply personal psychological motive to bring the body to the sexual experience, which I have alternately referred to as sexual willingness or motive. Sexual desire problems usually turn out to be matters of hidden motives to avoid or to engage in sexual behaviors. Motives are profoundly influenced by the quality of the nonsexual relationship, the compatibility of sexual identity, the influence of past experience with others on whom one was dependent, and the couple's skill at negotiating their sexual relationship. Motive is fed by both drive and the third component of sexual desire, wish.

Wish is the most difficult to understand because it blends imperceptibly with motive. But wish has to do with the influence of social experience on desire. Every person belongs to numerous social groups—family, ethnic, religious, racial, political, vocational, marriage—each of which may shape the expectations for how often we ought to behave sexually and what we should do. For example, 16-year-old religious Caucasian Baptist teenagers from the rural South are apt to have different values than some other teenage groups. In addition, we have evolving moral sensibilities which impact on our willingness to acknowledge that we desire someone or some behavior. These I consider social.

Desire, in summary, is the amalgamation of our three overlapping domains of existence—biological, social, and individual psychological. I have written about this model in several publications between 1984 and 1992 (Levine, 1987, 1989, 1992).

Finally, the editors requested a few more details about the case. About 12 years before the reported therapy, the couple sought me out after the wife refused to return for a third session to a therapist who suggested sensate focus. I worked with them conjointly for 4 months without being able to increase her willingness to behave sexually. I was unable to understand the meaning of their backgrounds and the actual causes of their interpersonal trouble. Most important, I could not help them to love each other. As I remember it, she was profoundly disdainful of his social behavior—"He works the crowds!" she said, meaning that he preferred others to her because they could gratify his narcissistic need for importance. He was recurrently angry at her sexual coldness and her haughty disapproval of most people in the universe. Both were sent to individual therapy; he went for 3 years. She came to consider his therapy a waste of time. She used numerous therapists over the years, including a few visits with me, to discuss why no one could help her obviously impaired husband. She then spoke briefly about her childhood but was disinclined to pursue the subject. His previous therapist, who had recently divorced, could not understand why he stayed married to her.

It was not my purpose to tell everything I knew about this couple. Far from it, I was concerned about confidentiality. Every case history is only a viewpoint, a product of the informant and the storyteller. The storyteller elects what to tell to the reader. This man and I regularly conversed for 2 years. It is beyond me to reduce this rich intimacy to a complete story. Stoller (1991) has written eloquently of the problem of subjectivity of gathering information.

REFERENCES

American Psychiatric Association. (1994). *Diagnostic and statistical manual of mental disorders* (4th ed.). Washington, DC: Author.

Kaplan, H. S. (1977). *Disorders of sexual desire.* New York: Brunner/Mazel.

Leiblum, S. R., & Rosen, R. C. (Eds.). (1988). *Sexual desire disorders.* New York: Guilford Press.

Levine, S. B. (1987). More on the nature of sexual desire. *Journal of Sex and Marital Therapy, 13*(1), 35–44.

Levine, S. B. (1989). The elegance of sexual desire. In *Sex is not simple.* Columbus: Ohio Psychology Publishing.

Levine, S. B. (1992). The paradoxes of sexual desire. In *Sexual life: A clinician's guide.* New York: Plenum Press.

Stoller, R. J. (1991). *Porn: Myths for twentieth century.* New Haven: Yale University Press.

Updike, J. (1993, June 20). The deadly sins/Lust: Even the Bible is soft on sex. *New York Times Book Review,* p. 3.

_____

6

_____

Integrative Therapy in a Woman with Secondary Low Sex Desire

HAROLD I. LIEF

INTRODUCTION

No clinical problem facing the sex therapist is as complex and confusing as is the diagnosis of hypoactive sexual desire disorder (HSDD). The revised third edition of the *Diagnostic and Statistical Manual of Mental Disorders* (DSM-III-R; American Psychiatric Association, 1987) rejected the term "inhibited" found in the previous edition (DSM-III); the phenomenologically based term "hypoactive" recognized that some patients are responding to biological processes rather than psychological ones. (HSDD is continued in DSM-IV; American Psychiatric Association, 1994.) Examples of biological factors are abnormally low levels of testosterone in both men and women, antidepressants, especially those that increase serotonin levels, and depression itself.

Psychological factors are almost always an intrapsychic and interpersonal combination. Even a celibate has fantasies of partner sex. To increase the complexity, a decrease in sexual activity or engaging in unwanted or undesired sex almost always affects the relationship, usually negatively. Obviously, reactions of the partner are also highly significant in modifying the sexual system.

To understand sexual desire, I have constructed a diagram of the trajectory of sexual desire (Figure 6.1) or, as Rado (1949) called it, the "sexual motive state."

Nonreporting (Outside Awareness) Brain Activity
(Hormones and Brain Neurotransmitters)
↓
Internal Scripting (Partial or Full Reporting
Brain Activity)
↓
Readiness to Respond to Sexual Cues and Stimuli
↓
Readiness to Generate Sexual Fantasies and/or to
Respond to Partner Stimulation

FIGURE 6.1. Trajectory of sexual desire.

A distinction can be made between desire *for* sex and desire *in* sex. This is one of my few points of disagreement with Schnarch (1991), who claims we must fuse the two. Of 52 women with HSDD whom I studied in one research project (Lief, 1991), 18 almost always were passionate and orgastic once the initial barrier to having sex was overcome. They had no desire *for* sex; mysteriously, they had no lack of desire *in* sex. It was as if once you thoroughly enjoyed savoring a steak, you never wanted another one. Cajoled or obligated to eat another, your pleasure the next time around was undiminished. Previously (Lief, 1981) I made a distinction between desire and arousal, as did Zilbergeld and Ellison (1980). To emphasize this, I created the acronym DAVOS, for desire, arousal, vasocongestion, orgasm, and satisfaction.

Desire must be distinguished from arousal. The excitement state is separated into two components, one psychologic (arousal) and the other physiologic (vasocongestion). The psychologic component of excitement is not always accompanied by its physiologic component. A classic example is impotence, in which there may be intense arousal and a diminished physiologic response. Conversely, it is possible to have a physiologic response without the full range of arousal. A case in point is that of a woman who is being physiologically monitored for perivaginal, uterine, and anal contractions during excitement and orgasm who shows the full range of sexual response, clearly indicating orgasm, but fails to label the experience as such. Heiman (1977) has reported that as many as 15 percent of women may fall into this category.

Just as arousal and vasocongestion are not always synchronized, and therefore have to be regarded as separate components of excitement, so too orgasm and satisfaction may be desynchronized—hence the need to have a separate component evaluating the quality of satisfaction. A person may go through the full range of human sexual response, and derive little satisfaction from it, usually because of negative feelings toward the partner or the situation in which sex occurs. On the other hand, it is possible to have a limited sexual response without orgasm and be well satisfied. This is often true of women who find their greatest satisfaction in the closeness and intimacy of the encounter. Much more emotional weight may be attached to the feeling of sharing and connectedness than to the erotic experience itself. Men, being more genitally oriented, are somewhat less likely to separate the total psychological experience from the quality of the erotic one. (Lief, 1985, pp. 61–62)

This case study demonstrates almost all the dimensions of HSDD discussed earlier. The interaction between biology and psychology is also fascinating, and ultimately I believe the case illustrates the validity of Schnarch's major thesis, in which the struggle between the goals of *differentiation* and *fusion* lies at the heart of psychopathology and our understanding of marital dynamics. It illustrates the most important battle each one of us must fight—the struggle between wanting to fuse with the "loved one" and our need to separate and to individuate.

What has this internal conflict to do with diminished or absent sex desire? If the adult retains highly ambivalent feelings toward self and projects the negative feelings to "the other" or "others," might this not modify profoundly the person's sense of self vis-à-vis the other? Nathanson (1992) puts it well: "If shame creates a sense of a defective self, it therefore creates in us a sense of *an other who sees us as defective*, no matter what that person really thinks of us" (p. 250). What if the protection against shame involves the need to do the *right thing* (fusion)? What if this need is in constant conflict with the need to do for oneself (differentiation)? Might not that person find it difficult to find let alone "follow his bliss," as Joseph Campbell put it?

I chose this case because it illustrates Levine's truism that "sex is not simple" (Levine, 1988). There were several Axis I diagnoses; a combination of personality patterns; biological, intrapsychic, and interpersonal dimensions; and many different therapies used: hormonal, pharmacological, behavioral, cognitive, and psychodynamic. In the latter category, there were several dynamic issues that sometimes seemed to compete with each other for primacy.

I have presented this case in a session-by-session format so the reader can accompany me on the rocky path of therapy. I took careful and fairly thorough notes during the course of treatment, which permit me to recapture my thoughts here.

DESCRIPTION OF PATIENT AND HER MARITAL PARTNER

The patient, Lil, is a 30-something-year-old housewife; she held a job involving mathematical skills before marriage. She is pretty in an all-

American, girl-next-door sense—more wholesome than sexy, more innocent than scheming, although she can be very clever. She wants to please;
the sense of "chutzpah" is foreign to her. Her sense of obligation is keen
and is in constant battle with her desire to be left to her own devices.
The aspect of life that she most desires is "space." She is about 5'4",
weighs about 115 pounds, and conveys a sense of petiteness, even of
fragility that is belied by her toughness and her standing up for what she
believes.

She has made a fortunate marriage to a professional who is laid back,
caring, and concerned and is in every sense of the word a competent man-
ager who seems to cope with any crisis big or small with patience and
equanimity. He seems to understand Lil well and if she is frightened, even
somewhat frantic, he is there for her and if she wants quiet or silence he
seems to sense that too. "With what other man could I ride for many
hours in complete silence, with both of us content?" she asked in one
session.

When Lil came into treatment, they had two small children. Now
there are three. The transition from romantic couple to parenthood
played a big role dynamically, as we shall see.

Although Lil seems to be the very essence of the professional middle class, she is somewhat upwardly mobile. Even her husband's
name, Newbold, seems to call attention to their different backgrounds,
but another admirable aspect of her husband is his lack of class consciousness.

SESSION-BY-SESSION ANALYSIS

Now let us go through the process of therapy, session by session. There
were 23 sessions before Lil gave birth to her third child. Most will be
highlighted or summarized with occasional quotations of the patient's
words. My thoughts or words are italicized; if spoken, they are in quotes.

Session I

Lil developed a depression approximately 6 months after the birth of
her second child but did not do anything about it. She sought help about
a year later from Dr. R who transferred her to Dr. S. Both of them made
the diagnosis of depression and prescribed Prozac (fluoxetine), which
she had been taking for a little over 3 months. She had responded within
6 to 8 weeks. Her symptoms of depression had abated and she felt well
in every way except sexually.

She had noted a gradual decrease in sexual desire. She is unsure which came first, although she has some suspicion that the problem with sexual desire preceded the depression.

At this point in the interview I was thinking about the connections between depression and loss of sexual desire. It certainly occurs often enough, in anywhere from 10% to 25% of depressed patients. The fact though that we do not know the prevalence with any greater degree of certitude indicates the need for more research with larger samples of depressed people. It is also common to see individuals with sexual problems who have become depressed as a consequence of those problems. Comorbidity in my clinic populations ran as high as 25% but we had not studied the direction of the vectors. Somehow, I almost immediately believed Lil was correct about the direction, namely, that the loss of desire had preceded the depression; this was a hunch, lacking proof. Yet, how to explain the fact that all her symptoms of depression had lifted save one, now her presenting problem?

She had a good sexual relationship before the first child. She noted that it took a while before her sexual desire returned after the birth of the firstborn and her lack of sexual desire became much worse after the birth of the second child. She does not think this was simply being overwhelmed by child care, but the major theme that emerged is her need for privacy, the time and space that are not occupied by anybody else. A sexual encounter seems to be an intrusion and an invasion of her space. It feels like a lot of work to become aroused and she has difficulty in becoming aroused even though she is orgastic more than half the time. Even when she is orgastic, the physical pleasure is insignificant because the negatives outweigh the positives. She does not want to participate and she feels that she is forcing herself to respond. There is no pressure from her husband; this is an inner feeling that she is obligated to do this. Last night, for example, she performed oral sex on her husband and because he did not touch her, it was much easier. She did not become aroused but, at least, there was nothing negative in that experience. She does say that oral sex is the way she usually achieves orgasm.

The thought I was having at that moment was a question. Does her resistance to the invasion of space also account for her preference for oral sex over intercourse? Does "space" have a double meaning?

Her background indicates there was a definite emphasis on privacy throughout her childhood. She recalls between the ages of 6 and 11 often playing by herself despite her mother's pressure to go outside to play with other children. Even now, on a nice day there is a vague feeling of guilt if she is inside rather than outside. She was the oldest of five children with three younger brothers and a young sister who arrived 15 years after

Lil's own birth. She says there was a reasonable degree of comfort in body touching. Her privacy is so important that she makes certain that she and her husband do not use the bathroom at the same time. They have a great respect for each other's privacy and she remarked that Newbold is the only person with whom she wanted to share her life.

Her depression was seen by both psychiatrists as biological and she had the vegetative earmarks of endogenous depression, with the exception of weight loss. She now believes that she had previous episodes of depression in childhood, as well as in her teen years, but she was not altogether aware of these because they were not as severe as the depressive spell she had recently. Her mother also had suffered from depressions and it was her mother who pointed out to Lil her more recent depression before she was even aware of it or had labeled it as such.

I mentioned to her the various ways in which we could deal with this, from pharmacological treatment to psychological and I recommended that we try to work this out psychologically because the inhibition of desire and arousal seems to be related to the central theme of feeling that sex is an intrusion, an invasion of her space.

Curiously, it is the only way in which she feels this intrusion. She and her husband are able to converse with each other easily, share thoughts and feelings, but she does not want to share her body.

Session 2

This was the first conjoint session but I spent a few minutes with Lil's husband and found him as I described him earlier. He was very anxious to get to the bottom of his wife's problem because it was clearly upsetting to his wife and, obviously, the more she was interested in sex, the better the quality as well as the frequency of sexual relations. During the conjoint session we went over the various options and I recommended the use of sensate focus. We discussed Lil's need for space and the need to ward off the intrusion of sex. She gets into bed, she takes a book, and she encloses herself away from the outside world. This is not to separate herself from her husband but to create a space for herself.

How could she do one without the other? Is this an attempt to deny its effect on her husband? I wondered whether they would be able to manage the sensate focus exercises given Lil's need for space and privacy and her feelings that sex was an intrusion on her space, including her body. I was also concerned that the Prozac might still be playing a role in maintaining her decreased sexual desire and responsivity.

Session 3

They reported that they had some reluctance to start sensate focus as if they were too sophisticated for this and had gone beyond it, a rather common reaction to the recommendation of these exercises. However, they said that they would attempt sensual massage during this next week. Lil said that she did not feel that her reluctance to carry out the exercises was part of maintaining her space. She made clear her feeling that something was missing; she has absolutely no sexual fantasies and no response to sexual stimuli on television, books, or movies. Because there was an absence of sexual fantasies or dreams, I decided to shift her from Prozac to bupropion (Wellbutrin), building up gradually to 300 mg a day while reducing Prozac.

Despite the fact that Prozac is a very effective antidepressant, many people report sexual dysfunctions while on it. It is my impression that somewhere close to 40% of female patients will have decreased desire and decreased arousability. In the male, the most frequent outcome is a marked decrease in the ability to orgasm, so much so that it appears to be an effective remedy for premature ejaculation. A recent specific serotonin reuptake inhibitor in the treatment of premature ejaculation is paroxetine (Paxil), as low as 10 mg a day. At any rate, the clinician treating a patient with sexual dysfunction who is also on Prozac often has a real problem.

Session 4

This was the third conjoint session. Lil avoided the sensate focus exercises until almost the last minute. She felt as if she *should* be doing this but, nevertheless, she did not want to carry it out. She was pleasantly surprised how much she enjoyed the pleasuring sequence and became aroused even though there was no direct genital stimulation and, because she was enjoying the experience, she felt closer to her husband. She is now taking Wellbutrin without any ill effects except for dry mouth. She reported an increase in sexual dreams since starting Wellbutrin but was really cheered and made more hopeful by her sexual response to what happened the previous night. They will continue with sensate focus.

Session 5 (Conjoint)

Lil and Newbold reported that a week ago they had intercourse and it was a very enjoyable experience. After that, Lil, however, began to get more frightened of intercourse. She began to have nightly nightmares with people chasing her. The dreams were violent; she felt unable to move, paralyzed, unable to get help.

During the week, she felt considerable pressure from various social obligations. She experienced the same need to be alone. When she has completed a social obligation successfully she feels as though she has gotten through with a chore. It became clear that she has the same feeling toward social obligations that she has toward sex. These are all intrusions on her time for herself. There is an obsessive need for time alone.

Before having children, she was able to have successful sex with Newbold because she was able to have enough privacy so that the time with him was not an intrusion on the available time. She recalled that as a child she was bored by school and cherished the time that she could go to her bedroom without being interrupted by anybody. That was the most delicious time.

We relabeled the problem. It is not a sexual problem so much as an obsessive need to be alone and it feels somewhat like a phobia. When she does not have the time to herself, Lil can feel her anxiety mount and become very overt. She feels that her tension increases unless she engages in some maneuver by which she finds time for herself. It becomes a defense against anxiety.

In view of the increased anxiety, she had the courage to suggest that perhaps she ought to "bulldoze" her way through this by having sex despite anxieties.

I said she could do this although there might be a very definite increase in anxiety. In view of my gradual appreciation that the search for privacy acted like a compulsive ritual to ward off anxiety, her suggestion to confront it head on made sense from a behavioral therapy point of view. Yet, as I warned her, there could be a definite increase in anxiety. At this point, we had two Axis I diagnoses—Depression in Remission and Hypoactive Sexual Desire Disorder. As far as Axis II is concerned, at times she acted as if she had an Avoidant Personality Disorder except that she was not afraid of people as such but of their demands; she was afraid of the loss of time. There were definite elements of Obsessive–Compulsive Disorder especially in her need to control time. At this point, she did not fulfill the criteria for any definite personality disorder.

Session 6 (Conjoint)

With her own injunction of "full speed ahead," Lil went through the three scheduled sexual encounters with responsivity and great pleasure. Once started, there was no trouble at all. She reported dreams in which she was being chased by *some* nameless person. In her dreams, she and her husband are trying to run away from *some* nameless terror and they are trapped; they cannot escape.

As Lil talked more, it became increasingly probable that the nameless terror represented her own conscience, probably personified by her therapist. She reports having great joy when she finishes a task. She is always under the tyranny of "shoulds" and "musts," so that any social engagement, finishing her bookkeeping, balancing her checkbook, and so on, is put in a category of a conscience-driven task. She puts sex in the same box of tasks to be finished, and this takes the joy out of it. When she is alone with a book or the newspaper, or even when she is with her children, who are part of her "self," in contrast to the others, there is tension relief.

I suggested to Lil that she was suffering from what the Jesuits call "overscrupulosity" and that when she is free of tension it is because "the self has successfully risen up against the conscience." So, what I have been labeling as a need for privacy all through the treatment has, in reality, been a place where she can find relief from her conscience-driven shoulds and musts. This is what Karen Horney (1935) labeled "the tyranny of the shoulds." When Lil has time alone, usually reading, she has escaped the prison formed by her own conscience, which has, in recent weeks, been demonstrated in her dream life where she tries to escape from this nameless terror but cannot. It is of interest that my prediction that she would have increased anxiety when she forced herself to have sex has come true. It is odd and perplexing to see Lil's dual attitude toward sex. On the one hand, it is a task and if she rises up against the conscience she wants to avoid it. On the other hand, when she has to do it, because her conscience tells her that it is time to have sex again, she does it, albeit reluctantly, and, then, when she is immersed in it she can enjoy it and when the task is completed enjoy the orgasm. Yet, following sex, which at some other level is regarded as pleasurable and thus self-indulgent, Lil once again is racked with "guilty fear," the emotional signal that one's conscience has been thwarted or defeated. Simply put, sex for Lil is both a task and a pleasure and with her there are two sources of guilt: one, when she does not appease her conscience and two, when she allows herself to receive pleasure. She is damned if she does and damned if she does not. I thought to myself, what a pretty picture of the id fighting the superego.

If only all of psychology could be reduced to several homunculi. Because Lil gets automatic thoughts about what she should do or must do, I asked her to keep a journal in which she would prioritize her tasks, some that are absolutely essential and some less so and some much less so, so that she can learn to postpone those tasks that were not essential without feeling guilty. She also agreed to come in for a number of sessions during which time we could try a variety of cognitive methods in the treatment of her obsessive–compulsive personality patterns. (Incidentally, Lil reported that the Prozac, which she had taken a few months earlier, had no effect on her obsessive–compulsive behaviors.)

At this point, a critical juncture in therapy had been reached, and I reviewed for myself what we had been through. At first, there was a psychodynamism that seemed to offer a lot in the way of explanation of Lil's sexual problem, namely, her need for privacy that had its roots in childhood. Later, we could see that that dynamic really involved a way in which Lil could have respite from her task-oriented or conscience-driven life. We set some behavioral tasks for Lil at the very beginning, mostly sensate focus, which had very modest effects. We shifted her medication from Prozac to Wellbutrin without any dramatic effect, although there had been several sexual encounters with intercourse and orgasm but no sustained pattern. Then, Lil herself suggested a sort of immersion therapy, that she go ahead despite her resistances and reluctance to engage in sex. That had been, essentially, a way in which we treated the symptom as a phobia and even though that worked in the sense that she was able to have intercourse and enjoyed the experience, and was orgastic, it led to a much higher level of anxiety. This higher level of anxiety exposed the nature of her primary emotion, namely, guilty fear, an alerting signal that lets the person know that she is not living up to her own expectations. It certainly was the signal to me that we were missing an important dynamic in the case. And it seemed to signal that she was guilty if she did not have sex (need to separate and foil her conscience) and guilty if she did have sex (please someone else).

Session 7

We had been conducting all the sessions, except the very first one, conjointly. Now, for the first time since that initial session, which had taken place about 14 weeks earlier, Lil came in alone. This session was devoted to how she could alleviate some of the pressures coming from her "shoulds." There is no doubt that she feels guilty when she is not toeing the line. She feels that she would be better off if external control was instituted by Newbold and if he insisted that they have sex. It would become an external rather than an internal "should" and it would be easier for her to comply. Because control is essential to Lil, I suggested that she suggest to her husband that he ask her to have sex. While osten-

120 Sexual Desire Disorders

sibly passing the control to him because she had, as it were, given the orders to him to order her, she would be secretly in control.

Whether this game playing would work, I had no idea, but I was trying to experiment with a variety of approaches. I thought to myself, this is the kind of trick that Jay Haley (1973) loves to use. In my hands, perhaps because it is in my hands, these tricks usually do not work.

Session 8

About 6 weeks had passed since Lil's last session. She had not been pleased with the progress in therapy but, as usual, in keeping with her overly strict conscience, tended to blame herself. We had never found a significant interpersonal reason for her sexual problem, although there was many a time when I wondered whether it would not have been a lot easier for her if her husband had been less of a nice guy and had really "smoked her," expressed his irritation and anger of which there was hardly any overt evidence. There was no smoke, let alone fire, but if Newbold had become angry at her it might have decreased Lil's own self-punishment. She could have turned some of the anger against him.

In this session, Lil hinted that something like that might be going on because she had spent about 10 days away from Newbold and felt a great release of tension.

We had tried a number of psychological methods, most of them falling into the cognitive-behavioral category. Lil tried to increase her time alone, increasing the amount of privacy. We tried to set up a method by which she would decrease the sense of oppression of the "shoulds" by prioritizing her tasks. We treated the inhibition of sexual desire as if it were a phobia with "immersion therapy." Each one of these worked for a time but had ultimately failed.

Lil feels as if sex is an awful effort, a chore, a burden despite the fact that she continues to be responsive. She cannot focus on the pleasure of sex; she can only focus on its burden.

She is happy to be away from her husband for a week or 10 days when she does not have the internal pressure to meet his unspoken demands. After 7 to 10 days, her conscience gets the better of her and then she submits to having sex and, at these times, interestingly enough, she is responsive and orgastic.

In the back of my mind, I was wondering whether testosterone would help. Over the years, I had been administering between 75 and 100 mg intramuscularly to premenopausal women with HSDD, giving them one injection a month for 3 months. This was not standard therapy, but I knew that it had been carried out in the United States by Greenblatt (1943) in Atlanta, who used testosterone pellet implants, and in the United Kingdom by Bancroft. Bancroft (personal communication, 1993) had used oral and sublingual preparations of testosterone undecenoate (unavailable in the United States) rather than injections. About 50% of my patients reported a significant increase in sex desire and in several cases it was a signal success, but one could not tell in advance which premenopausal woman would respond. In any case, I never gave more than three injections because it was not standard therapy. There was also the possibility that a woman, unknowingly, might be pregnant at the time she received the injection. I had never seen any adverse effects from the testosterone, not even hair growth, certainly not at the dosage I was using. These were the thoughts in my mind as I raised the possibility of biological therapy.

As I mentioned the possibility of testosterone, Lil told me that she had had low progesterone levels during her pregnancies causing two miscarriages at about 1 month postconception and that when she did conceive, she had been protected by taking progesterone prior to delivery.

Because progesterone is a mild androgen, I wondered whether there is something in the androgenic response situation. I asked Lil to get blood levels for testosterone, luteinizing hormone, and follicle-stimulating hormone. The thought occurred to me that the progesterone suppositories, which she took during her pregnancies, might have given her enough androgenic effect to have influenced her sexual desire. She did not remember any loss of desire during her pregnancies.

Session 9

Lil returned, 9 days later, after having blood levels, which revealed a very low testosterone, 16 ng/dl, with a free testosterone level of 0.2 ng/dl. (The normal range for testosterone in this lab is 15–110 ng/dl.) A decision was made to begin androgen therapy, and she was given an intramuscular injection of 100 mg of testosterone enanthate.

Session 10

About 5 weeks later, Lil called in to ask about her laboratory report. I reported that her "T" level was very high, namely 380 ng/dl, rising from its preinjection level of 16. The blood sample was drawn 11 days after the injection. She said on that same date, her sex drive returned and it had been wonderful all month. "It is as if a miracle has happened. It is back to where it was before I had all this trouble." I told her to get in touch with me if there was any change.

Session 11

Six weeks later, Lil came in for a second shot. The first positive response lasted a month, but for the last 5 or 6 weeks, Lil was without sex desire. It looks, from this evidence, as if her desire is hormone driven. Her last testosterone level dropped to 22 ng/dl.

Session 12

She came in for a third shot and reported that there was no change following the second shot except that it was "a little easier to get into it." Unlike her response to the first injection, nothing dramatic happened. Once again, each treatment works for a while—another placebo response?

It turned out that Lil was about 3 weeks pregnant when she got the third injection of testosterone. This is something that I have always been concerned about but I reassured her, as did her obstetrician, that the injection would have no effect on the fetus. Hormone-driven sexual brain programming occurs between the 50th and 150th day of fetal life, so the injection had taken place well before this process started.

Session 13

Lil decided to return for therapy when she was several months pregnant and had received reassurance that the testosterone injections could not possibly hurt her fetus.

I decided to shift the focus of treatment. We had tried cognitive-behavioral approaches. We had changed her medication. We had used hormone therapy and none of this had a lasting effect, although each technique, in turn, had a temporary fleeting success. I decided to return to the use of psychoanalytically oriented psychodynamic therapy—"return" in the sense that this was the therapy with which I had been most familiar and had enjoyed my greatest successes over the years.

Several themes emerged in this session:
1. Lil generally acts against something rather than toward something. She moves away from what is expected. At the same time, she does

not want to be the center of attention. She wants to keep her behavior quiet. For example, now, she does not want to tell anyone about the pregnancy. Instead of blurting it out, making a fuss about it, she wants to be different and part of the difference is keeping something like that quiet. Her kids do not watch television. That is another way she is different.

2. She repeated her need for solitude. "If I have the chance to be home alone for a few hours, I prefer being with myself. I like to go to the movies by myself. I even prefer that than to go with Newbold."

3. Although she likes being different and unique, the fact that she has this problem with desire sets her apart and that bothers her.

4. She gave much more detail about her school phobia. From kindergarten through the seventh grade she was very unhappy. There was a great fear of going to school and being left at school. Her home was perceived as safe. During those years everything was a chore, drudgery. There was a daily battle between herself and her mother to get her to go to school and about 25% of the time Lil got her way and would stay home. She was always relieved when she was sick because that gave her the excuse to avoid school. Once again, her home was a safe place. Her mother had the same feelings about home. Her mother did not want to socialize with anyone outside the immediate family. Even visits to the extended family were unsafe. Lil's mother did not want Lil to be like her. She wanted to push Lil out, Lil says. She goes on to say, "I cannot continue to live like this. Sex is an important part of me and I feel it is gone." Sex, somehow, drains Lil of emotions, but she has only a certain amount of reserve emotion and the children get that; her husband does not. Therefore, Lil prefers to be alone and not with her husband but that produces a lot of guilt. Because her husband is private too, their marriage can survive this. Lil says, "If the relationship weren't so good, it wouldn't survive this problem with sex."

Session 14

The major theme in this session was sexual guilt and guilty fear. She had had the usual Catholic upbringing in which her mother presented her values that sex was to be avoided premaritally. Lil wondered whether she had had any underlying guilt before she had sex. "There probably was but once I began to enjoy sex there was no guilt at all and there was never any guilt about birth control." She reported a dream. "I was in here with you. My mother was here and I felt very uncomfortable answering your questions about sex with her here." She also reported how oversolicitous and overprotective her mother had been and she was always favored.

Everything Lil did was okay except there was one occasion in high school when she was with her boyfriend downstairs in the parlor. They were watching television and not doing anything sexually but her mother came to the head of the stairs in a rage saying, "You might be able to do this in school but you can't do that sort of thing here." Her mother was in a frenzy and, of course, they were not doing anything. Lil was still a virgin at that point.

I was wondering at that point whether for Lil the role of mother was incompatible with being a sex partner; as a variant of the madonna–prostitute complex where she is seeing her role as a madonna incompatible with that of a sex partner, which then became that of prostitute. "Good girls do not." In other words, despite her feelings that she had not absorbed some of the guilt, were Lil's reactions at this point still driven by guilty fear and expressed in the dreams wherein she was being chased by a threatening figure?

The key to the psychodynamics in this case may well be the dream she presented in which she was in a therapy session with her mother present and she felt "very uncomfortable answering your questions about sex with her here." Being a parent increased Lil's identification with her mother and her mother's fear of the outside world, the fear of other people. Lil's mother represented safety but also repression and limitation.

Summary of Sessions during Remainder of Lil's Pregnancy

Nine more sessions took place before the birth of Lil's child. She broke off treatment 2 months before delivery and returned to therapy when the new baby was 4 months old. In this section of the chapter the nine sessions are summarized.

1. A definite increase in sexual desire occurred after the third injection of testosterone. Desire waned and returned to a 0 to 1 level (on a scale of 0 to 10) in the month following the last injection of "T." Additional injections of "T" were impossible because of her pregnancy.

2. The absence of sexual desire was uncomfortable. Lil felt trapped by her lack of interest as if her body and "self" were not integrated. She had really enjoyed sex a great deal before the first child arrived.

3. The mother's oversolicitous attitude and Lil's fear of leaving home had reinforced each other in creating the school phobia which lasted until the seventh grade. Only then did school become fun. Lil put it this way: "I was ready to go to summer camp, that is, I was emotionally about age 12, when I went off to college."

4. Lil was in conflict between her identification with her mother ("The outside world is dangerous and threatening") and the resultant dependency and her strong desire to be independent. Part of this rebellion included a now politically incorrect concept first termed by Alfred Adler (1956) "masculine protest" (majoring in math and physics and playing contact sports with zest). She did not tell her mother that she was pregnant until it was impossible to hide the evidence.

5. Part of Lil's obsessive need for organization, precision, and perfection (e.g., organizing her house, her activities, and her management of time) was in large measure a protest against the mother's disorganization, almost chaos in her daily life. Lil's identification with her mother included a similar pattern of carrying out obligations and then regarding them as impositions. Thus, the identification with mother included positive and negative identifications, similar and opposite features.

6. The change in Lil's attitude toward sex after she became a parent could hardly be coincidental. Her identifications, both positive and negative, were key elements. I would "give anything" to know whether this psychological change was paralleled by a reduction in testosterone levels following the birth of her first child.

7. Closeness created a sense of inadequacy and vulnerability. When they were constructing the house that they are now living in, Lil did not want to be touched by her husband. If she failed with any details of organizing the house, she needed to feel distant. "If I were closer I would feel even more inadequate." When I pointed out the negative psychological effects of closeness, namely, her increased sense of inferiority and her increased vulnerability, Lil responded by saying that her mother preached to never depend on anyone. "I see dependency as a negative thing. I couldn't stand the idea of vulnerability. As soon as a guy expected me to be around or that I needed him, I had to show them that I didn't care, that I wasn't dependent. The reason I married Newbold was that he never demanded that dependent feeling. He never minded my independence." In another session she put it this way: "We work together as parents so well, yet, I want to see myself as separate and I don't. I get a smothering feeling when I think about us as a marital unit."

8. Lil's need for space and aloneness is a phobic response to the fear of being engulfed. By keeping sufficient distance from her husband she could maintain the fiction of being a fully autonomous person.

9. When I pointed out the conflict spelled out above, Lil broke off treatment for 6 months until the new baby was 4 months old. I wondered whether I had been too close to pay dirt and that was why she broke off treatment when she did. (Realistically, it is not too comfortable to move around when 7 months pregnant and, no doubt, she was overwhelmed by the demands, including breastfeeding, of the newborn.)

Summary of Sessions following the Birth of the Child

Lil came in when the new baby was 4 months old and she certainly was frazzled. She had had little sleep. She thought she might be depressed but she did not look depressed. I thought she was just exhausted. Although Lil had been having some erotic dreams, there certainly was not any marked change in her desire for sex. She still varied her "time-outs." The dynamic issues were still the same. Everything is organized in terms of obligations to her children, to her husband, to the house. Her enormous sense of obligation stems from these sources:

1. Her mother's overprotective attitude when Lil was a small child.
2. The mother's critical approach to Lil even though there was concomitant favoritism (being the favorite and being criticized at the same time leads the child to seek constant approval).
3. Lil's fear of the children at school and the consequent school phobia which lasted until Lil was between 13 and 14.
4. The safest place was the house and the safest place within the safest place was her own room where she could get away from the other children of whom she was afraid and engage in a fantasy life with her dolls, fantasies she now cannot recall.
5. Lil was trained always to try to figure out what other people expected and to move to meet those expectations. In this way she remained a "good girl."
6. Lil really did not do anything for herself until she was in the eighth grade, when she was good enough to win a place in the orchestra.
7. Lil did not date during high school; she only had a few dates in college.
8. Lil had been able to have a very satisfying sex life for almost 15 years before the first child arrived.
9. After Lil became a parent, there was enormous identification with her mother and she acted toward her children the way her mother had acted toward her by imposing all kinds of obligations upon herself and then resenting them.
10. Unlike most people who are dependent, Lil is more comfortable when she is alone. Her most pleasurable periods are the times when she has no one to take care of and no one whose expectations she has to guess at. It is only then that she feels in control. If she has to do things for others, her sense of control is threatened, for, she imagines, they may be critical. If she has to make a choice, she may make the wrong choice and be criticized.

11. Sex is best for Lil if she does not have to make a choice. If she feels the situation demands it and she has no room to maneuver, unlike a truly autonomous person who would value the choice and whose free choice would truly bring a sense of intimacy, sex usually does not bring a sense of sharing. However, it must be pointed out that that sense of sharing at least, up to a point, was present before she became a parent.

Lil never really fought back or rebelled, so the psychological separation from her mother was never completed. To this day, there is a symbiosis between the two of them as if they were mirror images. Each can see her own behavior in the other and they often get angry with each other when they can recognize themselves in the behavior of the other. Lil cannot even substitute her husband for her mother and try to fuse with him, the ordinary adaptation of someone who is still highly dependent. Paradoxically, to all outward appearances, Lil is an independent and self-reliant person.

To summarize: Lil had three internal struggles. One was against her dependent needs, out of which arose her behavior that appeared to be autonomous and concealed her dependency. The need for and fear of fusion is the central core of this internal struggle. She struggles against her conscience but usually loses. The third struggle, which revolves around Lil's sense of inferiority and shame, comes into play with her husband and inhibits her freely choosing to be close to him. Lil said in one session that her husband "does everything so well and even though he never lords it over me, the effect is very much there." Whatever her husband does is done so well that despite his practically never being critical, Lil is always aware of his appraisal. That was why she had to be such a good parent. She could not bear to have Newbold criticize her for doing a bad job.

THEORETICAL CONSTRUCTS

Conflict Theory

The three inner conflicts—dependence versus independence (fusion vs. differentiation), conscience versus self, shame versus pride—are interlocked.

Object Relations Theory

The libidinal ego and the antilibidinal ego are locked in battle, so much so that the central ego is diminished in effectiveness and ease (Scharff, 1988).

I see little place for the other two major theories, namely, trauma theory and deficit theory. There was no evidence of physical or sexual abuse or of neglect (actually the opposite was true; her mother was over-protective and oversolicitous). Lil's identification with her mother is a key to much of her adult psychopathology.

Systems Approach

Key factors are:

1. The advent of parenthood, increasing the obligations created by Lil's conscience and identification with her mother.
2. The awe in which Lil holds her husband; his success and per-fectionism are additional facilitators of her conscience-driven behavior. On the positive side is Newbold's tolerance for Lil's sexual inhibitions; this still remains a good marriage despite the sexual problems. Paradoxically, if her husband were less perfect, the marriage would improve. Lil's awe and intimidation would decrease and her self-reproaches would diminish.

FINAL WORDS

I think I selected this case because I was puzzled that deepening the patient's understanding did not seem to change much. I am also frustrated that here is a person who outwardly has everything going for her, an adoring successful husband, lovely children, more than enough money to be comfortable, some close caring friends, and in this one realm of her life she remains baffled, as baffled as I am that nothing seems to change the equilibrium. This is the hard part of therapy when you work hard and you have, from all appearances, a very cooperative patient, and nothing seems to work.

At the point I am now, the patient's laboratory report (she was breastfeeding her infant) indicates a normal prolactin and a testoster-one level under 20 ng/dl. Would anyone suggest another round of "T" (she stopped breastfeeding the day she went to the lab) or to continue with psychotherapy alone, or do both? With the advent of health care reform, soon we may not have the luxury of having choices of therapy.

When Lil reported to me, after 4 months of therapy following the birth of her child, that she had had sex only four times in 8 months, I had to admit that psychotherapy had failed. I believe it was very helpful in terms of characterological changes, but it had not really touched the major symptom, the reason she had sought help in the first place. I resumed the injections of testosterone. Her total "T" rose to 340 ng% and her free "T" to 4.4 (normal values 0.1–2.8). Her sexual behavior changed commensurately. Her desire, responsivity, and orgastic capacity were at their preparenthood levels. At this point, her response following a second injection is undiminished. What next? There are no standards for this type of pharmacological therapy. Consultation with an excellent endocrinologist is essential, of course.

I am sorry to leave the reader dangling; that is the danger of selecting for reporting an ongoing case. The only thing I am really sure of is that Stephen Levine is absolutely correct when he says, "Sex is not simple."

REFERENCES

Adler, A. (1956). *The individual psychology of Alfred Adler* (H. L. Ansbacher & R. R. Ansbacher, Eds.). New York: Basic Books.

American Psychiatric Association. (1987). *Diagnostic and statistical manual of mental disorders* (3rd ed., rev.). Washington, DC: Author.

American Psychiatric Association. (1994). *Diagnostic and statistical manual of mental disorders* (4th ed.). Washington, DC: Authors.

Greenblatt, R. B. (1943). Testosterone propionate pellet implantation in gynecologic disorders. *Journal of the American Medical Association, 121,* 17–24.

Haley, J. (1973). Uncommon therapy. New York: W. W. Norton.

Heiman, J. R. (1977). A psychophysiological exploration of sexual arousal patterns in females and males. *Psychophysiology, 14,* 266–274.

Horney, K. (1935). The neurotic personality of our time. New York: W. W. Norton.

Levine, S. B. (1988). *Sex is not simple.* Columbus: Ohio Psychology Publishing.

Lief, H. I. (Ed.). (1981). *Sexual problems in medical practice.* Monroe, WI: American Medical Association.

Lief, H. I. (1985). Evaluation of inhibited sexual desire: Relationship aspects. In H. S. Kaplan (Ed.), *Comprehensive evaluation of disorders of sexual desire.* Washington, DC: American Psychiatric Press.

Lief, H. I. (1988). Foreword. In S. R. Leiblum & R. C. Rosen (Eds.), *Sexual desire disorders.* New York: Guilford Press.

Lief, H. I. (1991, December). *Women with low sex desire despite frequent orgasm.* Paper presented at the meeting of the American Academy of Psychoanalysis, New York, NY.

Nathanson, D. L. (1992). *Shame and pride: Affect, sex, and the birth of the self.* New York: W. W. Norton.

Rado, S. (1949). An adaptational view of sexual behavior. In P. H. Hoch & J. Zubin (Eds.), *Psychosexual development in health and disease.* New York: Grune & Stratton.

Scharff, D. E. (1988). An object relations approach to inhibited sexual desire. In S. R. Leiblum & R. C. Rosen (Eds.), Sexual desire disorders. New York: Guilford Press.

Schnarch, D. M. (1991). *Constructing the sexual crucible: An integration of sexual and marital therapy*. New York: W. W. Norton.

Zilbergeld, B., & Ellison, C. (1980). Desire discrepancies and arousal problems in sex therapy. In S. R. Leiblum & L. A. Pervin (Eds.), *Principles and practice of sex therapy* (1st ed.). New York: Guilford Press.

7

Joyce and Leonard:
Sexual Aversion
or Sexual Addiction?

CATHRYN G. PRIDAL
JOSEPH LoPICCOLO

INTRODUCTION

With the landmark publication of Masters and Johnson's *Human Sexual Inadequacy* in 1970, great optimism and excitement were generated for the effectiveness of modern sex therapy techniques. In large part, these techniques consisted of educational and behavioral interventions. Patients seen in the 1970s often showed ignorance about basic aspects of anatomy and physiology of sexual response, lack of knowledge about effective techniques for sexual stimulation, negative attitudes toward sex resulting from cultural indoctrination, and lack of familiarity with behavioral techniques for overcoming specific sexual problems. Therapists provided sex information, helped the individual or couple to reevaluate negative attitudes, and suggested specific sexual activities designed to increase arousal and reduce performance anxiety (LoPiccolo, 1977). Patients were generally responsive to these educational and directive techniques, and the effectiveness of modern sex therapy, as reported by Masters and Johnson (1970), was generally high.

Nowadays, the situation in sex therapy practice is quite different. Currently, sex therapy techniques do not seem to work as well with-

131

today's typical broad range of sex therapy patients. The reasons for the declining effectiveness of modern sex therapy procedures probably relate to societal or cultural changes, with resulting changes in the nature of the client population and the etiology of their problems. Our culture has become more accepting of sexuality, and sexual information is now widely available. Therefore, few patients appear for treatment at this time who suffer only from negative attitudes about sex, performance anxiety, and lack of information. Self-help books are widely available for most of the specific sexual dysfunctions, so many uncomplicated cases are able to self-treat and never appear for professional therapy.

Because sexual dysfunctions caused by simple negative attitudes, lack of information, and sexual skill deficits are less common today, the cases that do appear for treatment reflect a more complex etiology of their sexual problems. The simple educational, anxiety-reduction, and behavioral skill-training procedures of modern sex therapy are likely to be ineffective with such individuals, as these more complex factors are not addressed by such procedures. Currently, most patients do not complain of a specific symptomatic dysfunction such as premature ejaculation but rather of less focused sexual dissatisfaction, which often involves concerns about frequency of sex and quality of the sexual relationship.

The case presented in this chapter illustrates the evolution from modern sex therapy to "postmodern sex therapy" (LoPiccolo, 1992). In the postmodern approach, rather than simply prescribing behavioral procedures, a deconstructive formulation of the underlying causes of the sexual problem is undertaken. The underlying causes of each sexual problem can be conceptualized as falling into four partially overlapping content areas.

First, sexual issues may reflect couple systemic issues, with major influence exerted by such emotionally loaded areas as emotional intimacy, closeness, vulnerability, trust, power sharing, conflict resolution, and time spent together. Similarly, a sexual problem may be caused by individual psychodynamic issues, with the problem providing the means for the individual to ward off anxiety or depression, maintain self-esteem, or defend against awareness of unacceptable cognitions such as homosexual urges or paraphiliac arousal. Third, a sexual problem may be caused by unresolved family-of-origin issues, such as fears of closeness resulting from being raised in a family with an alcoholic parent of the opposite sex or sexual aversion resulting from incestuous sexual abuse. Finally, sexual problems may have an operant reinforcement dimension; for example, the financial success that comes to a man who works especially hard to compensate for his erectile failure.

In the case presented in this chapter, the patients' sexual problems focused around issues of frequency of sex and ongoing disagreements about particular sexual behaviors. While the husband was eager for treatment for what he considered low sexual drive, inhibited arousal, and orgasmic dysfunction in his wife, she conceptualized the problem as being one of "sexual addiction" in her husband. Along with extensive individual therapy, they had two brief trials of couple modern sex therapy, with negative results, before coming to us. Instead of accepting either of their formulations, a functional analysis was developed according to the postmodern deconstructionist model in order to identify the determinants of the sexual difficulties in each individual. These underlying issues were addressed from the perspective of cognitive, psychodynamic, and couple systemic interventions. This broadly focused therapy was combined with specific behavioral sex therapy in order to both prevent client resistance to behavioral procedures and allow the clients to make sense of why they were unable to resolve their sexual difficulties in the past (LoPiccolo, (1994).

PRESENTING PROBLEM
AND BACKGROUND INFORMATION

Leonard and Joyce were referred for therapy by Joyce's individual therapist, Dr. S. Leonard complained that Joyce suffered from low sexual drive. He described her as sexually inhibited, "frigid," and perhaps even "asexual." He felt that his life had been ruined by her sexual inhibition. Joyce stated that Leonard suffered from "sexual addiction," was obsessed with sex, and that she felt pressured by his constant sexual demands. She felt that Leonard's sexual demands were "ruining her life." The couple had engaged in many bitter, accusatory, and long-lasting fights over these issues, and had separated twice. One separation lasted about 3 weeks and the other lasted nearly 3 months. They were both receiving individual therapy during the second separation, and their individual therapists both recommended that they seek couple therapy when the extent of their sexual difficulties became apparent. Leonard and Joyce both wished to reconcile, and agreed to try couple therapy.

Leonard and Joyce are both in their late 40s and have been married for 28 years. They have three adult children, all living independently. Leonard is a vascular surgeon who invested successfully in real estate, as had Joyce. They report a joint yearly income in excess of $1 million. Joyce was educated as an elementary school teacher and was teaching in the community where Leonard was completing his residency when they met. Joyce did not work outside the home for a few years after their marriage; subsequently she worked as an office manager in her husband's real estate development office. She now manages her own investments and no longer works in the development office.

When they presented for treatment, both Leonard and Joyce had each received individual therapy for nearly 2 years. During this time, they also attempted couple therapy with each of their individual therapists, but they could not agree on which therapist would be most helpful to them as a couple, and, in fact, each developed a strong dislike for the other's therapist. Both individual therapists sent treatment summaries to us prior to the initiation of couple therapy.

Joyce's individual therapist, Dr. S, indicated that she entered therapy to focus on individual issues, specifically her feelings of always having been so controlled by her husband. She related that throughout the first 20 years of marriage she had given in to her husband's demands, including his sexual demands. During the 6 years prior to entering therapy, she had decided no longer to give in to Leonard and was responding to his sexual demands with anger and rejection. Her 2 years of individual therapy had focused on her needs to express herself in the marriage and had supported her self-exploration and growth as an individual.

Leonard entered individual therapy after he and Joyce had several sessions of couple therapy with Mr. F, a master's-degree-level counselor. Joyce felt that Mr. F was not sympathetic to her point of view and subsequently entered therapy with Dr. S. However, Leonard disliked Dr. S, and chose to return to Mr. F for individual counseling. In Mr. F's case notes, he indicated that Leonard had severe insecurity about whether anyone loved and valued him and suffered from low self-esteem. In a rather different formulation of his problem, Leonard stated that sexual acceptance was critical to his feeling valued and loved by his wife. He indicated that sexual acceptance meant that his wife wanted to engage in *all* the sexual activities he found appealing, with the same level of enjoyment. Both individual therapists felt that their sessions had resolved many of the individual issues for Leonard and Joyce but that their sexual relationship remained wholly unsatisfactory. At this point, a referral for couple sex therapy was made.

SESSION 1: ASSESSMENT AND INITIAL THERAPEUTIC STRATEGY

Because the couple resides in a city about 2 hours' drive from the therapist's office, we did not follow the traditional format of weekly 1-hour therapy sessions. Instead, the first session occupied an entire day and included both assessment and some initial treatment interventions. Following the first all-day session, we met at 4- to 6-week intervals for half-day sessions over the next 6 months, for a total of five meetings. Prior to the first session both partners completed the Locke–Wallace Marital Satisfaction Inventory (Locke & Wallace, 1959) and a Sex History Questionnaire (Schover, Friedman, Weiler, Heiman, & LoPiccolo, 1982). During the lunch break on the first day, the Sexual Interaction Inventory (SII; LoPiccolo & Steger, 1974) was completed (see Figure 7.1). The Locke–Wallace scores indicated a severely distressed relationship (scores of 72 for Leonard and 78 for Joyce). Locke–Wallace scores were reduced by conflict around sexual issues, and the SII indicated that some of their sexual difficulties resulted directly from miscommunication. The SII also showed that Leonard was dissatisfied with the current frequency of sexual interaction (he obviously wanted more), was unaware of his wife's actual sexual feelings and preferences, and was very unaccepting of her as a sexual partner. Leonard indicated that he was satisfied with his own

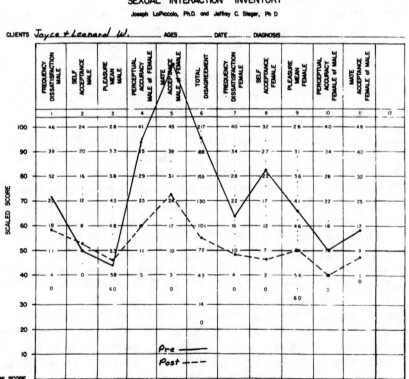

FIGURE 7.1. Pre- and posttreatment profiles for Joyce and Leonard on the Sexual Interaction Inventory.

sexual behavior and was about average in terms of the amount of pleasure he reported experiencing from sexual activities. Joyce was also dissatisfied with the frequency of sexual interaction (she also desired more)
and moderately unaccepting of Leonard as a sexual partner. She was quite
critical and negative about her own sexuality and reported experiencing
less pleasure from sexual interactions than average. However, she was very
accurate in her awareness of Leonard's likes and dislikes in the sexual area.

Despite their specific conflicts, the overall sexual assessment indicated that both Joyce and Leonard were within the normal range of sexual
desire and responsiveness. Specifically, she scored on the low end and
he on the high end of the sexual desire continuum. The therapists strongly
rejected their characterizations of each other as "frigid" and "addicted"
and suggested instead that while they differed in their desired frequen-
cies for sex, they were both in the normal range.

In addition to the paper-and-pencil measures, a detailed assessment
interview was conducted to explore their relationship history as well as
individual issues that related to their current problems. Their sexual interaction difficulties originated with miscommunications that began prior
to their marriage. Joyce revealed that prior to their marriage, she felt
sexually frustrated because she was determined to be a virgin on her
wedding night and yet felt a strong desire for sexual intercourse with
Leonard. She stated that she would frequently masturbate with thoughts
of Leonard when she returned home after a date with him. Leonard responded with amazement to this information; he had perceived Joyce as
sexually repressed and thought her refusal to engage in premarital sexual
intercourse was evidence of her lack of desire. Joyce reported that her
parents had specifically told her that she was responsible for maintaining her virginity and avoiding pregnancy. Both Leonard and Joyce described family-of-origin issues in their sexual and emotional development,
so genograms were constructed as part of the assessment.

On his genogram, Leonard identified himself as one of six children.
His father was a physician whose first wife had died, leaving him with
four children. Leonard's father subsequently married his receptionist and
had two children, Leonard being the older. Leonard described his father
as strong willed and hard working. As a child, Leonard was strongly
resented by his older half-siblings and they were covertly hostile and cruel
to him. They resented their stepmother, whom they perceived as "be-
neath" their father, and were even more negative toward their step-
siblings. These undercurrents were not expressed openly; instead the family presented a facade of loving harmony to the outside world. Leonard
therefore learned to distrust *statements* of love and acceptance and instead focused his needs for love and acceptance into sexual expression.
He engaged in parallel and occasional mutual masturbation with his

younger brother (15 months younger) during his early teenage years, in spite of his mother's statements about masturbation being sinful. Leonard's mother was not physically affectionate with her husband or her children, and Leonard felt sorry for his father, assuming that his father felt as rejected by her as he did.

Joyce s family-of-origin genogram placed her near the middle of seven children born to a farming family. She was raised traditionally, with the clear delineation of "men's work" and "women's work." She learned that it is the duty of the female to do the caretaking—emotionally and physically—in the family. She resented the rigid expectations for social conformity held by her parents and felt that they perceived her as "bad" because she occasionally rebelled. On the positive side, her parents were appropriately affectionate with one another and with their children. Joyce observed little conflict between her parents and felt that they had a warm, close marriage. She learned about menstruation from an older sister, and after hearing another sister discussing masturbation with a friend, tried it with positive results. The family messages about sex were mostly focused on female virginity and avoiding pregnancy before marriage.

During the initial interview, it became clear that Leonard was markedly depressed and drinking to excess as a form of self-medication. We referred Leonard for a complete medical examination to rule out any physiological factors in his sleep disturbance, low energy level, fatigue, and dysphoric mood. He was then prescribed Prozac (fluoxetine) by a psychiatrist colleague. Both Leonard and Joyce expressed relief that his depression was finally acknowledged directly and being dealt with, and that he was beginning a course of pharmacological treatment. Leonard was originally prescribed 20 mg daily of Prozac, and when he failed to show a positive response, the dosage was increased to 40 mg daily. He did show a good clinical response to this dosage, with his sleep disturbance, fatigue, and energy level markedly improving. There was less improvement in his mood in response to the medication as he remained very distressed by the sexual issues between him and his wife until these issues were dealt with in psychotherapy, as described later in this chapter.

Although the sexual assessment indicated that both Leonard and Joyce were within the normal range of sexual desire and responsiveness, their sexual interactions were confused by miscommunications, misperceptions, and misattributions. Leonard had entered the relationship with limited sexual experience (masturbation beginning in his early teens) and expected that marital sex would be all-consuming and all-satisfying. He was most disappointed to discover that his wife did not desire sex more than once a day, nor was she as vocally or physically expressive as he wished her to be. Leonard admitted freely that he needed his wife to be wildly sexual to feel confident that she accepted his sexuality and therefore loved him. He was unable to believe that she could love him and accept him if she did not want sex in exactly the same manner he did, so he became highly critical of her sexual performance over time.

Joyce was easily aroused and experienced orgasm during their sexual interactions in the first few years of marriage. However, she heard Leonard's complaints as indicating that she was failing in her caretaking role. She therefore made efforts to change her sexual performance when Leonard was critical, and even accepted his description of their sexual interactions as being unfulfilling to both of them. She questioned her own sexuality and sexual perceptions for the first part of their marriage. However, at some point, Joyce became more confident of her judgment in other areas of her life and began to resent Leonard's portrayal of her as sexually "frigid." As a result, she began to withdraw sexually and lost any feelings of sexual desire for him. She would only "accommodate" him a few times each week, but rarely experienced arousal on these occasions.

When Leonard and Joyce entered therapy, they were having sex about twice weekly. Leonard indicated that he would prefer to have sex three to four times per week, whereas Joyce stated that she wished to have sex only once a week. Ideally, she would have preferred sex about twice a week, but only if it were freely experienced with no pressure or expectations. They both indicated that although they were engaging in foreplay for up to 30 minutes and 2 to 4 minutes of intercourse, they found their overall sexual relationship extremely unsatisfactory. Leonard reported no difficulty in achieving or maintaining an erection or in ejaculation. Joyce reported perceiving little or no sexual arousal, but she indicated that she did not have difficulty with vaginal lubrication. She had not had an orgasm with Leonard in many years, nor did she masturbate.

Based on the initial assessment, we conceptualized the case as a desire discrepancy case complicated by faulty communication and emotional overloading on the sexual interaction. The desire discrepancy was magnified by the systemic structure in which Leonard took the role of the fully functional sexual person and Joyce was pushed into the role of dysfunctional and nonsexual partner. She was out of touch with her own sexual desire because Leonard was so sexually demanding. Instead, she reacted negatively to his pressure for her to be sexual in a specific way and consequently lost contact with her own sexuality.

Because the couple had serious communication difficulties, we focused part of the initial session on strategies for improving communication. We identified problematic communication styles, based on the interactions that we observed during the assessment interview and subsequent discussion. After these issues were identified, we described strategies for dealing with these problems. For example, we demonstrated and practiced paraphrasing and "I statements" in the therapy session.

Another problematic communication style was labeled "side comments." This pattern involved making several positive statements followed by a critical or negative comment, resulting in confusion for the receiver about whether he/she could believe and trust the positives. We suggested that it was most important that disagreements be dealt with independently from positive comments or supportive statements.

Another maladaptive communication pattern occurred when Joyce or Leonard was feeling vulnerable, confused, or strongly in need of resolving a problem. Each would tend to attack the other rather than simply sharing their feelings of distress. The partner then felt pressure to concede, or to come up with an answer, whether realistic or not, to alleviate the distress. The couple was instructed instead to search for the feeling behind the desire to attack the other and, rather than criticizing, to express that feeling directly. If one of them felt attacked by the other, he/she should label the situation and inquire about the cause of the other's upset rather than responding with anger or hurt feelings.

The final part of the initial session returned the focus to the couple's sexual interactions. We gave them reading assignments from *Becoming Orgasmic* (Heiman & LoPiccolo, 1988) and *The New Male Sexuality* (Zilbergeld, 1992). We advised both Leonard and Joyce to read the same chapters in both books and to do the same accompanying exercises. We also assigned sexual interactions two to three times each week. The structure of these "homework" sessions was that one day was designated as Joyce's day, on which she was to be wholly in charge. She was to decide how she wished Leonard to please her physically. It was emphasized that whether or not she became sexually aroused was not important, and that Leonard was not to try to "make" her become aroused. Instead, Joyce was to try to experience sexual feelings in her own way and for her own pleasure, without the fear that Leonard would pressure or evaluate her.

The second sexual day was to be Leonard's day, with Joyce bringing him to a climax in any way that was comfortable for her, most typically manual stimulation but possibly intercourse as well. Leonard was to explore ways to receive pleasure and to move away from a focus on his penis as his only sexual organ. On the third day, sexual activity was optional. However, we instructed the couple to engage in a mutually pleasurable activity, such as going out to dinner or taking a walk together. Both Joyce and Leonard had to agree before any sexual activity could occur.

As the next therapy session was scheduled for 5 weeks hence, we instructed Leonard and Joyce to keep a diary of each sexual encounter. The diary entries were to be mailed once a week so that we could evaluate them prior to the next therapy session.

Diary Reports

The sexual diaries indicated that Joyce did experience some degree of sexual arousal on "her days," and also occasionally on "his days." However, she was reluctant to express this arousal so Leonard was generally unaware of her feelings. He found himself confused much of the time, unsure of how he was "supposed" to be feeling or acting. Whenever Joyce became upset or angry, he felt convinced that the marriage was ending, or at least that things could never improve to a tolerable level. At this point, Leonard began to experience erectile difficulties, which he attributed to not performing the sexual activities that he desired.

SESSION 2

In the second treatment session, we discussed the information contained in the sexual diaries. Leonard was pleasantly surprised to learn that Joyce was actually experiencing a degree of sexual arousal, and we encouraged her to express her arousal to Leonard in ways that felt comfortable. Leonard became extremely emotional when discussing his feelings of being "put on the shelf" in the sexual area. He had accepted the therapeutic rationale of not coercing Joyce sexually so that she could connect with her own sexual feelings. However, in practice he was finding this situation very difficult. He expressed the sentiment that Joyce had to be totally accepting of his sexuality. He then explained that he wanted her to enjoy deep kissing, being kissed all over her body, his ejaculation in her mouth, and anal stimulation.

Joyce angrily stated that they had fought about these particular sexual activities for years. She explained that she did not enjoy anal stimulation, deep kissing, or oral ejaculation. She found these activities repulsive and resented being expected to perform them to make Leonard happy. She indicated that she would not mind the all-over kissing if it were done in a loving, gentle fashion instead of in a way that felt sexually demanding. She actually enjoyed fellatio, provided she was not pressured to have Leonard ejaculate in her mouth.

We responded to this exchange by suggesting that Leonard was narrowly focusing his definition of sexual happiness on those few activities that Joyce had already indicated she did not enjoy. Instead, he was encouraged to notice that she enjoyed many different types of sexual activity, such as giving and receiving oral sexual stimulation, different positions for intercourse, and various locations for sexual activities. Leonard then stated that he would never be happy in his life unless he could satisfy his needs for "sexual creativity." Upon questioning, however, it became clear that Leonard was using "sexual creativity" as a euphemism for anal stimulation, oral ejaculation, and deep kissing. At this point, we suggested that linking his life happiness to performing these few activities was like thinking that all his problems could be solved if Joyce would only allow him to put a dead mackerel on his head while making love. We made the interpretation that Leonard had never felt loved or accepted in his family of origin except when mutually masturbating (a forbidden activity) with his brother. As an adult, he would only feel secure about Joyce's true love for him if she would perform these taboo activities with him. There followed an extensive discussion of the overdetermined nature of sexual activity for Leonard. For him, sex was not just a way of expressing love and of giving or receiving pleasure; rather, it was a litmus test of Joyce's true feelings about him.

The issue of trust was the other major focus of the second therapy session. Leonard and Joyce stated that they loved each other and were committed to the relationship. Accordingly, we explored miscommunications throughout their marriage from the standpoint of identifying each person's attempts to make the other happy, rather than from the standpoint of who was "right" or "wrong." Joyce and Leonard both began to see the other in a new light, as someone who was participating in a relationship *with* the other rather than *against* the other.

Sexually, we instructed Leonard to express his desire for Joyce as a reflection of his love and regard for her instead of as though he thought of her only as a sexual object. Joyce also noted that Leonard's insistence that either they would have sex or he would be devastated led to her viewing him as emotionally crippled rather than as a sexually desirable man whose need for her made her feel sexy and desirable. We then instructed Leonard in more appropriate and effective ways to initiate sex. We instructed Joyce to accept or reject Leonard's initiations as she desired. However, when declining sexual interaction, she was to state that while she wanted a "rain check" on sex right now, she did enjoy making love with him. Joyce was then to project a time in the near future when she expected that she would be able to respond positively to his initiation.

Sexual assignments were to continue with the Joyce day/Leonard day/free day arrangement, but with instructions not to follow this structure too rigidly. Instead, the arrangement was to be used as a "safety net" if Leonard and Joyce encountered serious difficulty with initiating and declining. Leonard was now to ask for what he wanted, with the understanding that Joyce was free to decline. The couple was also to continue their reading, performing the accompanying exercises, and writing about them in their sexual diaries (Heiman & LoPiccolo, 1988; Zilbergeld, 1992).

Diary Reports

Joyce continued to experience more sexual arousal and enjoyment but still felt unable to reveal her reactions to Leonard. Leonard found himself becoming tentative when initiating sexual interactions, as he was fearful of rejection. This fear persisted despite Joyce following our instructions to decline gently and to suggest an alternative time when she would be receptive. Leonard usually did not follow up on her suggestion; rather, he felt anxious and was fearful of approaching her. Several times Joyce gently initiated a sexual interaction at the time she had suggested, only to be met with hesitancy and fear on Leonard's part.

SESSION 3

After mailing the sexual diaries, and prior to the third session, Joyce experienced orgasm during sex with Leonard for the first time in many years. They were both delighted with this occurrence and more openly affectionate in the therapy session. The session focused primarily on the issue of initiating and declining sexual interactions. Leonard was to focus on his love for Joyce, to foster closeness with her in other contexts, to be more affectionate in general, and to specifically state that he was interested in making love with her at a particular time. Joyce, in turn, was to decline by prefacing her refusal with a statement that directly addressed Leonard's concerns; for example: "I love you and love to make love with you. However, I'm feeling very tired and would really rather talk with you about my tough day now, and make love later, when I am more relaxed."

We instructed the couple to prioritize their relationship while understanding that they each also had needs for separateness and independence. They were to attempt to engage in multiple activities together so that sex was not their sole focus and only avenue to closeness. We instructed them also to focus on the positive feelings they had for each other and to express those feelings frequently.

We encouraged Joyce to express her feelings of sexual enjoyment to Leonard. He agreed that he would not place demands on her or overreact to her expressions of pleasure. She acknowledged that she did need to know that he desired her sexually as well as in her role as a partner in other areas of their lives.

We also addressed Leonard's difficulties with erections. We discussed the irony of this situation in that Leonard now felt under pressure to perform similar to the way Joyce had felt earlier in their marriage. He was able to see that he could look forward to ("count on") having sex with Joyce, but that he did not *have* to have sex with her at any particular time if he did not feel comfortable doing so. Joyce validated his option to decline, or to change the plan, at any time. We also instructed Joyce and Leonard to finish reading *Becoming Orgasmic* (Heiman & LoPiccolo, 1988) and *The New Male Sexuality* (Zilbergeld, 1992), doing the final exercises and writing about them in their sexual diaries.

Diary Reports

Joyce did not write about angry or resentful feelings toward Leonard and was able to express her sexual arousal and enjoyment while engaging in sexual activities. She experienced several orgasms during the intervening 4 weeks between sessions 3 and 4. In turn, Leonard began to feel less desperate about their sexual interactions and began to be able to hear Joyce's verbal statements of love and acceptance as genuine. He continued to have occasional erectile difficulties, especially when they planned to have sex at a specific time.

SESSION 4

This session began with a focus on Leonard's emotional needs. It had become clear that he often attempted to deal with feelings of loneliness, depression, job anxiety, and so on, by having sex with Joyce. Over the course of their marriage, alcohol and sex had served as a means of self-medication for dealing with these feelings. Sex allowed him to feel loved and accepted, without having to experience or examine his needs for closeness and acceptance. Both Leonard and Joyce agreed, after discussion, that it would be preferable for Leonard to express his emotional needs directly so that she could respond appropriately rather than framing these needs as sexual overtures.

We addressed Leonard's erectile difficulties similarly in the context of his fear of acknowledging essential needs for emotional intimacy and acceptance. His sexual difficulties were thus seen as an indication of developing emotional vulnerability in their relationship. If he began to count on having loving sexual interactions with Joyce, he would become acutely aware of how important she was to him and how disappointing it would be if sexual relations were not possible. Fortunately, Joyce was able to reassure Leonard that she loved him fully, was committed to their marriage, and wanted to have pleasurable, loving sexual interactions with him.

We also discussed creativity in their sexual interactions. Both partners expressed a desire for creativity in terms of location, position, and "props" (music, candlelight, massage oil, etc.). Joyce was concerned that Leonard would expect her to engage in the same activities that she had formerly found repulsive, but he was able to reassure her that his main desire was for loving exploration of mutually enjoyable sexual creativity.

Diary Reports

Both partners wrote about continued increasing comfort and enjoyment in their sexual interactions. Leonard still noted concerns about Joyce ever being "totally free" in her expression of sexual arousal and pleasure. Joyce indicated feeling more accepted by Leonard as herself; however, she was still aware of occasional pressures from Leonard to be more "wildly passionate."

SESSION 5

Because this was the final therapy session, the focus was on gains achieved and areas for further growth. Both Leonard and Joyce expressed satisfaction with the progress made so far. They felt that their communication was much improved and that they were consistently able to resolve interpersonal difficulties as they arose. They also stated that their sexual interactions had become mutually enjoyable and that they were both developing confidence in their abilities to please each other as sexual partners.

Joyce had made considerable improvement during the course of therapy. She reported that she was now experiencing orgasm on nearly every occasion that they engaged in sexual intercourse. She also reported being aware of renewed sexual desire and enjoyment of physical affection and sexual expression with Leonard. Joyce further stated that she felt emotionally closer to Leonard than she ever had in their relationship, which she attributed to their improved communication style. She said that she could trust Leonard to pay attention to her feelings and to be honest about his own feelings in a way that was neither demanding nor demeaning.

The issue of "exploring creativity" continued to be a sensitive one. Leonard still seemed to have some need for Joyce to match his definition of a creatively sexual person (one who will engage in anal stimulation, etc.), which she continued to resist. After some discussion, it was agreed that this would likely be an ongoing issue for the couple. It was hoped that Leonard would be able to value Joyce for who she was sexually. Using a tactic from acceptance and commitment therapy (Kohlenberg, Hayes, & Tsai, 1993), we instructed Leonard simply to accept his feelings of regret regarding missed sexual experiences rather than translating these regrets into demands for Joyce to change. We pointed out to Leonard that allowing his regrets to control his behavior was self-destructive, as his demanding that Joyce engage in particular sexual activities had the effect of suppressing her drive to engage in the wider range of sexual activities that she did enjoy. With some difficulty, Leonard accepted this interpretation.

Prior to attending the fifth session, the couple completed the Locke–Wallace and SII again. On the Locke–Wallace, both Leonard and Joyce received a score of 99, reflecting a net improvement of 27 points for Leonard and 21 points for Joyce. We discussed these scores as reflecting the improved communication and increased general happiness in their marriage. On the SII, the scores also improved dramatically, as indicated by the posttreatment profile on Figure 7.1. Leonard was much more satisfied with the frequency of their sexual interactions and was much more accepting of Joyce's sexuality. The continued mild elevation of his mate acceptance score indicates that there is still some room for improvement in this area. Joyce also was happier with the frequency of sexual interactions, was much more accepting of her own sexuality, was experiencing more sexual pleasure, and was more accepting of Leonard as a sexual partner.

According to Leonard's report, and Joyce's confirmation, his depressive symptoms had almost completely abated. He still experienced episodes of insomnia while out of town on business, but he attributed this difficulty to the stress of business meetings and sleeping in a strange bed and bedroom. He continued to drink wine occasionally with dinner but had discontinued the excessive consumption of alcohol. Leonard also occasionally felt pessimistic about the future but was able to talk with Joyce about his feelings, and these talks typically improved his mood. In consultation with the prescribing psychiatrist, it was decided that Leonard would continue to take Prozac for a few months and would then have a period of a lower dose and finally a trial of no medication, to see whether there was a major biological component to his depressive symptoms.

DISCUSSION AND SUMMARY

In retrospect, several issues addressed in therapy seem to have been critical to the process of change in this case. One issue was the question of the actual frequency of sexual interaction, as opposed to the ideal frequency as stated by each member of the couple. At the onset of therapy, the couple perceived themselves as extremely disparate on ideal frequency— Joyce thought Leonard wanted sex every day, while Leonard thought Joyce never wanted sex. In actuality, they were having sex about twice a week, which turned out to be slightly below his ideal of three to four times per week and at the top end of her ideal range of once to twice a week. Another issue was their shared belief that certain specific sexual activities defined each partner's identity as a sexual person. Because Leonard wanted to engage in anal stimulation, deep kissing, and oral ejaculation, Joyce considered him to be a sexual addict or pervert. On the other hand, because Joyce was unwilling to engage in those activities, Leonard considered her to be repressed and even asexual.

The major turning point in therapy occurred with the "dead mackerel" interpretation. When Leonard gained insight into how his desire for Joyce to engage in these specific activities was overdetermined and related to his family-of-origin issues, he began to be less demanding of her sexually and to make more direct requests regarding his emotional needs. Joyce responded positively to this change and readily expressed her feelings of love and acceptance toward Leonard.

During the course of treatment, we were faced with two important dilemmas. The first difficulty was resisting the pull to align with one or the other member of the couple. At times it was easy to perceive Leonard as demanding and immature and to see Joyce as a long-suffering victim of his neediness. At other times, Joyce appeared to be withholding her sexual expressiveness as a power ploy, and Leonard could easily be seen as a confused, lonely victim. We strongly resisted the pull for alignment and the tendency to be polarized into one or another of these viewpoints.

The second key therapeutic issue was to avoid becoming arbiters of what constituted sexual health or normalcy. Both Joyce and Leonard frequently raised the issue of what was normal in terms of sexual frequency, enjoyment of, or aversion to certain activities, and so forth. Often, these requests were framed as apparently innocent intellectual curiosity about what the latest research had revealed on a particular topic. We reinterpreted such questions in the context of the relationship distress and pointed out that rather than relying on external norms or therapeutic expertise, the couple would need to develop their own individual solution. The acceptance therapy-based intervention of having Leonard note, but not feel compelled to act on, his longing for taboo sexual activities allowed him to see how much richer his sexual life had become. In essence, he learned to focus on the nearly full glass of water rather than on the few ounces that were missing.

This case illustrates the increased complexity of current sex therapy cases. The couple's problems were not caused by the negative attitudes, information deficits, and poor sexual techniques that the sensate focus-based techniques of modern sex therapy address so well. Indeed, each of their previous therapists tried sensate focus exercises during their brief courses of couple therapy with negative results. Rather, this couple's problems reflected complex family-of-origin issues, individual psychodynamic and cognitive issues, and systemic issues in their relationship. By addressing these multiple factors in a broad-spectrum, postmodern fashion, therapy was successful in improving their individual happiness, their emotional relationship, and their sexual adjustment.

REFERENCES

Heiman, J. R., & LoPiccolo, J. (1988). *Becoming orgasmic: A personal and sexual growth program for women.* Englewood Cliffs, NJ: Simon & Schuster.

Kohlenberg, R. J., Hayes, S. C., & Tsai, M. (1993). Radical behavioral psychotherapy: Two contemporary examples. *Clinical Psychology Review, 13*(2), 579–592.

Locke, H. J., & Wallace, K. (1959). Short marital adjustment and prediction tests: Their reliability and prediction. *Marriage and Family Living, 21,* 251–255.

LoPiccolo, J. (1977). From psychotherapy to sex therapy. *Society, 14*(5), 60–68.

LoPiccolo, J. (1992). Postmodern sex therapy for erectile failure. In R. C. Rosen & S. R. Leiblum (Eds.), *Erectile disorders: Assessment and treatment* (pp. 171–197). New York: Guilford Press.

LoPiccolo, J. (1994). The evolution of sex therapy. *Sexual and Marital Therapy, 9*(1), 5–7.

LoPiccolo, J., & Steger, J. C. (1974). The sexual interaction inventory: A new instrument for assessment of sexual dysfunction. *Archives of Sexual Behavior, 3*(6), 585–595.

Masters, W. H., & Johnson, V. E. (1970). *Human sexual inadequacy.* Boston: Little, Brown.

Schover, L. R., Friedman, J., Weiler, S., Heiman, J. R., & LoPiccolo, J. (1982). A multi-axial diagnostic system for sexual dysfunctions: An alternative to DSM-III. *Archives of General Psychiatry, 39,* 614–619.

Zilbergeld, B. (1992). *The new male sexuality.* New York: Bantam.

8

Childhood Sexual Trauma
and Adult Sexual Desire:
A Cognitive-Behavioral Perspective

BARRY W. McCARTHY

INTRODUCTION

Conceptualization of the causes and treatments for sexual problems has come full circle. Traditional psychoanalytical beliefs held that sexual problems were rooted in individual intrapsychic childhood conflicts. In contrast, a key concept of the Masters and Johnson (1970) model was the view of sexual dysfunction as primarily a couple problem. Subsequently, Kaplan (1974) presented her triphasic model, with an emphasis on sexual desire as the first phase of sexual response. The past decade has seen an extraordinary upsurge of interest in the role of childhood sexual trauma as the core issue in sexual dysfunction, especially inhibited desire. Once again, the role of childhood sexuality and intrapsychic causes of sexual dysfunction is predominant. Does this serve the needs of clients?

According to current clinical lore, if a couple presents with a problem of inhibited sexual desire and individual histories uncover a pattern of sexual abuse or trauma for one (or both), this must be addressed before dealing with the couple issues. Maltz (1991) has argued that couple sex therapy is the treatment of choice for inhibited sexual desire even when there is a history of sexual abuse or trauma. McCarthy (1990) has further argued that treating a couple sexual dysfunction with "benign neglect"

148

while addressing childhood issues can have iatrogenic effects by building frustration and resentment, which may in turn exacerbate the couple's sexual problems.

Sexual dysfunction, especially inhibited sexual desire, can be viewed as multicausal and multidimensional, involving a wide range of individual and couple issues. This presents a particular challenge for the clinician in terms of both assessment and treatment and compounds the difficulty in building a scientific knowledge base. The field is vulnerable to the whims and fancies of new therapy movements and treatment approaches, often with little empirical support and unreplicated findings. This trend is accelerated when approaches such as "adult child" and "victimization" garner public attention and acceptance. The pendulum has swung strongly away from denial and minimization of sexual trauma to the belief that many, if not most, sexual dysfunction clients come from a dysfunctional family and have been sexually victimized. This overemphasis on sexual victimization sensationalizes and trivializes the issue (McCarthy, 1992).

ASSESSMENT ISSUES

The "stock-in-trade" assessment technique of sex therapy is the individual sex history. Sex therapy is best conceptualized as a couple process. The initial interview is with the couple, followed by individual sex histories and then a couple feedback session. The skilled clinician assesses psychological, sexual, developmental, and relationship factors. He/she asks open-ended questions about sexual trauma, negative sexual experiences, and sexual secrets to elicit a comprehensive history of sexual sensitivities and vulnerabilities. Clinicians are more likely to pursue sexual trauma with female patients. It is critical to examine this issue with males, as well as exploring whether there is a history of sexually compulsive and/or abusive behavior. If the clinician asks, "Have you ever been sexually abused?" the answer will generally be "No." A more productive, less judgmental phrasing is, "A significant number of men have had negative, confusing, or traumatic sexual experiences. What was your most negative or abusive sexual experience?" Even if he does not respond at the time, he is aware that these issues can be discussed and explored. At the end of this session, another open-ended question is asked: "Is there anything else I should know about your sexual feelings or experiences?" which provides an opportunity to discuss difficult issues. Trauma is particularly important to assess in sexual desire cases. In the spouse's sexual history, it is important to ask whether there is problematic sexual behavior and/or sexual secrets.

TREATMENT STRATEGIES AND TECHNIQUES

Cognitive-behavioral sex therapy takes an optimistic view of sexual problems. According to this approach, sexual dysfunctions are caused by inappropriate cognitive, behavioral, and emotional learnings, which can be relearned. Approaching the problem as a couple is optimal. Each individual takes responsibility for his/her sexuality. To avoid guilt and blaming, the task is conceptualized as developing a couple sexual style that is functional and satisfying for both partners. The focus is on working together as an intimate team to develop a couple style based on comfort, pleasure, and satisfaction. Sexuality is seen as cooperative, sharing, and pleasure oriented, not as a goal-oriented performance where each individual is trying to prove something to self or partner. The prescription for satisfying sexuality is emotional intimacy, nondemand pleasuring, and erotic stimulation. This is an active therapy that emphasizes *in vivo* learning "homework assignments." Reading and cognitive restructuring are important, but the crucial element is sexual exercises organized in a semistructured manner to build comfort and skill (McCarthy & McCarthy, 1993b).

In conceptualizing treatment strategies, childhood sexual abuse is an area to be carefully assessed. Interventions are designed to deal with past and present sexual attitudes and feelings. A major clinical trap, however, is focusing therapeutic attention on resolving childhood issues and postponing dealing with couple issues. This strategy of benign neglect may result in sexual avoidance, inhibited sexual desire, and increased partner frustration and resentment.

My conceptualization and treatment strategy focuses on resolving present sexual issues within a couple format. The client and sexual partner are made aware of vulnerabilities and anxieties due to trauma or abuse, as the therapist assists the individual and couple in designing coping strategies to deal with sexual trauma and its aftermath. The cognitive theme is that the person deserves to be a survivor, not to play out the victim role. The person owns his/her sexuality, enjoying desire, arousal, and orgasm, so that sexuality comes to enhance his/her life and intimate relationship. Sexual trauma is integrated into sexual self-esteem as the client is viewed as a survivor, not a victim. (McCarthy, 1993) The appropriate cognition is, "Living well is the best revenge."

Sexual trauma issues are particularly difficult for males. The literature focuses on abuse of female children and the image of males is primarily that of perpetrators. Males with a history of sexual abuse usually treat it as their "shameful secret." Boys suffer the breaking of three taboos—sex between an adult and child, the need for a boy to be strong and able to protect himself, and the stigma of male–male sexual activity. The questions the boy asks are, "What's wrong with me that he picked me to abuse? Does it mean I'm gay?" Boys are afraid to reveal the abuse because they will be blamed and labeled. Over time, the sexual secret becomes more powerful and distorted, controlling the boy's self-esteem. There are few therapeutic and self-help resources for sexually abused boys, especially those who are not perpetrators. Although a significant percentage are likely to use the "macho" strategy of becoming perpetrators themselves, most do not (Becker, 1988). The majority feel embarrassed, stigmatized, and guilty, which interferes with sexual functioning. It is a shameful secret, revealed to no one, especially not his intimate partner.

PAUL AND RACHEL

Paul and Rachel were referred by a marital therapist who had seen them in therapy for 1½ years. The therapist felt they had made good progress on understanding family-of-origin issues and couple communication skills, but Rachel was becoming increasingly frustrated by their poor sexual life. Low frequency of sex sabotaged the goal of starting a family. Paul valued Rachel and their marriage but was frightened and avoidant of sexuality. His strategy was to placate Rachel rather than developing a viable sexual relationship.

The first session generally includes both spouses. Rachel was very enthusiastic about seeing a sex therapist, but Paul was quite reluctant. He preferred to continue marital therapy. I resisted Rachel's desire to make an early individual appointment—having both people present reinforces the importance of thinking and talking about sex as a couple issue.

The first session was highly anxious and disjointed. Paul raised four or five different issues. Rachel and I were reacting to Paul's fears, anxieties, and ambivalence. As Paul's anxiety heightened, Rachel became increasingly angry and critical. They were a couple highly adept at the guilt–blaming cycle and in diverting clinical issues. I kept them focused on the assessment contract and suggested they maintain monthly contact with the marital therapist. This reduced Paul's anxiety enough to schedule an individual sex history appointment. They left with a copy of *Couple Sexual Awareness* (McCarthy & McCarthy, 1990) and an agreement to discuss the chapter on inhibited sexual desire.

I saw Rachel first individually. She was verbal and forthcoming. Rachel reported a very active sexual life as an adolescent and young adult, driven by a strong desire to prove her attractiveness and worth. She had an unwanted pregnancy which was terminated at age 20 and two bouts of sexually transmitted diseases which she dealt with effectively. When Rachel met Paul at age 26, she felt ready to marry and saw him as a healthy partner choice. She had been in group therapy for 2 years and felt her self-esteem had improved and she had chosen an appropriate partner. Currently, Rachel felt enraged and sexually betrayed. She wanted satisfying sex and a baby and felt Paul had purposely lied and was punishing her. The therapist was taken aback by the intensity of Rachel's feelings. Her sense of being victimized by Paul was powerful. She saw no value in moderating her emotional reactions. She felt that only by keeping an intense confrontative tone would Paul break through his denial and begin to resolve his sexual problems. Rachel had little understanding or empathy for Paul's concerns and took no responsibility for changing her cognitions or behavior.

When asked whether there was anything Rachel wanted kept secret, she revealed that if therapy did not work in 6 months, she would leave the marriage. Rachel vehemently stated that sex and a baby were more important than Paul and the marriage. This session left me drained and worried that the prognosis for this couple looked poor. I asked whether Rachel was willing to engage in bibliotherapy to broaden her perspective. She agreed and I gave her *The Dance of Anger* (Lehner, 1985).

Adding to concerns about the prognosis, Paul canceled his first individual appointment and arrived 20 minutes late to his second. Paul's anxiety was palpable, especially in discussing guidelines for disclosure of sexual secrets. It was obvious he had major worries about confidentiality and sharing information. I spent some time conveying examples of other clients, how shame over secrets had inhibited their desire, and how problems had been resolved in therapy. I gave Paul the option of writing out the secret or discussing it as part of the sex history. He chose the latter and made an appointment he vowed to keep. Between sessions he agreed to read chapters on inhibited sexual desire and marital sex in *Male Sexual Awareness* (McCarthy, 1988). Before leaving, Paul reaffirmed his desire to preserve his marriage and have children. Paul came to the next session prepared to self-disclose. He was the oldest of three children, and was 7 when his father moved out of state for a job. This served as a convenient way to end the marriage. Paul had few memories of his father but knew his mother was very bitter. After the separation, his mother began drinking heavily and had a series of affairs, some of them abusive. Paul felt confused and distressed by the sexual displays. He liked some of the men but avoided attachment because they would disappear in weeks or months. Most of the boyfriends did not treat his mother well and were often drunk or angry. Usually, Paul and his sisters were ignored, but on occasion mother's boyfriend would become angry and threaten to discipline or beat the children. Paul felt protective of his sisters. If there was a violent incident, he took the brunt of it. As Paul became older, he remained supportive of his mother but increasingly began to pity her, viewing her as weak and sad. In junior and senior high school, Paul was the target of jokes and teasing about his mother's promiscuous behavior. Paul tried to ignore it but internally seethed.

There were two specific traumatic incidents involving different boyfriends. The first occurred at age 10 when the man would come into Paul's room and anally stimulate him through his pajamas. Paul pretended to be asleep and nothing was said. Paul felt confused and violated by these incidents which occurred in an intermittent pattern over 2 months. The second incident occurred when Paul was 13 and involved a live-in boyfriend. He would get Paul alone and spank him for some misdeed (usually concocted) and then fellate Paul to orgasm. Paul was humiliated by the spanking and agitated and ambivalent about fellatio. The man said Paul was a "bad boy" who wanted both the spanking and sex. Over time, the spanking became more severe and painful. Paul hid the welts and treated this physical and sexual abuse as his secret. He remembers locking himself in the bathroom, vomiting, and crying. Paul felt the man continued to date his mother so he could have access to Paul. Paul had never revealed these incidents but was very angry at his mother for having men like that in their home. He felt she should have intuited that something was wrong and been protective of Paul.

After disclosing this incident, Paul looked drained and I felt drained. There were 15 minutes remaining in the session. I asked whether Paul was willing to disclose this to Rachel. Paul feared Rachel would be repulsed, see him as hopeless, and abandon him. Paul blamed himself for the sexual abuse and felt humiliated. It was a source of shame and he felt like a fraud who was about to be exposed. I assured Paul it would not be disclosed without his permission.

I asked Paul to do a written homework task. He would record each incident in the first column; in the second column, the perpetrator's responsibility for the incident; in the third column, his mother's responsibility; and in the final column, his responsibility. A second task was writing his fears about how Rachel would respond to this secret in one column and in the second column how he would like Rachel to respond. A follow-up individual session was scheduled as well as a couple feedback session for the next week.

Two days later, I received an urgent call from Rachel. She said Paul was tearful and agitated, but would not tell her what was wrong. I focused on Rachel's response rather than her suspicions or worries about Paul. I advised Rachel to encourage Paul to complete his therapeutic homework and to assure him she was his intimate spouse. These were Paul's issues, and she was not to make them her own.

At Paul's individual session he reported not doing the first task, but he did complete the second. He had decided to share the sexual secret with Rachel. As we reviewed what he had written, his fears were clearer and more specific than what he wanted from Rachel. Paul's fear was that Rachel would view him as gay, a wimp, and damaged goods and would pity him, find him unattractive, be turned off sexually, and abandon him. Although anxious, Paul was feeling overwhelmed by his sexual secret. He had felt some relief from the sexual history and was willing to take the risk and share this with Rachel. Most of the session was spent in discussion and role plays. Paul wanted Rachel's help in completing the homework task of sorting out issues of responsibility, guilt, and shame. I suggested that Paul ask Rachel to be objective and nonjudgmental. Paul said he hoped she would but that was asking too much.

The feedback session was scheduled as a double session (100 minutes), which lasted 115 minutes. I structured the session by saying it was not unusual for secrets and fears to inhibit sexual desire.

Paul valued Rachel and their marriage. This feeling gave him the courage to disclose his history of sexual trauma. Paul was anxious and tearful in discussing his abuse but was clear and articulate. Midway through Rachel began crying, and as he finished, she hugged him and both cried. Rachel's most poignant words were, "You were a good son, you didn't deserve that." Paul was amazed by the strength of her support. Rachel was relieved, not angry or rejecting. She had assumed the secret involved her (e.g., that she was not sexually desirable, that Paul was not attracted to her, or that the secret involved an extramarital affair with a woman or man). Understanding the prime cause of his inhibited sexual desire reduced Rachel's distrust and anger significantly. Revealing his secret and receiving support and empathy rather than revulsion and abandonment were healing experiences. Rachel's anger was directed at the perpetrator, not at Paul.

I was impressed by the therapeutic power of revealing secrets. For Paul, the abuse had become more distorted and powerful over time, so it controlled his self-esteem. Paul's fear that Rachel would discover his secret and abandon him motivated sexual avoidance. They were ready to deal with issues as a team for the first time in the relationship.

As with any marriage, problems are multicausal and multidimensional. Dealing with Paul's history of trauma was necessary but not sufficient to resolve inhibited sexual desire. Rachel's anger interfered with desire and she, too, had to change her attitudes and behavior. They needed to work together and develop sexual scenarios and techniques to increase comfort and confidence. Paul needed Rachel's help in learning ejaculatory control and both needed to improve sexual communication skills.

The assignments at the end of the session were (1) to process the feedback session, (2) to do the writing tasks about responsibility for the abuse, and (3) to develop a trust (vulnerability) position to use with sexual exercises. They left the session tired but upbeat. I believed sex therapy was off to a good start. They were reminded they had the option of calling during the week if there was something they were confused about or experienced an unexpected roadblock.

When I saw them in the waiting room the next session, I was aware of tension, especially from Rachel. She had left the previous session unrealistically buoyed by discovering a sexual secret she was sure could easily be remedied. It was clear to Rachel that the boyfriend had been the evil perpetrator, Paul's mother was the incompetent caretaker, and Paul was the hapless victim who was blameless. Rachel tried to lobby this view, but Paul was not buying. Rachel reverted to criticizing Paul and feeling angry. This provided an excuse for Paul to avoid his written task and the trust position.

I commented how easy it was for them to fall into "old traps" and suggested Rachel initiate the trust position. Rachel was encouraged to assume the role of Paul's intimate friend, not his angry critic. Rachel's sexual interest, arousal, and orgasm were friends to the sexual relationship, not a demand for performance. Rachel had to learn to personalize her desire for Paul, not just a physical need to be sexual.

Why had Paul relinquished his responsibility? Paul needed to overcome his confused, ambivalent, passive approach to sexuality. Rachel had to back off so she provided less of a target to react against. Paul needed to act instead of react. He was given the task of completing the homework about responsibility for abuse and to initiate the exercise about establishing comfort talking and touching clothed in the bedroom and nude outside the bedroom. Paul was asked how he would react if it had been Rachel who was sexually abused by her mother's boyfriend. Paul was clear how he would support Rachel. Could he reverse roles and be kind to himself?

Rachel's empathy increased when she realized that Paul believed "real men can't be abused." When Rachel was gentle and tearful, she could communicate with Paul in a way she was unable to when she was angry and confrontational. Paul and Rachel had their monthly session with the marital therapist who felt the system was becoming more flexible and was enthusiastic about the movement she observed.

The change process continued to be rocky and uneven. Rachel and Paul established two trust positions and the comfort exercise in the bedroom went well. However, Paul reported feeling anxious about being nude outside the bedroom. The couple agreed to conduct all exercises in their bedroom. Paul made progress in the abuse writings but remained ambivalent about whether he was really a survivor. I suggested four individual sessions with Paul. Couple sessions focused on building desire, which was conceptualized as a couple issue. The couple task was the attraction exercise where each takes turns describing the psychological, physical, interpersonal, and sexual aspects they find attractive about their spouse. Each then makes up to three requests of what would increase their attraction to the spouse (McCarthy & McCarthy, 1993b).

Paul made progress in his individual sessions. Cognitive restructuring was the most valuable technique, but he also benefited from guided imagery and reworking the traumatic incidents. Cognitive restructuring focused on pride at being a survivor, appropriate anger at the perpetrator (including writing a letter outlining the abuse and his feelings), and acknowledging his mother's deficiencies as a caretaker without negating her value as a person and parent. Especially important was the cognition, "Living well is the best revenge." Paul benefited from reading selected passages from *Victims No Longer* (Lew, 1990) and *Confronting the Victim Role* (McCarthy & McCarthy, 1993a).

Paul explored his pattern of masturbation and sexual fantasies. Masturbation frequency is an important measure of sexual interest. Paul masturbated three to four times a week, a fact he had kept from Rachel and the marriage therapist. He was ashamed of his masturbation frequency and was surprised that I viewed it as a positive prognostic sign. Paul's fantasies were varied and did not involve abusive incidents—another good sign. Paul read about positive uses of sexual fantasies (McCarthy, 1988) and engaged in stop–start ejaculatory control exercises with masturbation (Zilbergeld, 1992). Appreciating masturbation and using a variety of sexual fantasies in a guilt-free manner were empowering. Paul found it relatively easy to practice and improve ejaculatory control during masturbation, which increased his confidence about transferring these skills to partner sex.

The couple sessions continued to be difficult and stressful. Although motivation and awareness improved, the trap of Paul's avoidance/passive–aggressive behavior combined with Rachel's anger and blaming was a powerful, overlearned pattern. It was easy to get off track and become discouraged. Assigning specific exercises between sessions and processing positive learnings before discussing problems were helpful in nurturing Paul's sexual self-confidence and confirming Rachel's role as the intimate spouse. However, they slipped off track and fell into a destructive cycle of attacking, counterattacking, and avoiding with great frequency. The intervention to break this pattern was that any participant could call a "time out," saying the discussion had gotten off track. After three time-outs per session, any subsequent off-track comments would result in a couple fine of $10. The money went to a charity both disliked.

It is not unusual for sex therapy to have a rhythm of "one step forward, two steps back," especially from sessions 7 through 12. The desire and pleasuring exercises set a solid base to develop a functional, satisfying sexual relationship. However, integrating scenarios and techniques into Paul and Rachel's sexual repertoire was not easy. Maintaining a rhythm of sexual contact two to four times per week was difficult. The "ping-pong" system of initiation did not work so Rachel agreed to be the prime initiator, with Paul taking the lead at least twice a month. For Paul, anticipatory anxiety was the biggest hurdle. He much preferred being sexual at Rachel's initiation, especially when her scenarios were sensual and prolonged. Rachel was creative and inventive in initiating but wished Paul would develop sexual self-assuredness.

Ejaculatory control exercises are more than a repetition of stop–start practices (McCarthy, 1989). They involve the couple's becoming an intimate team who appreciate a broad-based pleasure-oriented approach to touching and stimulation. Developing a clear communication system is as important as prolonging arousal. The woman must be an involved partner who enjoys giving as well as receiving. The male must learn how to discriminate the point of ejaculatory inevitability and not to overreact to mistakes. The quiet vagina exercise, which utilizes the female-superior intercourse position, with her guiding intromission and utilizing minimal movements, is the first step in integrating intercourse with the pleasuring. Gradually, the couple introduces other intercourse positions and thrusting speeds.

Paul's learning ejaculatory control was not to perform for Rachel but to make intercourse and orgasm a functional, satisfying experience for both. Rachel had been easily aroused and orgasmic and now became orgasmic with intercourse. Paul was shocked that this was not a "big deal" for her. I reminded Paul that he had learned ejaculatory control for himself. Paul's comfort and confidence with arousal, intercourse, and ejaculatory control gradually but significantly improved.

Afterplay and emotional satisfaction were particularly important. Conceptually, sex therapy has focused too much on arousal and orgasm and not enough on desire and satisfaction. Afterplay was crucial in closing the sexual loop for Paul, acknowledging the value of the sexual connection. Before sex therapy, sex ended with Paul's orgasm and he emotionally withdrew. To counteract that pattern, they developed afterplay scenarios. One third of the time Rachel requested additional manual stimulation for more orgasms (this was true whether or not she had an orgasm during intercourse). Although he was not sexually aroused, Paul enjoyed giving stimulation and did not view it as "mechanical servicing." Afterward, Paul would make a pot of tea and they would sit and talk, especially about the possibility of buying a house and having a baby.

Sometimes Paul would turn on their favorite music and they would dance. It was easier for Paul to talk about feelings and share when there was another activity.

A major mistake sex therapists make is to terminate therapy when the couple has achieved their initial goals. Paul and Rachel came to the 13th session in a buoyant mood. They had had three fulfilling sexual experiences during the week, one initiated by Paul. Rachel reaffirmed her commitment to the marriage by abandoning the use of her diaphragm. Both were excited by the possibility of becoming pregnant. I acknowledged their progress and shared their happiness but cautioned that it was important to develop an active program to maintain and generalize individual and couple gains. I suggested that each schedule an appointment to assess changes, explore remaining issues, and develop a maintenance program. After the next couple session, visits would be reduced to biweekly.

Rachel told me what she was reluctant to say in front of Paul. Although she was extremely pleased with the sexual progress, had mastered anger control skills, recommitted to the marriage, and was excited about getting pregnant, Rachel worried about Paul's reluctance to sexually initiate. She felt badly that sexual pleasure and arousal were so much easier for her. Rachel agreed to raise these issues in the context of requests and enhancement rather than seeing Paul as the deficit spouse.

Paul was ready to terminate therapy. He was pleased the marriage was on solid footing and wanted to have a child. I focused on two issues: (1) reviewing the sexual trauma and determining whether there were still "demons" active, identifying traps Paul had to monitor, and what to do if he began to regress into silence and inhibition; and (2) determining how important Paul wanted sex to be in his life and marriage, especially in terms of initiation and quality. Paul became defensive and tears welled. He asked, "What will be enough for Rachel?" I reasserted my respect and caring for Paul and what he had survived as a child. Paul's growth over the past 6 months was reinforced. However, I suggested that Paul do a writing exercise (he responded well to specific tasks, especially involving a concrete action). I gave Paul an option to schedule an individual session before the next couple session.

Paul called the day before the couple session, saying he had discussed this with Rachel and wanted to come alone. Paul had written a letter to his mother expressing anger about the abusive incidents, their effect on him, and his desire for her to apologize and affirm the value of his life, marriage, and sexuality. It was a powerful, clear, and healthy six-page letter. I made suggestions and clarifications and urged Paul to share the letter with Rachel. Paul agreed that further work and exercises to enhance the quality of their sexual life would be of value. He was satisfied with the initiation pattern and wanted that to stand.

At the couple session, Rachel (who liked Paul's mother) agreed with the feelings and content of the letter and concurred with Paul's decision not to mail it. Writing had been therapeutic. His mother's anguish and guilt would not be healthy for Paul (or his mother). His mother had acknowledged Paul as a good person and son and was very supportive of their marriage. Rachel was enthusiastic about pursuing sexual exercises involving arousal and eroticism, special turn-ons, and enhancement. She was aware that Paul's desire and arousal pattern was different from hers and that sex need not be a competition.

Biweekly sessions continued for 2 months, followed by monthly sessions for 2 months and then 6-month follow-up sessions, which have continued for the past year and a half. Both partners value these sessions and continue to schedule them.

CLOSING THOUGHTS

Life is meant to be lived in the present with planning for the future, not controlled by the trauma of the past (McCarthy & McCarthy, 1993a). Paul and Rachel are each complex individuals, dealing with a number of personal, couple, and sexual issues. Disclosing and coping with the secret of Paul's sexual abuse was a necessary, but not sufficient, component of their sexual functioning. Without couple sex therapy and Rachel's active involvement, inhibited sexual desire would not have been resolved. Although this marriage was in danger of ending because of the sexual dysfunction and its side effect of preventing conception, once Paul and Rachel committed to being an intimate team, threats of marital dissolution stopped. My empathy for Paul's dilemma yet continuing to promote the sexual growth process was a helpful model for Rachel to follow with Paul. To Rachel's great credit, she was able to modulate her anger and criticalness. My belief that they could become a viable sexual couple remained a consistent motivator during the more frustrating weeks.

Most therapy reports involving sexual trauma focus on the woman who had been abused, but it is crucial to realize that men have histories of abuse that inhibit and control their sexual self-esteem. A therapeutic approach that respects the man's self-esteem while confronting the harmful effects of the sexual secret and shame is crucial. Bibliotherapy can reinforce and elaborate on the verbal messages of the therapy sessions. Paul developed the cognition of himself as a survivor who deserved a gratifying sexual life. Although most sessions were conjoint, focused individual sessions with Paul were a vital element in moving the therapy toward a successful resolution. Sex therapy must address dysfunctional attitudes, behavior, and feelings but cannot stop there. In order to maintain relationship and sexual gains, healthy attitudes, behavior, and feelings need to be nurtured so the couple's relationship is robust enough to prevent relapse (McCarthy, 1993).

REFERENCES

Becker, J. (1988). Adolescent sex offenders. *Behavior Therapist, 11*(9), 185–187.

Kaplan, H. S. (1974). *The new sex therapy.* New York: Brunner/Mazel.

Lehner, H. (1985). *The dance of anger.* New York: Harper & Row.

Lew, M. (1990). *Victims no longer.* New York: HarperCollins.

Maltz, W. (1991). *The sexual healing journey.* New York: HarperCollins.

Masters, W. H., & Johnson, V. E. (1970). *Human sexual inadequacy.* Boston: Little, Brown.

McCarthy, B. (1988). *Male sexual awareness.* New York: Carroll & Graf.

McCarthy, B. (1989). Cognitive-behavioral strategies and techniques in the treatment of early ejaculation. In S. R. Leiblum & R. C. Rosen (Eds.), *Principles and practice of sex therapy* (2nd ed.): *Update for the 1990s* (pp. 141–167). New York: Guilford Press.

McCarthy, B. (1990). Treating sexual dysfunction associated with prior sexual trauma. *Journal of Sex and Marital Therapy, 16,* 142–146.

McCarthy, B. (1992). Sexual trauma: The pendulum has swung too far. *Journal of Sex Education and Therapy, 18,* 1–10.

McCarthy, B. (1993). Relapse prevention strategies and techniques in sex therapy. *Journal of Sex and Marital Therapy, 19,* 142–146.

McCarthy, B., & McCarthy, E. (1990). *Couple sexual awareness.* New York: Carroll & Graf.

McCarthy, B., & McCarthy, E. (1993a). *Confronting the victim role.* New York: Carroll & Graf.

McCarthy, B., & McCarthy, E. (1993b). *Sexual awareness.* New York: Carroll & Graf.

Zilbergeld, B. (1992). *The new male sexuality.* New York: Bantam.

9

Sexual Desire Disorder in a Lesbian–Feminist Couple: The Intersection of Therapy and Politics

MARGARET NICHOLS

INTRODUCTION

It is obvious to therapists experienced in working with both heterosexual and homosexual couples that in most cases sexual orientation is irrelevant to the course of treatment. There are striking exceptions to this rule, however, especially in the treatment of sexual problems. It is therefore appropriate that this chapter be devoted to a case that typifies the "signature" sexual problem of gay women, an affliction so common that lesbian comics crack jokes about it and it has been colloquially named "lesbian bed death." Mickie and Cheryl came to sex therapy for help with low sexual desire and low sexual frequency—three to four sexual episodes per year—in a long-term monogamous relationship.

Certainly lesbian couples have not cornered the market on low sexual desire; it may be the most common sexual problem for all couples. But two things make this disorder stand out in the lesbian community. First, data suggest that sexual frequency may be lower normatively for lesbian couples than for any other type of gender pairing (Blumstein & Schwartz, 1983). Moreover, this may not be a recent phenomenon. The lesbian historian Lillian Faderman has written extensively about the existence

161

of lesbian relationships devoid of genital sexuality in the 19th century (1981) and lesbian relationships where sexuality was greatly deemphasized in the 20th century (1991). And Faderman (1991, p. 304) quotes the French author Colette (1930), "who wrote about lesbianism from her firsthand experiences":

> In living amorously together, two women may eventually discover that their mutual attraction is not basically sensual. . . . What woman would not blush to seek out her amie only for sensual pleasure? In no way is it passion that fosters the devotion of two women, but rather a feeling of kinship.

Second, sexual desire problems among lesbians are discussed widely within the lesbian community in political terms, a phenomenon unparalleled among heterosexuals or even gay males. This is part of a broader tendency of lesbians to politicize all sexuality and indeed most aspects of day-to-day living. The feminist movement of the 1970s coined the phrase, "the personal is political," and lesbians in the latter 20th century have taken this belief very much to heart. Indeed, Faderman's history of 20th-century lesbianism, *Odd Girls and Twilight Lovers* (1991), includes an entire chapter titled "Lesbian Sex Wars in the 1980's," and much of this chapter is devoted to ideological conflicts touching upon the issue of low sexual frequency among lesbians.

Because even experienced sex therapists may be unfamiliar with the political meanings of sex within the lesbian community, it is useful to preface this case presentation with a brief discussion of both clinical and cultural aspects of low desire in gay women. For a more thorough exposition of clinical and therapeutic perspectives, the reader is referred to my chapter in *Sexual Desire Disorders* (Nichols, 1988).

There seems little doubt that low sexual desire is more common among lesbian couples than among other couples, and that most low desire is secondary, rather than primary, in nature. That is, lesbians, whose predominant form of sexual behavior is serial monogamy, seem to begin relationships with about as frequent sexual activity with their partner as do heterosexuals or gay men. But within 1 to 2 years, sexual activity drops dramatically: In the Blumstein and Schwartz study (1983) only about one third of lesbians in relationships of 2 years or more had sex once a week or more and 47% had sex once a month or less. By contrast, among heterosexual married couples two thirds had sex once a week or more and only 15% had sex once a month or less. Most lesbians report strong sexual desire in the beginning of their relationships—in other words, their dysfunction is not primary—although many report that the rapid and extreme decrease in activity is a pattern in all their long-term relationships.

Therapists within the lesbian and bisexual community have discussed this issue widely and proposed various theories for the relative diminution of sex in lesbian relationships (Burch, 1987; Loulan, 1985; Nichols, 1987). Some causes seem fairly obvious. Because women are culturally socialized to be less sexually assertive than men, lesbian couplings suffer from the lack of a "trained initiator"; one might hypothesize that frequency in heterosexual couples is often determined by the male partner. Because women are similarly socialized to be less attuned to their own sexual needs and even the physiological indicators of arousal, they simply may not experience desire in the same visceral way. Indeed, one lesbian sex authority has suggested that women should not expect to feel desire as a physical phenomenon; Loulan (1985) encourages lesbians to focus on their willingness to have sex rather than on their desire to have sex. Moreover, many women appear to have intimacy needs fulfilled by physical, nongenital affection rather than genital contact. Indeed, the stereotypical low-frequency lesbian couple exhibits an abundance of cuddling, touching, and other expressions of nonsexual closeness.

Women in this culture also seem to be more conflicted and guilt ridden about exhibiting strong sexual drives, and, again, pairings of two women double this possible source of sexual inhibition. Because women are sexually assaulted far more frequently than are men in contemporary society, lesbian relationships also double the probability that at least one partner will have a traumatic history of incest, molestation, coercion, or other sexual abuse. So, simply based on gender and cultural experiences, female–female pairings are more likely to be "sexually disadvantaged." Within the lesbian community, this problem is often compounded. Lesbians themselves have sometimes labeled certain sexual desires "bad," especially desires for men or sexual desires that seem to resemble male sexual preferences (ranging from an interest in pornography to an interest in penetration). Thus, the lesbian "sexual unconscious" contains not only the injunctions against sex taught to all women and traumatic memories of sexual abuse suffered by many women, but additional injunctions against homosexual behavior inculcated at an early age and proscriptions learned upon entry into a "supportive" lesbian community. For some lesbians, the unconscious is a virtual minefield, which may ultimately be simply too dangerous to enter. Inhibitions against sex may be a parsimonious way of avoiding conflict-laden fantasies, images, and desires.

Finally, most therapists within the lesbian and bisexual community have agreed that lesbian relationships are often characterized by what is variously called fusion or merging, an extreme degree of intimacy in which individual identity seems almost to be lost. It is possible that within the context of already excessive closeness, the act of sex, characterized by even greater union, may be too threatening. For all these reasons, then, lesbian relationships may inherently be "loaded" for low sexual frequency.

Some lesbians have argued that the definition of sex—that is, what we literally "count" in studies of frequency—is skewed to a heterosexist standard (Clunis & Green, 1988). For example, neither researchers nor subjects themselves are likely to consider nongenital touching that does not lead to orgasm to be "sex." Yet this type of contact, very common in lesbian couples, may fulfill the sexual needs of the women involved as well as does intercourse in a heterosexual couple. Hurlbert and Apt (1993) found lesbian women in couple relationships to be just as satisfied with their sex lives as were heterosexual women in relationships despite the fact that the lesbians had less frequent sex. And it may be that nonorgasmic sex is satisfying to lesbians in part because when they have sex that is directed toward orgasm, they seem to be more successful at it. While no comparable statistics exist, the clinician working with lesbians notices the infrequency of anorgasmia as a complaint among gay women. One can speculate that lesbian sexual techniques, primarily digital and oral stimulation, are more likely to reliably result in orgasm for women than is heterosexual intercourse. One might even wonder how the frequency of sex for heterosexual and homosexual women would compare if the only episodes sex researchers "counted" as sex for heterosexuals were ones that culminated in orgasm for the female partner.

Treatment of a lesbian couple complaining of low sexual desire is complicated by the subcultural context within which the couple is supported. This is particularly true of lesbian "baby boomers," those most likely to have been affected by the lesbian–feminist movement of the 1970s and the "sex wars" of the 1980s. Faderman (1991) begins her chapter on the latter with a quote from T. G. Atkinson: "I do not know any feminist worthy of that name who, if forced to choose between freedom and sex, would choose sex" (p. 246). Because feminists in these decades often saw sex as primarily a tool used in male hands to oppress women, they also saw freedom and sex as diametrical opposites. A decade ago, the lesbian community's polarization around sexual issues reached such heights that gay women could often be described as belonging to one of two camps, cultural feminists and the much smaller group of lesbian sex radicals. Cultural feminists tended to have fairly rigid views about which sexual behaviors, acts, and attitudes were or were not "politically correct." Their ideology was an extension of the 1960s and 1970s feminist critiques of sexual mores that served to oppress women, from the use of makeup and dress to transform women into sexual objects to the glorification of sexually violent/rape-like images. These critiques led some feminists to become suspicious of sex itself, at least of all sex between men and women. Andrea Dworkin (1980) probably epitomized the ex-

treme with her statement that heterosexual sex in the missionary position —man on top—was inherently rape. Thus, cultural feminists within
the lesbian community came to cast a critical eye on all sexuality that
seemed to resemble heterosexual sex, labeling it "patriarchal" and "male
identified." These women eschewed pornography, penetration, "butch–
femme" roles, and rough sex. The sexual ideal proposed by these lesbians appeared to be that of total mutuality, sensuality rather than overt
genitality, and complete "naturalness"—no toys, props, costumes, or
roles. While this brand of sexuality may have represented the actual
preferences of many gay women, it by no means included the preferences
of all. Moreover, by codifying sex—labeling some acts "p.c." (politically
correct) and other acts "p.i." (politically incorrect)—the cultural feminists, without meaning to, added to the already heavy burden of sexual
acts proscribed for women.

Not surprisingly, some lesbians rebelled against these restrictions,
and a few, the lesbian sex radicals, took their rebellion to breathtaking
extremes. Borrowing heavily from the gay male sexual liberation of the
1970s, the sex radicals started S/M (sadomasochistic) clubs, butch–femme
support groups, pornography magazines, and video companies and engaged in all manner of unusual sex acts from vaginal "fist fucking" to
public sex orgies. Although the number of lesbian sex radicals was small,
their ideas and practices became widely known and hotly debated within
the community at large by the end of the 1980s. Variously denounced,
banned, and lauded, the sex radicals created vociferous and continuous
dialogue about sex. Of utmost importance to the sex therapist treating
lesbians born before 1975 is the fact that most of this generation of gay
women have opinions, one way or the other, about the political implications of their sexuality.

Still another aspect of lesbian sexuality affects the baby-boom generation. Unlike gay men, many lesbians of this era view themselves as
having chosen their sexual orientation for feminist/political reasons. As
we shall see in the case discussion that follows, this factor can influence
not only the etiology of sexual desire disorders but also the course of
treatment.

A CASE OF LOW DESIRE AND LOW FREQUENCY

Initial Presentation

Mickie, a 44-year-old chemist, and her partner of 10 years, Cheryl, a
47-year-old social worker, called for sex therapy after referral by the
therapist whom they had seen for couple counseling. This colleague, with

whom I had worked closely in the past, thought that the couple could effectively work on sexual issues while they continued to work with her on their relationship, and I agreed to take on this somewhat unusual referral. From the beginning we all agreed that I would consult with this couple no more frequently than once every other week, to alternate with my colleague's sessions.

Our initial interview was cautious and tentative. Far from treating me with the deferential respect some clients display in facing a "professional," Cheryl and Mickie interrogated me and challenged my credentials—my credentials as a feminist and activist, that is. I was frank about being bisexual rather than lesbian; my frankness earned me some points that compensated for those I lost through bisexuality. My activist history and obvious familiarity with feminist theory, combined with the recommendation they had received from their couple therapist, whom they trusted, allayed their initial suspicions.

From the very first session my clients' political orientation toward the world determined therapeutic interventions. The women presented as prototypes of lesbian–feminists who had come of age during the 1970s women's movement: both cultivated an androgynous look, wearing no makeup, "practical" clothing (slacks, unisex shirts, boots), short unstyled hair, and little jewelry besides an occasional political button. Just as prototypically, they reported a couple history of relatively frequent, satisfying sex at the beginning of the relationship diminishing to sex three or four times per year during the last few years. Untypically, however, they also described a continuously high-conflict relationship. They had been in some variety of relationship counseling for most of their 10 years together and fought frequently and painfully. A few of their fights had degenerated into physical violence and most included mutual accusations of betrayal that included every incident of discord for the entire duration of their marriage.

Both women initially agreed that Mickie was the source of the sexual problems. Cheryl was characterized as "the passionate one" who had patiently and often not so patiently waited for Mickie, characterized with her WASP background as "the sexually repressed" member, to overcome her asexual heritage. After our initial sparring and rapport building and after eliciting some history of the relationship and sexuality within the relationship, I spent the remainder of the first session "training" the two women in a particular view of sexuality, especially regarding low desire in lesbian couples.

I used the rhetoric of the feminist, lesbian, and gay movements to do this training. First, the view was presented that much female sexuality was not so much nonexistent as undiscovered, quoting Mary Jane Sherfey, an early feminist who believed that women were inherently more sexual than men but had been repressed in the service of patriarchy. The possibility was offered that Mickie might not necessarily be as asexual as both women believed. Next, the theories of C. A. Tripp (1975) regarding the need for a "barrier" to create sexual desire were discussed and related to women's tendency to rely on romance to create a barrier, thus experiencing waning sexual desire once the limerance phase of a relationship is over. Low sexual frequency among lesbians was considered in light of counterarguments that many lesbians are satisfied with nongenital relationships. This allowed Cheryl and Mickie to assert that they were not satisfied with only hugging and cuddling. It was suggested that sex might be separated from other conflicts in their relationship and that their sexual relationship might be potentially dependent on some factors—such as creating time for sex, structuring mood, and learning technique—that were mechanical rather than psychological or even political in nature. The women were presented with the view that sexual preferences might be a matter of style or personal taste rather than "right" or "wrong." Both women were given some reading material—copies of my articles and suggestions of lesbian sex books—and questionnaires to complete and return before the next session, which was scheduled for 2 weeks later.

The questionnaires, three extensive documents each covering symptom complaints, personal/family background, history of sexual orientation development, and descriptions of sexual behavior within the current relationship, were received before the second meeting. Several items were noteworthy in the women's responses. Mickie's self-report revealed an active childhood and adolescent sexuality, all with males, as well as frequent masturbation from an early age. Although she wrote that she felt guilty about sex, her guilt had not inhibited her behavior; she had had more than 20 male sexual partners with two marriages and, after "coming out" at age 33, six female sexual partners. Her ratings on a series of scales fashioned after the Kinsey continuum scales placed her in the bisexual range, and she viewed herself as a rather militant lesbian by choice: "I think in this society it is easier and more comfortable for me to be exclusively lesbian. . . . I feel I clearly chose to be a lesbian. . . . I think it's unnatural that heterosexual women chose to relate to the person they have sex with, since most of them would rather relate to women." Mickie's questionnaire on the current sexual relationship also conveyed some interesting responses: Several times she reiterated the feeling that sex in general, and particularly her sexual desires, were "dirty"; she admitted to sexual fantasies that included "torture"; she acknowledged desires for S/M sex, "dressing up" in roles during sex, dildo use, bondage, and the use of enemas—all of which the couple had actually enacted, at least occasionally. Mickie reported that she was "sometimes aroused, sometimes disgusted" by pornographic materials, and that she preferred "my turn/your turn" sexual encounters over attempts at simultaneous arousal. In general, Mickie reported a combination of guilt and shame over her own sexual desires, high performance anxiety surrounding her encounters with Cheryl, an expectation of criticism from Cheryl of her sexual functioning, and a sense that Cheryl's criticisms of her were appropriate. She acknowledged that she usually rejected Cheryl's advances toward her and that when the couple did have sex, it was because Mickie girded herself for the anxiety of a sexual encounter and initiated sex herself. Not surprisingly, Mickie's predominant feelings about sex with Cheryl were of dread and anxiety.

Cheryl displayed the same stance in her questionnaires that she had in the first session—that Mickie was the source of the couple's sexual problems. She characterized herself as on the verge of leaving the relationship because of the lack of sexual activity and expressed great frustration about not being able to initiate sex with Mickie. Her own sexual history, while also "bisexual" (10 lifetime male partners, 18 female), was more clearly lesbian oriented. She recognized her lesbianism at age 16, when she fell in love with a girlfriend, and after several years of turmoil over her identity that included a suicide attempt at age 21, she became positively lesbian identified through the feminist movement of the late 1960s–1970s. All her romantic relationships were with women and she had had a number of monogamous pairings as an adult, although none had lasted more than 3 years. In fact, in her only acknowledgment of concern about her own sexuality, Cheryl admitted that she had encountered low sexual desire in her other partners but had always left the relationship without attempting to work out the sexual difficulties. Moreover, she expressed worry that her sex drive might be "too high" and that this made her "like my father," who had been a womanizer. Cheryl reported that sex was a primary outlet for her not only for intimacy but for tension, relief from boredom, and so on. She displayed clear negative judgments about Mickie's sexual style. She felt Mickie was "not spontaneous," "not capable of mutual sex," and too interested in sadomasochism and other atypical sexual acts. She deplored in general Cheryl's "slut mentality" toward sex.

The following hypotheses were generated after reading the women's questionnaires:

1. That Mickie was in fact capable of being quite sexual but that her sexuality had become ego-dystonic not only because of guilt inculcated in her childhood but because of ongoing criticism of her sexuality by Cheryl.

2. That Cheryl had, in a sense, too much "riding" on sex; she viewed sex as a panacea and relief for a variety of different frustrating feelings, and that this made low sexual activity much more problematic for her than it might have been otherwise.
3. That Cheryl's high need for sex combined with her rigid views of what was sexually appropriate and inappropriate (basically, her sexuality was "right" and Mickie's "wrong") created overwhelming pressure on Mickie leading to insurmountable performance anxiety around sexual activity.
4. That the two women had distinctly conflicting sexual styles/ scripts.
5. That both women had built up years of resentment about the sexual difficulties—Cheryl, because she felt she had been denied sex; Mickie, because she felt she was criticized and pressured for sex—that would be hard to diffuse.

The Course of Treatment

During session 2, these hypotheses were offered to Cheryl and Mickie. Two things were emphasized in this initial feedback session: the idea that Mickie might be inherently a sexual person but simply frightened of her own sexual desires and the concept that the stylistic conflicts between the women might be merely differences, rather than right and wrong. Mickie had a dramatic reaction to the first hypothesis; she cried in relief that there might be hope for her to recover a joyful sexual expression. The second hypothesis drew a mixed response: Both women were somewhat disbelieving of the reframing of their differences as normal variations of sexual preferences. This was true not only because Cheryl had tapped into Mickie's underlying guilt about sex to convince her that her sexuality was wrong. It also appeared that the couple was fused in a very special way. While they were capable of having some separateness in job, friends, and other aspects of daily life, they were not capable of having different beliefs or values and respecting each other's beliefs as valid. At later points in treatment this problem came up repeatedly; the couple could never "agree to disagree," and all differences had to be argued until one conceded to the other. The women had other reactions to the hypotheses as well. Mickie, as might be expected, was heartened by the ideas while Cheryl was predictably suspicious of me. Because Cheryl saw her form of sexuality as "genuinely" lesbian and Mickie's as "male identified," my defense of Mickie was at first attributed to my bisexuality. About one third of this session was spent in dialogue between me and

Cheryl in which I described the position of the lesbian sex radicals in order to support my view, quoting extensively from Pat Califia (1988), a controversial but impeccably lesbian writer and radical. Cheryl tentatively agreed to reserve judgment on the issue of sexual political correctness and the first sensate focus exercise was assigned as homework. The couple was asked to reserve 2 hours of "prime time" to be together and to use some of this time relaxing and setting the mood for intimacy. They were instructed to take turns as toucher and touchee and to engage in sensual stroking, avoiding contact with breasts and genitals.

Cheryl came to the next session angry. While Mickie had very much enjoyed and even been aroused by being touched, she had experienced conscious performance anxiety ("Am I doing this right? Will Cheryl be mad at me?") while touching Cheryl. Cheryl, on the other hand, initially was able to articulate only her criticisms of the exercise itself: Because sensate focus is by nature "my turn/your turn," and because Cheryl prefers mutuality, she felt the assignment of the exercise was a tacit disapproval of her preferences. Her anger was allayed somewhat by acknowledging the artificial nature of the exercise and explaining in more detail the reasons for its structure. Ultimately, Cheryl, who over the course of treatment displayed great capacity for self-awareness, was able to admit that she had been very uncomfortable being touched by Mickie because it made her anxious to receive pleasure without at the same time giving in return. As we explored this feeling, it emerged that Cheryl placed an enormous emphasis on her own ability to be a good lover and felt undeserving of a partner's total attention ("it's selfish"). In fact, it was her discomfort with purely receiving that probably made her so adamant about the necessity for sexual encounters to be completely mutual. Homework for session 4 was a sensate focus exercise with "guided touch," that is, with each woman guiding her partner's hand while being touched. In addition, the couple was asked to talk to each other after the sensate focus, using a couple dialogue they had learned in relationship counseling, and to express only their positive feelings to each other. This was done in part to begin to change a destructive aspect of their relationship. In the name of honesty, Mickie and Cheryl had a tendency to blurt out every negative feeling they had toward each other without reflection. I wanted to reinforce the idea that it was not necessarily "dishonest" to focus on positive feelings and keep some criticisms private.

At session 4, both women expressed some anxiety over being touched and guiding, although for different reasons. Mickie was concerned that her guiding of Cheryl would reveal "bad" sexual desires, and Cheryl became aware of a vague discomfort, although she was also surprised at how nurtured she could feel simply through nongenital touch. I was pleased at the latter because I hoped it would begin to teach Cheryl that she did not always need genital sex to feel intimacy. Both women were put in trance in this session so that they could explore the anxiety they felt during the homework more deeply; light hypnosis often allows clients to experience emotion more vividly and to make connections not easily accessible in the fully awake state of consciousness. Cheryl emerged from trance in touch with her own feelings of unworthiness while Mickie was overcome with the terror she felt at being criticized by Cheryl. Both women related these fears to issues they had been exploring in their relationship counseling; Cheryl to her awareness of her role as caretaker and Mickie to her insight that criticism evoked a fear of abandonment in her. The women's homework for session 5 was to repeat the same exercise concentrating fully on receiving pleasure when they were being touched.

The women appeared at session 5 without having carried out their assignment. Cheryl reported that shortly after the last session, she had fallen into despair about the relationship and become consumed with thoughts of leaving. It was conjectured that perhaps she had gotten too close to areas of intense anxiety; Cheryl rejected this hypothesis. Little was resolved and the previous homework assignment was repeated. For the next few sessions, the women completed assignments without great resistance.

During sessions 6 through 9, conducted over 3 months, Cheryl and Mickie progressed through sensate focus exercises that included genital touching, alternating who would initiate the homework assignments. In treatment, a core power struggle issue emerged: the conflict over which woman would control the structure of the sexual encounters. As Mickie lost much of her performance anxiety and guilt about sex and became able to be approached as well as to initiate sex, Cheryl became increasingly aware of how vulnerable to hurt she felt when she did not have total control. In general, these sessions went smoothly with a high degree of insight in both women and few accusations between them.

The couple arrived at session 10 in high spirits. They had gone on vacation together and had sex several times. Although most often Mickie had initiated sex and the sex had been brief, somewhat rough, and sometimes one-sided, Cheryl reported that she had enjoyed the encounters and appeared to have become more flexible in her own sexual script. She did voice concern, however, that "this can't continue" and that she might be disappointed once again. Her expression of this worry frightened Mickie, who again voiced fears of "displeasing" Cheryl. In retrospect, the disaster that followed this session might have been avoided had a relapse been predicted.

Three weeks later the women reported no sexual activity and dissatisfaction with each other, but instead of discussing their conflicts turned on me and attacked my bisexuality. Because nothing fruitful was resolved in this session, another session was scheduled for 1 week later. No sexual contact had taken place but both women were able to acknowledge their fears about becoming more sexual, and they were "given permission" to go more slowly in their sexual relationship. Because Mickie still reported anxiety over whether her sexual desires were okay, they were invited to come up with private "wish lists" of sexual desires and fantasies and to bring them to the next session. Session 13 was spent in using the technique of couple dialogue for the partners to reveal and validate their sexual desires to each other. The pair continued to avoid sexual contact during this period, choosing not even to engage in the simplest sensate focus.

The couple produced another conflict that discouraged sexual intimacy during the next 6 weeks. Cheryl became outraged over Mickie's herpes, which Mickie had contracted before the two women met but which suddenly emerged as a reason why Cheryl feared sex with Mickie. Cheryl also revealed a deeper concern. She realized that even if she and Mickie succeeded in "reviving" their sex life, it was not going to resemble her private fantasy. Cheryl spoke of her desires to have the kind of intense, passionate, spontaneous sexual experiences found only in the limerance phase of a relationship. She readily acknowledged that as she had left all previous relationships after 1 to 3 years, she had no realistic concept of what to expect from sex in a long-term relationship. Moreover, Cheryl was acutely experiencing a midlife crisis that involved feelings of loss and failure in all aspects of her life, especially her career. The recognition that a good sex life with Mickie might involve satisfying sex but was unlikely to include episodes of weak-kneed, overwhelming passion was deeply upsetting to Cheryl. Mickie, on the other hand, having always felt some guilt over sex and feeling now more sexually free than ever, experienced no such sense of loss. This left Cheryl feeling more alone.

In sessions 17 through 19, sensate focus was reintroduced and the two women gradually became more sexual with each other again, with a frequency of about once a week. Nevertheless, Cheryl's depression deepened and she was referred for antidepressant medication. After some sparring about why a lesbian psychiatrist could not be identified, Cheryl accepted the consultation and was placed on Paxil (paroxetine hydrochloride).

The Paxil radically changed Cheryl. She attained a greater acceptance of her relationship with Mickie, both sexual and otherwise, with all its inherent flaws and imperfections. Most important, she became more accepting of herself. She likened this experience to experiences she had had in Tibetan monasteries, and she and I had some interesting conversations about Ram Dass, Buddhism, and accepting and enjoying "what is" in life rather than pining for what one cannot have. Over the next 4 months, follow-up sessions were conducted every 3 to 4 weeks. At termination, the couple enjoyed a regular and satisfying sexual relationship, although it was one that resembled Mickie's script more than Cheryl's "regular" script. That is, the couple had expanded their repertoire so that sex did not always have to be "equal" and mutual. Sometimes sexual encounters involved one woman pleasuring the other; sometimes sex was very brief; at times the women would engage in sensual foreplay and then bring themselves to orgasm in each other's presence with vibrators. In this couple's relationship, Cheryl had compromised more than Mickie, letting go of many cherished beliefs about how sex should be. It remains to be seen whether she will be satisfied in the long run, however, or whether she will ultimately decide to seek another partner whose sexual script more closely resembles her own. This may depend on the nonsexual aspects of their relationship. At this writing, the women are still receiving relationship counseling, and it is uncertain whether they can ever live together harmoniously enough to satisfy them both. Although the sex therapy was at least a partial success, it may not be enough to save the relationship.

CONCLUSIONS AND DISCUSSION

This case was typical of the kind of sexual issues presented by lesbian couples not only in the problem but also in interventions used and outcome. It was perhaps most atypical in the degree of suspicion the clients had of the therapist and their extreme politicization of sex. The case raises some interesting questions about lesbian sexuality and lesbian partnerships.

To begin with, the relatively low frequency of sex in long-term lesbian relationships should make us question our norms for sexual behavior. Although most of us like to think of ourselves as nonjudgmental about sex, of course, this cannot be true and all of us have an unconscious or minimally conscious set of expectations about what is "healthy" and "unhealthy," "normal" and "abnormal," and so on. But if, as almost all research shows, universally males in Western industrialized societies are more sexually active than are females, it is probable that our expectations of normal frequency are skewed toward male desire, and probably heterosexual male desire as well. Most of us tend to assume that long-term relationships "should include" genital, orgasmic sexual contact, but in fact we have little understanding of the functions, other than procreative, served by sex in relationships and whether other behaviors would serve as well. We might look to the behavior of many male couples to get glimpses of other ways of being, as well as to the behavior of lesbian couples who do not come to therapy (McWhirter & Mattison, 1984; Clunis & Green, 1988). For example, McWhirter and Mattison report that before AIDS the norm for gay male couples was nonmonagamy, with perhaps less genital contact between the long-term partners than with their outside sexual contacts. Moreover, many urban gay men in the 1970s experimented widely with less common forms of sexuality: dominance and submission, bondage, manual–anal penetration ("fist fucking"), sexual use of enemas and/or urine, as well as various types of group and public sex. These sexual techniques often deemphasized genital contact and orgasm. For example, much public S/M sex involves no oral or genital contact whatsoever, and orgasm is not the goal. And even after HIV greatly decreased gay male sexual activity, a new form of group sex emerged: the "J/O" ("jerk-off") party in which many men looked at and touched each other but brought themselves to orgasm through masturbation. Thus an urban gay male accustomed to sexual practices of the 1970s and 1980s might not define sexual contact in the same way as would a sex researcher or sex therapist or the average heterosexual. "Sex" between partners might consist of watching a porn movie together, touching each other a little, and self- or mutual masturbation. It is interesting to consider how such broadening of the definition of sex might affect sexuality in long-term couples—or how it might affect the technique and approach of sex therapists. Many lesbian couples seem to find that our genital–orgasm focus on sexuality does not fit their needs or practices. It may be that, for some couples, two or three satisfying genital–orgasmic contacts per year, lots of cuddling, and some masturbation might be perfectly sufficient for quality relating.

In fact, in many cases of low sexual frequency in lesbian couples, it becomes difficult to tell the source of the couples' dissatisfaction. The cultural feminist critique of sex therapy may have some merit, after all. Perhaps we should be working harder with couples such as Mickie and Cheryl to normalize less frequent sexual contact, to expand definitions of sex to include nongenital and/or nonorgasmic arousal, or self-masturbation, as an orgasm technique. As sex therapists, we may need to do more psychoeducation to help our clients break free of unconscious heterosexist models of sexuality. This would benefit all clients, not just lesbians. For example, consider the heterosexual couple whose complaint is that the women cannot reach orgasm through intercourse. For some couples, the wisest course of treatment might be to help free them from their intercourse focus and their belief that orgasms must be produced by their partner's efforts. Perhaps as sex therapists we should be more aggressive in challenging clients' requests for change. Most of us would automatically challenge a gay client who asked to change her sexual orientation. Perhaps we should also consider questioning the request of "increase desire," or at least stop accepting this therapeutic contract at face value.

REFERENCES

Blumstein, P., & Schwartz, P. (1983). *American couples*. New York: Morrow.

Burch, B. (1987). Barriers to intimacy: Conflicts over power, dependency, and nurturing in lesbian relationships. In Boston Lesbian Psychologies Collective (Ed.), *Lesbian psychologies: Explorations and challenges* (pp. 126–142). Chicago: University of Illinois Press.

Califia, P. (1988). *Macho sluts*. Boston: Alyson.

Clunis, D. M., & Green, G. D. (1988). *Lesbian couples*. Seattle: Seal Press.

Colette (1930). *The pure and the impure*. New York: Farrar, Straus, & Giroux.

Dworkin, A. (1980). Why so-called radical men love and need pornography. In L. Lederer (Ed.), *Take back the night: Women on pornography*. New York: Morrow.

Faderman, L. (1981). *Surpassing the love of men: Romantic friendship and love between women from the Renaissance to the present*. New York: Morrow.

Faderman, L. (1991). *Odd girls and twilight lovers: A history of lesbian life in twentieth-century America*. New York: Columbia University Press.

Hurlbert, D. F., & Apt, C. (1993). Female sexuality: A comparative study between women in homosexual and heterosexual relationships. *Journal of Sex and Marital Therapy*, 19, 315–327.

Loulan, J. (1985). *Lesbian sex*. San Francisco: Spinsters Ink.

McWhirter, D., & Mattison, A. (1984). *The male couple*. Englewood Cliffs, NJ: Prentice-Hall.

Nichols, M. (1987). Lesbian sexuality: Issues and developing theory. In Boston Lesbian Psychologies Collective (Ed.), *Lesbian psychologies: Explorations and challenges* (pp. 97–125). Chicago: University of Illinois Press.

Nichols, M. (1988). Low sex desire in lesbian couples. In S. R. Leiblum & R. C. Rosen (Eds.), *Sexual desire disorders* (pp. 387–411). New York: Guilford Press.

Tripp, C. (1975). *The homosexual matrix*. New York: McGraw-Hill.

10

Sexless Marriages and Sex Therapy: The Many Factors in Sexual Avoidance

DOMEENA C. RENSHAW

INTRODUCTION

Many couples perceive sexual relations as a barometer of the relationship. In this modern era of improved contraception and high-technology fertility assistance, choices about offspring have a wide range with greater human control. In today's pursuit of novelty, excellence, and achievement, coitus easily can become routinized and may reflect stasis within a coupleship or a lack of spontaneity in one or both partners. A vague personal discontent may set in with self-doubt: "Is the passion gone?" or "Am I in love?" For most couples, at times of stormy conflict there is no intercourse, simply because it is difficult to make war and love at the same time. It is a rare couple who can use intercourse to make peace. Both, or at least one after a fight, will withdraw to nurse hurt or angry feelings, feeling pain due to rejection or persistent criticism. Forget and forgive takes perspective and time to attain. For example, 3 days later a dent in the car or a forgotten laundry pickup is no longer the major crisis or personal injury that one individual felt at the earlier moment of discovery.

More persons than will admit to it use sex for bargaining. "Give to get" is a commonplace social behavior, not only at gift-giving days but in daily home and workplace negotiations. In a pair-bond relationship, coitus consciously or unconsciously may be "given" to achieve material gain, an exotic trip, a job, affection, approval, attention, touching, tenderness, tension release, cooperation, pregnancy, status, or power.

176

From the dawn of time, sexual exchange has also been used as a battleground. Dominance and control needs may take the form of crude claims of masculine superiority, provocative feminine seduction, or immovable resistance in deliberate withholding of affectionate or sexual contact. These and a variety of other dynamics are often at play in marriages in which a couple's conflicts lead to lack of sexual relations.

However, despite apparently blatant interpersonal conflicts, sexual avoidance may have more than one underlying determinant. Thus, biological factors also must be considered.

Medically, a differential diagnosis must include the following.

1. *Physical causes.* Coital pain, discomfort, or distress may occur because of illness, such as acute prostatitis, endometriosis, or vaginitis, or a lesion, such as Peyronie's disease of the penis or an abscess at the vulva. These are evident on examination and treatable. Other physical causes come from generalized illnesses resulting from energy depletion, heart failure, renal dialysis, cancer, chemotherapy, anorexia, bulimia, and so on. Hormonal imbalance, particularly (low thyroid) myxedema, pituitary problems, or low testosterone, must be ruled out, as well as, quite commonly, chemical suppression of neurohormones leading to sexual side effects caused by needed medications (antidepressants, tranquilizers, etc.), over-the-counter analgesics, antihistamines, and so forth, or acute or chronic overuse of alcohol or street drugs. Peripheral neuropathy has numerous causes and may make coitus difficult, so negative interpersonal reactions may arise. Arteriosclerosis with vascular compromise of the flow of blood to the penis may result in erectile failure or partial erections. This is not "all in your head" but due to lessened penile blood flow, which has only been measurable in recent years.

2. *Emotional causes.* In men, fear of erectile dysfunction may lead to sexual withdrawal. Sustained sexual avoidance may also be traced to intrapersonal anxiety or ignorance about sexual anatomy, responses, coital techniques, or the importance of shared intimacy. Severe inhibitions (shyness or religious orthodoxy) or experience(s) of sexual trauma, difficulty with trust, pregnancy or impregnation fears, anxiety about pain (receiving or inflicting), unresolved anger at the partner, depression, or a need for control are intervening factors in someone presenting with apparent sexual apathy. Individual therapy may be of value for self-understanding and growth.

3. *Interpersonal causes.* Unresolved conflicts often build up over months or years, so that these resentments affect what goes on in the bedroom. Communication skills can be taught and then applied in sex or marital therapy to allow each partner to develop a better understanding of the other and the ability to express thoughts, desires, needs, and

feelings openly and honestly. Such open dialogue can remove barriers to sexual relations.

4. *Stress reactions.* Environmental realities such as war, danger, pollution, illness, or death of a family member or close friend; job loss, or financial pressure may all represent severe relatively chronic external factors that can disrupt bedroom harmony. In contrast, loving, unconflicted couples frequently use sexual intimacy or affectionate togetherness as a stress reducer or a valued social support, like a safe harbor in a storm. Couples should be counseled to collaborate in order to cope with evident external stresses as these unfold in the course of therapy.

How do couples adapt to years of sexual distance? In various ways. Sometimes coital absence is accepted by a couple who constructively build togetherness in other areas of a shared activity such as a business, individual higher education, home projects, volunteer or church work, or side-by-side cycling, exercise, sports, or hobbies. Compensatory nonsexual but creative outlets (sublimation) may be sought domestically (e.g., in cooking, gardening, home construction, or art work). Accumulating a fortune may function as a shared substitute for sex by some couples who can so create a luxurious lifestyle for themselves.

For many persons, masturbation is a conflict-free form of normal sexual expression. For others it is laden with anxiety and taboo (Masters, Johnson, & Kolodny, 1986; Renshaw, 1976). These beliefs need to be discussed and respected. Information regarding the prevalence of masturbation from infancy to late age should be shared with the patient so that attitudinal changes may be encouraged. Consultation with a religious adviser can be recommended in some instances. When a sexually deprived partner, faithful to marital vows, can comfortably self-release sexual tension, dramatic change may result. The intense interdependence (therefore, resentment) may be reduced and the buildup of sexual tension lessened, freeing emotional energy for positive exchange in the relationship.

Brief sex therapy has been remarkably effective at times in reversing inhibited sexual desire, psychogenic impotence, and other sexual symptoms related to anxiety—sometimes with the concomitant use of medications and always with prior assessment to exclude underlying physical causes (Kaplan, 1987; Masters et al., 1986; Renshaw, 1988). At times, under threat of divorce, one partner will coerce the sexually apathetic partner into therapy. However, the compliant one may present with a hidden agenda: "Not even sex therapy will change me, and then you'll finally leave me alone," or "Fix him/her. I'm fine."

The alert therapist should gently confront such behavior: "It is not possible to shake sexual desire from someone like pennies from a piggybank. Each can only change oneself. Your relationship has several positives that you both value and recognize [give examples]. Mary/John realizes she/he has a quite normal sexual drive but feels lonely when he/

she masturbates. Could you hold and be close to her/him in bed? It could be a positive alternative to feeling isolated from each other."

Another issue of concern is whether "sexless" marriages are on the rise in the 1980s and 1990s, following the sexual openness and enthusiasm of the 1960s and 1970s. While this makes for a good newspaper headline, there are no credible statistics to date. An informal answer regarding how many individuals prefer to remain sexless came in early 1980 following a "Dear Abby" letter from a 50-year-old Nebraska woman who said, "I'm tired of sex, and could live without it." The subsequent deluge of 227,000 replies was divided into 114,000 who agreed with "tired" and 113,000 who did not. The large number of affirmative responses to this letter suggests that there are many persons who, by choice, prefer to control or ignore their sexual urges through abstinence and have little sexual interest or appetite. Celibacy itself is normal.

It is also clear that issues of sexual avoidance are an increasing concern in couple therapy. Results have generally been positive. Those motivated to seek sex therapy, according to one study, achieve approximately 80% symptom reversal inas few as seven in-depth weekly sessions (Renshaw, 1988). What comments do couples make after the restoration of sexual intimacy? "We just got lazy and let other things get in the way of lovemaking." "We had a baby, bought a house and he got a new job all at one time." "We knew all the techniques, but neither would make the first move after a huge fight about in-laws. Looking back it seems so insignificant an issue." "If only we had not stopped touching, even when we were tired, the whole avoidance thing wouldn't have happened."

Some case illustrations follow.

CASE I

Deb, a petite attractive redhead of 22, married for 4 years, presented for sex therapy with her 26-year-old husband, Ron, in a final attempt to salvage their marriage. Both had completed high school, and Ron worked as a train driver on a local run. Theirs was a rebound marriage for Ron. His previous fiancée, Joan, was killed in an accidental fire at work a month before the planned wedding—5 years earlier. Deb had known both Ron and Joan, as they were all raised on the same street in a rundown section of Chicago. Deb felt sorry for both. She was the third of seven children. Her alcoholic father was shot to death when she was 6 years old. Joan (an only child of elderly parents) was the only child on the street with a father at home. He was an elderly amputee and he openly welcomed Ron as a future son.

Deb went over to sympathize with Ron after the wake. He was devastated by the tragedy, and Deb was greatly impressed by his deep devotion to Joan. It was a totally new and admirable emotion for her to observe in him. They drank many cups of coffee together in the following days. He stared; she sat. Sometimes Deb patted Ron's shoulder, feeling motherly toward him although she was newly 18 and he 22. As months passed, they began to go out for an occasional beer. Deb worried that Ron was drinking too much, and told him so. He would often hold on to her, and sigh deeply on her doorstep when he took her home.

Then Ron landed his train driver's job, and Deb graduated from high school. "Let's get married next month," he said, and they did. They spent the first weekend fixing their tiny new efficiency apartment. "We were so broke we laughed. Most of our gifts were 'early garage sale,' but we worked together to clean it all up. We got some drapes from a friend's attic. I was proud of every inch of it and we were so exhausted I didn't worry that we hadn't made love. I was a virgin. I knew Ron needed a little more time to get over Joan. He cried a lot and I let him. We were on our own, I began to waitress nearby, but was looking for a secretarial job and found one. Ron also had regular hours. We saved and got a used car and felt we were on an adventure together.

"But six months went by and we had sex only once. I began to worry. I read books and tried to approach Ron but he withdrew. I could only hug him when he was half asleep. We couldn't talk about it. I got depressed and must have been mad with him but I didn't know it, yet my body did. I developed sudden episodes of gut spasms and with such rapid breathing and heartbeats I would think I was having a heart attack and almost faint. The family doctor I found said they were panic attacks and asked for my husband to come in. I had told the doctor I was worried my husband didn't love me. Ron told him he did. I think the doctor must have told him to show it more and he tried. We went bowling and joined a church. Ron would hug me and kiss me like a brother, but still did not touch me in bed.

"After two years, I told him I was going to try a separation for a few months. He was upset and asked me not to go. He agreed to counsel for five visits with a pastor, but sex didn't get better. I felt I was to blame. I then went to my sister's for two months. When I came back I had an affair with my boss, which taught me a lot about sex and lies. I got really scared when I heard he was married. I went to Ron asking to try again with lovemaking. He was willing. For a year we had sex once a week and it seemed to me we were even having fun. He had found and fixed a motorcycle. We would go riding with a cyclist group. There was beer, pot and music and we had more friends than we had before. We have never fought or yelled. We're two different types. He's quiet, I'm active. But for the last year it's back to zero sex. I have had panic attacks, use medication and twice I left him again. I have no anxiety attacks when I leave him. I really don't think he is cheating. Can a man of 26 years really be sexless? If this therapy doesn't work I want a divorce."

Therapist's Comments

Both partners were in a transitional stage of "normal" life crisis when they impulsively decided to marry. Ron was beginning his first job and had unresolved grief at the tragic sudden loss of his fiancée Joan—and of Joan's parents (his loving surrogate parents) when she died before their marriage. He never met his own father, and his mother refused to discuss her past. His twin sister left home pregnant at 17 years old, and they had had no contact since then. In contrast, Deb, was a bright young high school graduate, ready to move out and up in the world. She was compassionate, kind, caring, and trustworthy—like the sister he lost. However, she did not substitute for Joan, his beloved. In their marriage there seemed two distinct phases to consider: first respectful collaboration and stability, which was relatively asexual unless Deb seduced Ron. Then, Deb left for some months, had a secret affair, but subsequently returned. With the help of counseling there was some improvement sexually and socially during the second phase. Ron had partially resolved his grief but periodic memories inhibited his sexual desire. Distraction by longing for his lost love would cause sadness, self-pity, and turbulent distress that he had no right to be alive or that he was disloyal to have married. Over time these episodes were less frequent.

Therapeutic Issues to Be Addressed

Issues and questions that were raised for me at this point in the therapy process were as follows: (1) Why had the regression occurred 2 years ago to a second phase of asexuality for Ron? (2) Had Ron and Deb returned to the old neighborhood in an emotional, if not a physical, sense? (3) Was the "ghost" of Joan still coming between them? (4) Most important, was there some primary physical problem that might have impeded Ron's sex drive even had he married Joan?

The last question was answered first. In fact, no physical abnormality was identified after thorough physical examination and blood tests were performed. Ron's levels of testosterone, prolactin, and thyroid were quite normal. His intake of beer was not excessive, but his marijuana smoking (by admission) was about two reefers per day. I gave him a firm medical reminder that marijuana reduces efficiency and eye–hand coordination, causes increasing errors, and made him a high risk to the public as a train driver. Marijuana also lessens the sperm count. It was an easy way to endanger lives and to get fired from his very satisfying train driver's job. Ron was, of course, using marijuana as an antidepressant. We discussed safer ways to cope with the grieving process.

When I asked Ron in an individual session about his feelings toward Joan, he freely talked. There was much self-blame that was clearly irrational. There had been an unusually heavy snowstorm so Joan and several others slept over in their office. The boiler exploded and six persons in the building were burned to death. "I should have fetched her from work." How? He had no car. Cabs were not moving. Most roads were not ploughed. He began to sob. Quietly he said: "She was pregnant, we hadn't told anyone. God punished us. I should have waited till we were married." The burden of his secret must have been exceedingly heavy. In his mind Joan had died for their (especially his) sexual sin. He "should" be punished by completely turning sex off. He said he was not aware until Deb left him for the first time that sex was so important to her. When she returned he made a conscious decision that his year of emotional numbness was sufficient punishment: "So I risked coming back to life for the next two years. If it wasn't for Deb, I might have killed myself in that first week after Joan's funeral. I wished I had died in the fire too. I wanted to be with her. Seeing her parents sorrow made me feel like a monster, because now their grandchild was also dead. Deb was so fresh and energetic, she gave me a reason to live. I know she's a great person. I don't deserve her." His grieving, therefore, had been aggravated by the secret pregnancy and the enormous emotional burden of carrying this secret alone. Yet the threat of losing Deb encouraged him to respond positively.

What then had happened two years ago to reverse the temporary improvement? The answer came: "For the first time in years we went to my mother's home for Thanksgiving. I decided to visit Joan's parents. There on the mantelpiece was a huge color photo of Joan and me. They said, 'Welcome, son.' It felt like something snapped in my head. We cried together. I couldn't tell them about the pregnancy. I wanted to, but I couldn't. This is the first I've told anyone. I thought I'd gotten over it, but it all came back." In other words, the therapist's speculation was correct—the ghost of Joan was evoked by that return visit. Ron's guilt and self-blame were resurrected. Once more his sexuality was punitively submerged. When I asked Ron whether he wished to share all this with Deb, he responded: "I owe it to her. If it was clearer to me before I might have, but I just did not make all the connections. I'm not a talker. My mind gets so blurred."

In a subsequent joint session, with my support, Ron told the full story. Deb began to cry: "How can I compete with someone who is dead?

I've always worried that he looks at me and wishes I was her. If it was an affair I'd go and tell her off," she began to sob and to breathe rapidly. Anticipating a panic attack, I instructed her: "Relax, Deb. Take a deep breath in, and hold it in while I count to four. Now breathe out and hold it out, I'll count again to four. Let's repeat that breathing exercise. Now listen. The Joan episode happened before you two got together. You, Deb, are not to blame. Ron, you are not to blame for Joan's death or her nonrescue. The Lord took her. Forgiveness even of yourself is *letting go*. That means also letting go of the self-blame. It's letting go of the past. For you Deb, it means letting go of the hurt of these past years. It's letting go of the noose Ron, that you've put around your own sexuality. You wanted to kill yourself in your state of shock. Deb seemed to be an angel of mercy and saved you, although neither of you were conscious of it at the time. Both of you have said that yours was not a romantic marriage. You liked and respected each other and still do. At this crossroads tonight, how do you want to proceed?"

Both opted to follow the program. They both seemed liberated, although tense. In the next 3 weeks the couple reported having "the best sex ever" in their relationship. Deb talked of having a baby. Ron's face whitened, his eyes glazed, he became withdrawn and could not discuss it. I suggested further individual therapy for him. He declined.

Outcome and Commentary

The sexual improvement for Ron was temporary. His griefwork was obviously incomplete, but he was not ready to continue. This decision must be respected. There are limitations to the pace and the direction of therapeutic change. Each individual is different. The therapist can only stand by and offer an open door. One year after the conclusion of therapy, Deb wrote that they were separated but "closer" than ever. She was not dating anyone else. She did not mention sex. There are many kinds of love and theirs is complex, unique, and very special to both of them.

CASE 2

"Bob is just a stick-in-the-mud. He doesn't drink or dance. All he does is smoke and work. I can't go on like this. I've given up faking interest in sex as I did before. For the entire last year I just say no. I'm not interested. I want a separation. I've had a short affair with Greg, his best friend. I told him about Greg and me, but he said nothing at all. Greg is actually a wimp yet he made me feel alive again, especially when we were keeping it secret, it was sort of romantic. I'm not serious with Greg, but now I think of freedom all the time yet I'm not sure. I never really had an adolescence because Bob and I married right after high school. I want a separation, just for ninety days, to be on my own and to see if I still love Bob but mainly I want first to find someone exciting."

Darlene was slim, attractive, and 30 years old. Bob was 33 years old, athletic, quiet, and bright. They met when she was 16, working at a hamburger stand, and he was in college. After 4 years of teen dating they were engaged. Bob completed his M.B.A. and was offered an executive position. The couple agreed not to have children until they had purchased a home. Darlene found employment in a hospital doing computer billing. Bob was stable and pleased with his job. Recently he had suggested that they try to have a child because they could now sacrifice one salary. Darlene refused.

Bob wished and asked for intercourse three times a week; Darlene agreed to once weekly. When Darlene confessed to her affair with Greg, who had stayed at their home for some weeks during the process of his recent divorce, Bob replied: "I can understand Greg. Darlene's so attractive and kind. Greg was really broken up at their divorce. I might have done the same. Darlene took him dancing to cheer him up. He is a good dancer; I am not. He apologized to me. Darlene will get over it."

Therapist's Comments

This couple presented for treatment at a sex therapy clinic—each with a separate agenda. Bob desired his wife to respond more frequently to his sexual needs. Darlene came in the hope that Bob could be encouraged to participate in a "90-day separation plan," which she was unable to implement independently. She was dependent both emotionally and financially on Bob, so she was afraid to risk a permanent separation or divorce. In their discussion of this topic at home, Bob had clearly spelled out, "If you go, it's for good," with a firmness unusual for him. The fact that their bedroom for at least the past 8 months had become a sexless "avoidance game" now threatened Bob's limitless patience.

It was evident that Bob still saw Darlene as the 16-year-old girl who attracted him so strongly with her vivaciousness, energy, and apparent independence. In many ways he seemed more like an indulgent father at a carnival, going along on "just one more ride" with his cute, tireless little girl. Darlene played into this role unconsciously, naively striving always to "run away from home." Their roles were entirely complementary. His thoughtful and calm posture provided her with the stability that had been missing in her chaotic and fatherless family of origin. She provided welcome animation in his overly serious lifestyle.

Therapeutic Issues to Be Addressed

A number of therapeutic issues and questions were raised at this juncture. These were specifically as follows: (1) How severely had the previous equilibrium now been threatened? (2) Were Bob and Darlene victims of the "sexual revolution"? (3) How could sex therapy assist this now sexless marriage? These issues could only be addressed gradually, over time. At first it seemed that the answer to question (3) was a clear no. Darlene kept up with her "I want a separation" theme although she had agreed to seven counseling sessions. At first she did not want to cooperate with suggested sensual home love play in the first week. She was childlike in her insistence that she was *not* seeking (by separation) a divorce or another sexual relationship. She said she had no specific man in mind. "I want freedom and a dance partner who is not a drinker" (her alcoholic father had deserted the family when she was 3 years old). Her "teenie bopper" earnestness that she was not searching for sex was convincing. Bob said he was also not looking for a new partner. In the second week of therapy Darlene, who was a most efficient computer technician, received an unexpected $1,000 end-of-the-year bonus. Bob always handled all finances. This check, however, she said was *hers*. This event signaled an end to the previous equilibrium. Darlene did not want to "mess up our investment plans, I'll still give him my paycheck as always. But before I decide to have a baby, I've got to get this [adolescent wild oats?] out of my system. All I want is freedom for three months." She was unyielding.

Bob sighed, shook his head, and turned to me. I responded: "What kind of a contract can you two come up with?" There was a change from his previous: "If you go, you go for good." Instead, Bob took a long time, then replied: "We can both date. Take what you need from the house and we'll meet here in the clinic three months from today." Darlene, wide-eyed, could not at first believe her ears. Then she stood up, "You can finish up here. I'll pack and be gone when you get home." Bob put his head down on the desk to cover his tears. "I could easily get drunk, but I have too much work to waste time feeling sorry for myself. I'll be alright, but will she? It's a jungle out there."

In addressing the effects of the "sexual revolution," it appeared that Darlene was influenced by seeing herself as left out of the glamour and romance of the "dating scene." She called the clinic 10 days later, stating, "Bob won't take my calls at the office. The answering machine at home is on day and night. Please ask him to call me." Bob declined to call but did agree to have a special therapy session with Darlene within a week. The resulting meeting was reminiscent of a scene from a television soap opera. Darlene apologized and pleaded to return. Bob shook his head unsmilingly: "I'm having too good a time. I've been asked out

almost every night since you left. I want to abide by the ninety-day deal."
Darlene told him she felt so bad staying at her hotel room that she had
bolted the door and refused to go dancing with her divorced girlfriend:
"All those long evenings after work, no housework, I really had time to
think. Californians go to a guru to teach them meditation. I thought things
out on my own. I didn't even watch television. How could I have been
such a child? I was longing for you. Let's forget that I wanted a separation, please. I feel it was all a bad dream." Bob, however, refused to
compromise. Having told one person at work about their separation, he
suddenly had female attention that he had not dreamed was possible.
He insisted he wanted more freedom: "Our deal was ninety days." They
left the clinic with Darlene planning to return home, fearing that Bob
might file for divorce. He did not indicate otherwise. They had not even
discussed sex.

Outcome and Commentary

The contracted 90-day appointment at the clinic was canceled by Bob's
secretary with no message. It seemed that these two were destined to join
the growing number of divorced Americans. However, about 8 months
later, Darlene called to say she was pregnant and that both were elated.
When I asked: "What was the magic?" She replied, "We both grew up."
That was all the explanation she could provide. Were the underlying
conflicts resolved? Probably not. Bob's "tit-for-tat" singles fling had
clearly affected Darlene in that when other women found him desirable
he became valuable, not dull at all. He was no longer someone to avoid
sexually, but she had to compete with several women for restoration of
their relationship. However, while babies are not glue, they symbolize a
special pledge and commitment. The test will be whether their primary
bond can be preserved, nurtured, and sustained.

CASE 3

An enduring stereotype is that of a wife's sexual avoidance by pleading
a "365-day headache" or menstrual cramps or bleeding, tender breasts,
vaginal discharge, pregnancy, and so on. Husbands reacted (again stereo-
typically) by saintly abstinence, guilt-ridden secret masturbation, or seeking sex outside the marriage because "no man can live without frequent
sex" (until he dies at age 99)!

However, in increasing numbers, couples (at the request of the woman)
seek sex therapy within a committed relationship for the male's sexual
apathy. When a careful history is obtained it is clear that the sexual problem is deliberate withholding or elective sexual disinterest.

Heidi, age 46, was a policewoman who called for help because her 54-year-old policeman live-in lover of 3 years (Pat) was "an unaffectionate slob who cannot get it up" for the past year. When they arrived for treatment, much unfolded. Heidi was previously married for 6 years to a businessman who threatened suicide if she did not give him a divorce (his fourth). She was bereft and angry with herself for being a poor judge of character. Pat was a Vietnam veteran, much decorated, a leader in many aspects of his career but recently disabled by two hip replacements and ankle surgery, which he felt were related to his exposure to Agent Orange, which had also caused gut pathology and a colostomy. Pat still had nightmares of the war. He worked full-time but now did a dispatcher desk job which he found to be a letdown after his exciting years in the Police Drug and Alcohol Department. Both of them were recovering alcoholics, dry for a few years and in Alcoholics Anonymous. Heidi was on Dilantin (phenytoin sodium) four times a day for job-related post-head-injury seizures. In addition, she was a survivor of breast cancer (mastectomy) which she minimized as insignificant. Both were intensely involved in restoring the 100-year-old home Heidi had bought several years ago. Both cared for their several pet dogs.

Pat's sexual history revealed no problems with erections and private masturbation twice a week. I asked why he did not include Heidi. "She's had herpes and the orthopedic surgeon warned me not to get any infection; it would give me problems with my hip operation. I don't want to hurt her feelings so I take the blame and say I'm not interested. Also, she has a fierce mouth and when she starts in on me, I retreat. You cannot cuddle a pitbull terrier, doctor." Heidi's sexual history revealed that she was menopausal and had both vaginal dryness and loss of libido, which she related to her Dilantin. The sexual disinterest was her projection onto Pat. Heidi would whine, plead, and blame Pat who then would take his walker and leave the house for several hours when he could not handle the hostile demands. On his return, he would work on walls or shelves silently while Heidi ranted and wept. Intercourse to her meant he cared; she could not see the "I demand, he retreats" hot-and-cold dance of anger between them (Renshaw, 1981).

Therapist's Comments

The individual physical disabilities were major for each partner, each presenting as tough and minimizing the pain, loss of mobility, posttraumatic stress disorder, seizures, colostomy, and so on. No self-pity in either. Pat was deliberately avoiding coitus because he feared contracting herpes. Heidi had not guessed this cause, nor had Pat tried to tell her. To save her feelings he unwittingly inflamed them.

Therapeutic Issues to Be Addressed

The therapeutic issues and questions were as follows:

(1) How could Heidi and Pat be so apparently mature yet so emotionally inept at the same time? (2) How big a role was played by their many physical problems and medications?

Again the last question is most easily answered. Heidi's disabilities of seizures, mastectomy, and dry vagina were real. Her explosive temper made for a stormy home whenever "strong, silent" Pat refused to react or to have the long discussions Heidi wanted as an index that he cared. The home was in her name, yet Pat quietly poured his long hours of labor and building materials into the project as his nonverbal messages of love and commitment despite Heidi's constant threats to throw him out when he displeased her. She needed much reassurance. He was a quick learner. "Just put your arms around this little five-foot volcano Pat. You will not be burned. She will subside. She will never become extinct. Heidi is like Mount Kilawayo. Expect periodic puffs." They both laughed. Humor is a personality strength that can facilitate change and growth.

Pat's pain was countererotic. His hip and ankle joints were a definite handicap and made coitus difficult or impossible, even with Heidi on top. They learned that coital alternatives could lead to orgasms for both. The closeness was enriching for each.

Regarding question (1), bright individuals may be superb with head and/or hands yet exceedingly inept socially and/or emotionally. Feelings feel; they do not think. Yet the pathway to feelings may often be through thinking and heavy petting (cognitive-behavioral techniques). For these two bright people, years of alcohol had stunted their relationship capacities. In their newly sober years, childlike frustration/temper/fearful withdrawal hampered mutuality until in the "nurturant holding pattern" of therapy they risked change. They attained another step forward in maturity. Mutual trust was being built too, within the "secure holding" of infrequent yet long-term contact with their therapist.

Outcome and Commentary

With sex therapy intervention, Heidi's explosions lessened as the "just hold her when she flies off verbally" technique began to be effective (7 days of trial did the trick). I asked them to do their mutual body massage without words (where Heidi truly could wound Pat) but to set up their favorite music (taking turns to select their favorites). A shower together and a bedroom picnic in week 4 was a turning point for this couple, who began to have fun. Although low-grade pain was persistent for Pat, the shower, toweling, and hand massages from Heidi were luxuries that he enjoyed and reciprocated, which she appreciated. I literally coached them to verbalize this appreciation to each other. A small vibrator helped Heidi attain orgasms with Pat alongside her while she helped him with oral stimulation. Learning to communicate was a major achievement. Their swing shifts and the corrosive politics of their jobs remained, but they were now able to cope. Their closeness was reassuring and gave perspective to the daily stressors. Neither wished to marry. Pat also had a traumatic first marriage. Both came from disrupted homes without display of affection. The opted for regular monthly follow-ups. "We still need a referee."

In summary, these three case studies illustrate both the variety and the complexity of male sexual avoidance, a previously neglected reality. Some therapists, even in the late 1990s, find it difficult to believe that so many have low libido due to enduring myths of powerful never-ending male libido and "liberated" females. Hypoactive sexual desire is an equal opportunity symptom. Also worth noting is that the "alleged symptom" is actually deliberate sexual avoidance and not a symptom at all but an interpersonal manipulation within the couple's negotiation to attain some compromise and need fulfillment. Intercourse is only one of many forms of sexual expression. Those who have no alternative ways of expressing intimacy are as handicapped by sexual ignorance as is a dyslexic with a new book. Learning from the therapist to accept and enjoy other forms of sexual exchange can open up new horizons of physical and emotional intimacy (Renshaw, 1995).

REFERENCES

Kaplan, H. S. (1987). *Sexual aversion, sexual phobias and panic disorders.* New York: Brunner/Mazel.

Masters, W. H., Johnson, V. E., & Kolodny, R. C. (1986). *Sex and human loving.* Boston: Little, Brown.

Renshaw, D. C. (1976). Understanding masturbation. *Journal of School Health,* 46(2), 98–101.

Renshaw, D. C. (1981). Coping with an impotent husband. *Illinois Medical Journal,* 159(1), 29–33.

Renshaw, D. C. (1988). Profile of patients treated at Loyola Sex Clinic between 1972–1987. *Proceedings of the Institute of Medicine of Chicago,* 41(2), 46–48.

Renshaw, D. C. (1995). *Seven weeks to better sex.* New York: Random House.

PART II

Sexual Performance Problems

Despite the widespread availability of educational and self-help materials on sexuality, many individuals continue to experience problems with sexual arousal and orgasm. Among women, the most common complaints are lack of orgasm or difficulties with penetration (vaginismus and dyspareunia), whereas men complain most frequently about erectile dysfunction or orgasmic disorders (delayed or premature ejaculation). Sexual performance difficulties vary greatly in the severity or chronicity of the problem, the presence or absence of organic factors, and the relative contribution of intrapsychic or interpersonal determinants. In recent years, increased emphasis has been placed on evaluating physical or medical contributions to these disorders, particularly in the case of male erectile disorder and complaints of sexual pain in women (vaginismus and dyspareunia). On the other hand, the cases in this section also illustrate the wide variety of individual and relationship issues that are commonly associated with sexual performance difficulties in both men and women.

Several themes are apparent in the case studies in this section. First, it is clear that treatment approaches have broadened considerably since the early days of sex therapy. Medical and surgical interventions are used increasingly, either alone or in combination with conventional sex therapy approaches. The case studies by Peter J. Fagan and Lois H. Blum (Chapter 11), Raymond Rosen (Chapter 16), Leslie R. Schover (Chapter 17), provide examples of the latter trend. Second, relationship issues and couple therapy approaches continue to play a major role in many cases. Therapists currently utilize an eclectic array of interventions for dealing with couple issues and conflicts, as illustrated in the case studies by Carol K. Lassen (Chapter 13), Sandra R. Leiblum (Chapter 14), S. Michael Plant (Chapter 15), and Bernie Zilbergeld (Chapter 18). Furthermore, unconventional treatment approaches are used, at times, for overcoming long-term effects of sexual trauma or abuse. For example, Julia R. Heiman (Chapter 12) describes the use of an unusual "healing ritual" in a fascinating case of vaginismus secondary to early sexual abuse. Issues of patient motivation or resistance to change are addressed by several authors, and Lassen provides an interesting example of "couple resistance" in sex therapy. Finally, treatment outcome is often mixed, even with those problems traditionally viewed as most amenable to treatment (e.g., vaginismus and premature ejaculation).

   Taken together, these chapters provide a stimulating and informative overview of current sex therapy approaches for performance difficulties in men and women. Among the distinguished authors in this section, Heiman and Zilbergeld have written extensively on female and male sexuality, and have greatly influenced our conceptualization and treatment of sexual dysfunction. Schover is a leading contributor to the literature on chronic illness and sexuality, while Fagan and Blum, Plaut, and Lassen are highly experienced and innovative sex therapists. Each of these authors brings a distinctive theoretical and clinical style to his/her case presentations, and the discussion of issues and outcomes is insightful and provocative.

11

Issues in the Psychotherapeutic Treatment of Sexual Dysfunction following Radical Retropubic Prostatectomy

PETER J. FAGAN
LOIS H. BLUM

INTRODUCTION

The message is abroad that if one is unable to achieve an erection, assistance is not far off. According to this view, medicine and technology have essentially solved the problem of attaining an erection. Intracavernosal injections (ICI), vacuum devices (Witherington, 1991), and penile prostheses have enabled even those men with biogenic erectile dysfunction to have erections sufficient for intercourse. Researchers at Case Western Reserve University have reported that vacuum devices were effective for intercourse for 87% of the participants who had a 20% dropout during the yearlong study (Turner et al., 1991). This compares favorably to ICI (Zorgniotti & LeFleur, 1985), which had a triple dropout rate (57%) and an 84% effectiveness rate (Althof et al., 1991). For decades penile prostheses have been employed with high satisfaction by men who report both confidence in the sexual functioning and support in their sense of masculinity (Tiefer, Pedersen, & Melman, 1988).

Thus, for most men and their partners, medical and technological assistance is sufficient to restore erectile functioning, and with it the emotional realities that existed premorbidly. For this group, being able to have intercourse again revives the emotional and interpersonal potency they once enjoyed. The path of treatment has been centripetal: from the peripheral (penis/erection) to the central (brain/cognitions and emotions).

For other men and their partners, however, the problem of erectile dysfunction is not quite so amenable to this type of treatment. For a variety of psychological reasons, simply restoring erectile function is not sufficient. The meanings and values they have attributed to sexual intercourse and sexual interactions are not supported by a chemically, mechanically, or prosthetically assisted erection.

Such couples face an impasse. The culture of medical science teaches that there need be no problem. The man can have an erection and the couple can continue to have intercourse. But, somehow, "things just don't work out." Penile injections are feared or overridden by the adrenergic effects of anxiety, vacuum devices are cumbersome interruptions, and prosthesis surgery is warily postponed. The spontaneity that was an integral part of the sexual experience has been lost. Sexual estrangement occurs as the sexual interaction, which was formerly a positive experience, becomes a source of anxiety and alienation.

There is one group of men and their partners for whom this scenario may be all too real—those who have undergone a radical retropubic prostatectomy (RRP). Usually involving the removal of a malignant tumor, until recent years the surgery typically left the man unable to achieve an erection because the cavernous nerves arising from the sacral center (S_2 to S_4) and the thoracolumbar center (T_{11} to L_2) were severed to remove the mass (Bergman, Nilsson, & Petersen, 1979). In the past decade, nerve-sparing surgical techniques have greatly increased the possibility of preserving erectile functioning (Walsh, Lepor, & Eggleston, 1983). For those whose cavernous nerves are spared, erections can still occur and orgasm be achieved, although emission does not occur postsurgically due to the removal of the seminal fluid-producing prostate and the seminal vesicles. There is a period of recovery (2 months to 4 years postsurgery) during which time enhancement of erectile functioning may occur. During this interim, the man and his partner must wait upon the silent healing process to determine how much of their former sexual life will return. While the biotechnical means of attaining an erection are available, the partners may experience anxiety as they await the return of "normal" functioning.

This chapter describes the waiting and healing process of one such couple. Spared the cancer through surgery, they expected medical science to make possible the resumption of the rich sexual life they had enjoyed the previous 33 years of their marriage. Presurgically, they expected that if the nerves could not be spared, there were always the injections, pump, or even implants. Postsurgically, what they experienced were the limits of technology and their own emotional difficulties in the "failure" of their sexual life together as they attempted to employ this new technology.

The purpose of this chapter is not to describe any special skills on the therapist's part but to elaborate the variety of intrapsychic and interpersonal issues that may arise as a psychologically healthy and sexually alive couple is confronted with a presumptively iatrogenic erectile dysfunction. While the specific therapeutic interventions described may be of some importance, it is the issues of the individual and couple dynamics that are of primary interest.

As the editors of this volume have written, given all the advances in the medical and technological treatment of biogenic erectile dysfunction, basic couple therapy must still occur (Leiblum & Rosen, 1991).

OVERVIEW OF CASE

Mr. and Mrs. Smith, ages 57 and 53, respectively, are an upper-middle-class couple who had been married for 33 years. They enjoyed a full sexual life together with no previous sexual dysfunction history. One and a half years prior to evaluation, Mr. Smith underwent a radical prostatectomy for the removal of a malignant tumor. No specific sexual counseling was offered to the couple presurgically. They were advised of and agreed to the surgical priorities: (1) remove the cancerous tissue, (2) preserve bladder control, and (3) preserve sexual function. Following the surgery, Mr. Smith was both incontinent and unable to achieve an erection. The couple reported that initially they were discouraged from seeking psychological assistance, as the urology team judged that the problem was primarily physiological. Ultimately the couple was referred for psychological help by the Women's Health Clinic where Mrs. Smith sought help.

During the initial evaluation, the couple's chief complaints were erectile dysfunction and an emotionally painful sexual estrangement, which had persisted for the past year. Mr. Smith reported decreased sexual desire and general difficulties with intimacy between his wife and himself. He stated, "I don't expect that this clinic will be able to help us very much." Mrs. Smith complained, "I was given the erroneous impression that potency would not be lost and that no nerves would be cut, but my husband has no potency. The pump has not been effective. Dr. X gave us injections and they did not work either. I am extremely upset and disappointed because of this unanticipated issue. I think I was misled a good deal. I am personally disinterested in sex, totally turned off." Aside from the sexual estrangement, the couple appeared to have a stable, loving, and committed marriage.

The Smiths were in couple therapy for 19 weekly sessions over 6 months during which the following issues were addressed:

1. The unexpected, unanticipated loss of their sex life.
2. Mrs. Smith's hurt and anger at the loss of her husband's ability to continue to be her lover, and presumptively her displacement of this anger onto the medical profession.
3. Mr. Smith's profound embarrassment at his incontinence and its integration into their sexual life.
4. Sexual rapprochement after the cessation of all sexual contact for the past year.
5. Integration of vacuum pumps and ICI into their lovemaking.
6. Mrs. Smith's sexual performance anxiety and her exaggerated sense of responsibility and control.
7. Learning to trust their own abilities to have a sexual relationship that was emotionally similar to what they had experienced presurgically.

The outcome of therapy was the reestablishment of the erotic pleasuring and ICI-assisted intercourse with mutual orgasm during intercourse at a one-to-two-times-a-week frequency consistent with their presurgical pattern. Communication level of the couple was good at onset; the therapy allowed them to address the issues listed above.

INITIAL EVALUATION OF THE COUPLE

A thorough evaluation is necessary to obtain knowledge sufficient to generate hypotheses about the factors that may cause sexual dysfunction as well as those that may be sustaining it. A comprehensive assessment provides data on which treatment approaches can be chosen and a prognosis can be made. It is important for the therapist to have a realistic expectation of treatment outcomes so that all involved in the process can give an informed consent to the effort and expense required, as well as the limitations of the intended therapy.

Evaluation Procedure

The setting in which this case report occurred is the Sexual Behaviors Consultation Unit, an outpatient unit in the Department of Psychiatry and Behavioral Sciences of the Johns Hopkins School of Medicine. The evaluation of couples is initiated with psychiatric residents interviewing the couple to assess how they interact and how they attribute causality to the sexual dysfunction. Following this couple interview, the residents (usually matching genders to partners) obtain a comprehensive psychiatric history and mental status examination in separate interviews. The couple is then interviewed by the supervising psychiatrist or psychologist.

Couples with sexual dysfunction are asked to complete the following psychological inventories: Dyadic Adjustment Scale (DAS; Spanier, 1976, 1979), the NEO Personality Inventory—Revised (NEO-PI-R; Costa & McCrae, 1992), the Golombok–Rust Inventory of Sexual Satisfaction (GRISS; Rust & Golombok, 1986), and the Michigan Alcohol Screening Test (MAST; Selzer, 1971).

There is a follow-up session about 1 week later in which the results of the evaluation, including the psychological inventories, are reviewed with the couples and the recommendations for sexual–marital therapy are given. Concerning the Smiths, the senior author (PJF) was the therapist at the follow-up session and provided the therapy, although he was not involved in the initial evaluation.

Mr. Smith's History

Mr. Smith came from a lower-middle-class merchant family. Immigrants from eastern Europe, his parents worked in the family retail store and lived into their eighth and ninth decades. His father had prostatic cancer; his mother a variety of cardiovascular diseases. There were two other siblings: an older sister who had manic depressive illness and committed suicide 20 years prior and a younger sister with no remarkable medical, psychiatric, or legal history and with whom Mr. Smith enjoyed a good relationship. The only other significant family history note was the suicide of a maternal aunt in years past.

Having achieved normal developmental milestones with no remarkable behavioral problems or unusual illnesses, Mr. Smith stated that he had been a moderately active, independent boy who did well in school and enjoyed his peers. After graduating from college, he enrolled in professional school and has worked in that profession continuously since then.

Mr. Smith used to smoke tobacco but quit years ago. He drank rarely but not to intoxication.

Mr. Smith's cancer was in remission since the RRP, and repeated prostate-specific antigen values had indicated no recurrence of the cancer. In addition to the prostatectomy, Mr. Smith's medical history was significant for borderline hypertension (130/90) for which he had been taking a low dose of ramapril for the past year. He also suffered from mild sleep apnea, which was exacerbated when his weight exceeded 195 pounds. He exercised regularly to keep his weight at or below 190 pounds.

On mental status examination, Mr. Smith was dressed in suit and tie and appeared relaxed, calm, and sincere. He became tearful once when discussing his sexual difficulties and their effects on his marital relationship. However, he described his mood as "good" and stated, "I don't expect that this clinic will be able to help us very much." His mental status was otherwise unremarkable. He was given a diagnosis of male erectile disorder of probable biogenic origin.

Mrs. Smith's History

Mrs. Smith's father was still alive but suffering from a dementia at age 91. Mrs. Smith's deceased (at age 75) mother was an insulin-dependent diabetic as long as Mrs. Smith could remember. As a young girl she administered the injections to her mother and recalled feeling responsible for her health and making efforts to spare her stresses and worries. The mother was in her late 40s (Mrs. Smith was not exact) when Mrs. Smith was born.

Other than growing up with an elderly and chronically ill mother, Mrs. Smith's youth was unremarkable for developmental, behavioral, or medical problems. She was a good student and enjoyed the company of friends. She graduated with a bachelor's degree and worked full-time for the past 20 years in a human services agency, in which she held several leadership positions. Work outside the home brought her a great deal of personal satisfaction.

Mrs. Smith's medical history was significant for ulcerative colitis and a sleep disorder for the past 10 years for which she took triazolam 0.125 mg at bedtime two to three times a week.

On interview, Mrs. Smith was conservatively dressed. She was an attractive woman who was quite forthcoming about how distressed she was about the couple's sexual problem. There were no neurovegetative symptoms other than her chronic sleep difficulties. She was given a diagnosis of adjustment disorder with mixed emotional features and sleep disorder on Axis III.

Marital History and Presenting Problem

The Smiths met as young teenagers and dated for 4 years before marrying. First intercourse for both occurred shortly before they were married. There was no history of sexual dysfunction. Intercourse occurred two to three times a week. While each initiated sex in the early years of marriage, since then Mrs. Smith usually took the sexual initiative. Mutual oral sex was integrated into the couple's foreplay. Describing their sexual life prior to the surgery, Mrs. Smith stated, "[Sex was] very easy, never any problems, no issues about it. I didn't know how lucky we were."

Over the years the marital relationship was reported to be satisfying and stable until the recent distress attributed to the sexual problems. The only previous psychological treatment occurred about 8 years earlier when they were in family therapy briefly (three sessions) adjunctive to a son's depression. Mr. and Mrs. Smith felt this treatment was beneficial.

Following the RRP, the couple did not attempt to be sexually intimate with each other for 6 weeks to allow healing from the surgery. In the months that followed they attempted to use both the vacuum device and penile injections about once a month, and on two occasions they had intercourse with ICI. Two weeks before the evaluation they had had intercourse using both the pump and injections with papaverine and phentolamine. However, the sex was not satisfying to them. While they pointed to the mechanical and chemical aids as the culprits behind the demise of their sexual satisfaction, the couple was unable to identify what was wrong with the assisted intercourse other than "something was missing" from the sexual life they had enjoyed for the past three decades. Mr. Smith felt sex was like "suiting up" and "lacked spontaneity." He avoided situations that might lead to sex, because "it will ultimately lead to a situation that is going to be disappointing." Mr. Smith believed that his wife was far more disappointed than himself with the erectile problems. While he felt sad about the loss, he was more concerned about his decreased desire for sex. He denied masturbating prior to surgery. Now he would do so rarely, with some partial erection resulting, but not sufficient for vaginal penetration. His motivation for masturbation seemed more to test his ability to achieve erection than driven by sexual urges.

For Mrs. Smith, sex was now "so much work" with "plastic, injections, lubricant which smells to high heaven, and rubber bands." She did not want to think about their marriage without a good sexual life, but separation was not an option. She stated plaintively, "I'm so young ... [not to have sex]."

Mr. Smith's incontinence was a major problem. It consisted of a fairly constant urinary leak with occasional spurts and necessitated wearing an absorbent pad at all times (six to seven changes a day) and also at night. He expressed reluctance at having his wife touch his penis as he was highly embarrassed at the urination. The result was that while they continued to sleep together and cuddle, there was no caressing of the breasts or genitals unless the couple was attempting intercourse with the vacuum pump or injections.

Psychological Inventories

On the NEO-PI-R (Table 11.1) Mr. Smith described himself as a calm, secure man for whom displays of anger were rare. He enjoyed social interactions and experienced a full range of enthusiasm and pleasure. He was sensitive to beauty and open to his feelings and the feelings of others. A tolerant man, he tended to seek compromise and was sensitive to the needs of others. He was also dutiful and conscientious.

Mrs. Smith's NEO-PI-R (Table 11.1) suggested a woman who while generally not prone to negative affect and usually secure under stress, was likely to experience episodes of angry hostility. She was an assertive, active woman who preferred a certain distance and formality with associates. Mrs. Smith had a high degree of esthetic appreciation and openness to her feelings and the feelings of others. A pragmatic woman, she tended to look out for her interests and was not shy in speaking about her achievements. Mrs. Smith had a high appreciation of her personal and professional competence, but there were some areas in which she felt she was exempt from some of the general norms of conduct. She was a diligent worker but not likely to strive for higher career positions.

The NEO-PI-R profiles suggested a generally positive prognosis for sexual–marital therapy. Mr. and Mrs. Smith were trusting and open to their own and each other's feelings and emotions. Neither had such a high degree of neurotic affect that the pace of couple therapy and the sharing of the therapist's attention would pose a narcissistic challenge. They were a conscientious couple for whom behavioral assignments would be diligently attempted. Mrs. Smith's anger and Mr. Smith's low (repressed?) anger would be a discrepancy in the couple's style that would have to be acknowledged and dealt with in the therapy. Mrs. Smith's low openness to ideas would demand a pragmatic approach to the sexual problem and the issues involved. Achieving rapid results would be important for her.

The GRISS combined profile for Mr. and Mrs. Smith is seen in Figure 11.1. With the cutoff of 5 or above indicating a problem area, Mr. Smith's GRISS scales indicated that impotency, male avoidance, and sexual infrequency were problems for him. Mrs. Smith's GRISS scales indicated that infrequency and nonsensuality (giving and receiving sensual pleasure) were areas of distress for her. Thus the GRISS profile con-

TABLE II.I. NEO-PI-R *T*-Scores for Mr. and Mrs. Smith

Factor (facets)	Mr. Smith	Mrs. Smith
Neuroticism	39	47
Anxiety	45	53
Angry Hostility	27	61
Depression	43	41
Self-consciousness	44	46
Impulsiveness	54	47
Vulnerability	36	35
Extraversion	66	55
Warmth	54	43
Gregariousness	74	56
Assertiveness	60	58
Activity	52	66
Excitement Seeking	58	41
Positive Emotions	67	57
Openness	59	59
Fantasy	40	54
Aesthetics	75	63
Feelings	58	58
Actions	38	45
Ideas	51	25
Values	58	66
Agreeableness	52	37
Trust	49	50
Straightforwardness	58	36
Altruism	63	39
Compliance	59	52
Modesty	40	27
Tender-mindedness	45	44
Conscientiousness	56	52
Competence	53	67
Order	49	54
Dutifulness	61	34
Achievement Striving	51	36
Self-discipline	55	64
Deliberation	53	52

firmed the data provided by the Smiths in their interviews. It also provided a baseline for charting the outcome of therapy.

The DAS assesses the relative presence or absence of marital conflict in areas such as marital satisfaction, cohesion, consensus, and affect expression. The DAS indicated a marriage that was satisfying to both, with Mrs. Smith's total score being 120 (mean = 114, standard deviation = 18) and Mr. Smith's a very high 142.

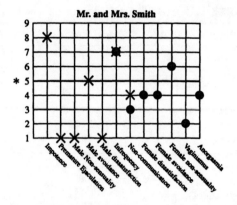

FIGURE 11.1. GRISS scales for Mr. and Mrs. Smith at initial evaluation.

The MAST is a screening instrument for alcohol abuse and dependence. A score greater than 6 indicates possible present or past alcohol abuse. Both Mr. and Mrs. Smith scored in the nonalcoholic range.

TREATMENT GOALS AND PROGNOSIS

The goal in the psychological treatment of primarily biogenic sexual dysfunction was to maximize postsurgical sexual function. For many couples this entails expanding their typical (and perhaps routinized premorbid) sexual script. In the main, this was the goal of treatment for Mr. and Mrs. Smith. Their past sexual life had not included pumps, injections, or even recalling a failure now and then to give them the experience of some minor sexual problems as normal. If sex were to be a part of their marriage in the future, these realities would have to be integrated into their sexual life together.

There were some biogenic factors in Mr. Smith's history that may have played a minor role in retarding the postsurgical return of erectile functioning. His antihypertensive medication, ramapril, is an angiotensin converting enzyme (ACE) inhibitor and as such one of the more benign antihypertensives regarding sexual dysfunction (Croog, Levine, Sudilovsky, Baumer, & Cleve, 1988; Ohman & Karlberg, 1984). Mr. Smith was on a low dosage and it was unlikely that there were negative sexual side effects. This would remain a hypothesis, however, because a drug holiday was never attempted.

The second possible biogenic factor for decreased return of function is the sleep apnea, which Mr. Smith experienced for the past 3½ years when he gains weight. Although the causality has not been established, an association has been reported between erectile dysfunction and sleep apnea (Quittell, Schidlow, & Goldberg, 1990). The oxygenation of corpus cavernosum has been the focus of recent studies of nitric oxide (Azadzoi et al., 1992; Burnett, Lowenstein, Bredt, Chang, & Snyder, 1992). It can be hypothesized that in men with chronic sleep apnea there may be negative effects on the cavernosal tissue secondary to disrupted rapid-eye-movement stages and normal nocturnal erections (periods of oxidation of penile tissue). Fortunately, Mr. Smith was below the weight at which he was likely to experience significant sleep apnea and so the possible effects on sexual function were remote.

Mrs. Smith was clearly the more distressed of the two. She was the initiator of sex in the marriage and now that the sex was "failing" in some sense she was experiencing a disproportionate feeling of responsibility for the failure. While it was his prostatectomy and his penis, it was her intercourse in which there was "something missing." Success of treatment lay in being able to assist the couple to identify the missing "something" and then to reintegrate this into their sexual life together.

Finally, although it was only three sessions, the Smiths had had a positive experience in family therapy. Many referrals from urology, for a variety of unspecified reasons, do not make a successful transition to mental health professionals (Schoenberg, Zarins, & Segraves, 1982). This couple seemed to be able to use cognitive-behavioral suggestions to profit from psychological interventions.

COURSE OF PSYCHOTHERAPY TREATMENT

To establish a therapeutic alliance marked by candor and collaboration, it is helpful to review with couples the psychological inventories that are completed during assessment. The profiles are presented as beginning points of discussion rather than indisputable scientific realities. Presented in this way, the inventory data usually generate more self-revelation and provide constructs for understanding both behavior and personality traits.

The Smiths took two sessions to review the inventories. Discussion of the NEO-PI-R was helpful in establishing good rapport. This was a particularly sensitive issue considering his low expectations of help and her anger at previous health professionals. In the discussion of their personality traits, Mr. and Mrs. Smith provided concrete examples of the salient traits while the interpretation of scales supported their budding sense of my (PJF) competency to handle their sexual problems and to provide a holding environment for their relationship.

At the onset, Mr. Smith expressed feelings of great embarrassment because of his incontinence. He had not given this aspect of the postsurgical deficits much thought as his greatest concern at the time had been his fear of the cancer and whether it could be successfully excised. Now he felt he had regressed to infancy as he was forced to wear a "diaper."

My first suggestion was to begin what is known as sensate focus exercises, starting with pleasure giving "touching exercises." Genital and breast areas were off limits in the first week. In these exercises Mrs. Smith reported that she had felt sensual and erotic pleasure for the first time since the surgery. Mr. Smith, on the other hand, was still extremely concerned about his possible incontinence during their lovemaking and his lack of sexual arousal. His anxiety was keeping him from feeling sensations of pleasure and tendering.

However, within the next few weeks, the couple began to try their own innovative approaches, with encouragement from me. In the bathtub together body touching took away the stigma Mr. Smith felt about the possibility of his wife coming in contact with any drops of his urine.

As Mrs. Smith took more control of their lovemaking, she felt more comfortable, conscious that this was the role she had held before and enjoyed. This aspect of her personality had been acknowledged earlier in their sessions. Her anger began to subside and she saw there was hope for a sexual life between them, even if somewhat compromised. Correspondingly, Mr. Smith was more able to speak openly of his own sense of loss and of his fears when he learned he had cancer and then of his subsequent impotency.

Having been able to speak openly of his own worse fears, the couple was able to move on and more fully embrace the range of possible solutions to their sexual problems, now being viewed in a different light. They had come up from the impact of cancer, even of death. Mrs. Smith could see her characteristic anger, a familiar emotion for her, and was able to deal with it in her familiar manner, by taking control of the situation. A solution, even if a mechanical one, began to seem like an acceptable possibility.

The couple took the vacuum pump from the box in which they had hidden it away and began to experiment with it. The couple took my suggestions seriously and generally attempted them. I stressed, using the couple's own words, the idea that the goal was not orgasm but the reestablishment of satisfying sexual intimacy. Mr. and Mrs. Smith were able to see that that was what they both missed and needed.

Mr. Smith slowly began to lose his sensitivity and embarrassment at his possible incontinence, feelings that had kept him from allowing his wife to fondle his penis. Mrs. Smith, who since childhood had seen herself as the goal-oriented caregiver who was responsible for her diabetic mother's insulin therapy as well as her emotional well-being, now was struggling with her need to be "successful" in this new phase of her marriage. Her performance demands that her husband remain tumescent and that she be orgasmic were openly discussed in the sessions. When Mrs. Smith recognized that even with the pump, tumescence was not guaranteed, her confidence flagged and her anxiety escalated. The couple further experimented using the pump as well as the ICI concurrently.

Now feeling more comfortable with the goals as they themselves had defined them, Mr. Smith was able to return to some extent to the role of lover as he had been perceived before his surgery. Oral stimulation had been an integral part of their lovemaking for many years. He now returned to this and they both found it familiar and satisfying.

When a sexual encounter was something less than perfection, Mrs. Smith's spirits fell. It was difficult for her to understand because she had always seen herself as the responsible one, the one in control. Then in one important session (14) Mrs. Smith connected her sense of responsibility with the "mothering" she had exercised over her own insulin-dependent mother. The fact that needles were involved both then and now further enriched her ability to identify the similar emotions toward her husband. During this same session, Mrs. Smith said that she had allowed a colitis condition to persist for 5 weeks. In effect, her mothering was directed to the "illness" of the other at the expense of caring for herself. Finally, as the sessions continued and the patterns emerged, Mrs. Smith was able to surrender some of this exaggerated responsibility. Together they dealt with the mechanical aids available to them, eventually giving up the pump and using only the ICI. Injections, frightening and therefore repugnant to Mrs. Smith at the beginning of treatment, became a familiar "friend" to her.

The couple began to gain their sense of humor, which had carried them through hard times throughout their lives. When, at a time of lovemaking, urine squirted in Mrs. Smith's face, this ultimate of embarrassments was dealt with with humor and mutual kindness.

Finally, the couple brought into the sessions other minor family problems. They no longer had the need or desire to talk of the mechanics of their encounters. They had regained the intimacy and wanted it for their own. As their therapist, I recognized that they had achieved the goals they had set for themselves at the beginning of therapy.

RETROSPECT

The Smiths began therapy faced with significant problems. In their 50s, they had been given the diagnosis of prostate cancer that had taken Mr. Smith's father's life. Following his surgery, Mr. Smith had become incontinent, a condition which, although not life-threatening, was a constant irritant and a threat to his feeling of security, socially and sexually. In addition, sexual intercourse, one of the great pleasures in the couple's life, had become a cumbersome, anxiety-provoking encounter with vacuum devices and needles. They were sexually estranged. Their condition was similar to many couples referred for sexual problems following cancer treatment (Schover, Evans, & von Eschenbach, 1987).

One of the tasks of the therapist is to examine the strengths and weakness of the couple and to judge what type and how much intervention is most likely to be helpful. What defenses have worked for them in the past? How have they dealt with narcissistic injuries? How have they handled loss?

The Smiths had processed their life together in a practical, forthright way. Delving into unconscious conflicts had not been foremost in their lives, and they did not seek this now. What they desired was a restored sexual intimacy. I decided that the interventions would be limited to the emotions and cognitions that were elicited in the course of sensate focus therapy. I would not attempt to explore issues classically associated with a more analytically informed psychotherapy.

Paradoxically, in addition to the gradual desensitization to the use of the vacuum pump and the ICI, the single most significant curative factor was the connection of Mrs. Smith's relationship to caring for her mother's illness (and her denial of her own). This interweaving of personal history, interpersonal homeostasis (Mr. Smith not wanting to hear about illness), and sexual problems gave the Smiths the understanding necessary to achieve confidence about future sexual expression. Their future sexual expressions may not be without problems, but they would be faced by the Smiths with emotional and interpersonal skills that would help them work through, not withdraw from, these issues.

The Smiths had gotten from therapy what they had sought: restored sexual intimacy. As is seen in their GRISS pre- and posttreatment profiles (Figure 11.2), all scales (with the exception of Mr. Smith's Infrequency scale), were in the unproblematic range (1–4). This contrasts with the five scales in which the Smiths indicated sexual problems 6 months earlier (Figure 11.1).

Perhaps the most compelling lesson I learned during this course of therapy was the reminder that ostensibly biogenic sexual dysfunctions are not without psychological and interpersonal effects. Regardless of

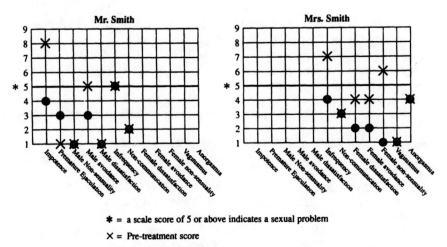

FIGURE 11.2. Pre- and posttreatment GRISS scales for Mr. and Mrs. Smith.

the progress of biomedical technology in the area of erectile dysfunction, sexual expression will be incomplete for most couples unless it includes a sense of affective pleasuring, mutuality, and intimacy. These realities cannot be given by technology alone. They must be achieved in the crucible of the sexual relationship.

REFERENCES

Althof, S. E., Turner, L. A., Levine, S. B., Risen, C. B., Bodner, D., Kursh, E. D., & Resnick, M. I. (1991). Sexual, psychological and marital impact of self-injection of papaverine and phentolamine: A long-term prospective study. *Journal of Sex and Marital Therapy, 17*, 101–112.

Azadzoi, K. M., Kim, N., Brown, M. L., Goldstein, I., Cohen, R. A., & Saenz de Tejada, I. (1992). Endothelium-derived nitric oxide and cyclooxygenase products modulate corpus cavernosum smooth muscle tone. *Journal of Urology, 147*, 220–225.

Bergman, B., Nilsson, S., & Petersen, I. (1979). The effect on erection and orgasm of cystectomy, prostatectomy, and vesiculectomy for cancer of the bladder: A clinical and electromyographic study. *British Journal of Urology, 51*, 114–120.

Burnett, A. L., Lowenstein, C. J., Bredt, D. S., Chang, T. S., & Snyder, S. H. (1992). Nitric oxide: A physiologic mediator of penile erection. *Science, 257*, 401–403.

Costa, P. T., Jr., & McCrae, E. R. (1992). *The Revised NEO Personality In-*

ventory (NEO-PI-R) and NEO Five-Factor Inventory (NEO-FFI) Professional Manual. Odessa, FL: Psychological Assessment Resources.

Croog, S., Levine, S., Sudilovsky, A., Baumer, R. M., & Cleve, J. (1988). Sexual symptoms in hypertensive patients: A clinical trial of antihypertensive medications. *Archives of Internal Medicine, 148,* 788–794.

Leiblum, S. R., & Rosen, R. C. (1991). Couples therapy for erectile disorders: Conceptual and clinical considerations. *Journal of Sex and Marital Therapy, 17,* 147–159.

Ohman, K. P., & Karlberg, F. E. (1984). Enalapril and atenolol in primary hypertension. *Scandinavian Journal of Urology and Nephrology, 79*(Suppl.), 93–97.

Quittell, L. M., Schidlow, D. V., & Goldberg, R. (1990). Obstructive sleep apnea's effects on sexuality. *Medical Aspects of Human Sexuality, 24,* 38–43.

Rust, J., & Golombok, S. (1986). *The Golombok–Rust Inventory of Sexual Satisfaction (GRISS).* Odessa, FL: Psychological Assessment Resources.

Schoenberg, H. W., Zarins, C. K., & Segraves, R. T. (1982). Analysis of 122 unselected impotent men subjected to multidisciplinary evaluation. *Journal of Urology, 127,* 445–447.

Schover, L. R., Evans, R. B., & von Eschenbach, A. C. (1987). Sexual rehabilitation in a cancer center: Diagnosis and outcome in 384 consultations. *Archives of Sexual Behavior, 16,* 445–461.

Selzer, M. L. (1971). The Michigan Alcohol Screening Test: The quest for a new diagnostic instrument. *American Journal of Psychiatry, 127,* 1653–1658.

Spanier, G. B. (1976). Measuring dyadic adjustment: New scales for assessing the quality of marriage and similar dyads. *Journal of Marriage and the Family, 38,* 15–28.

Spanier, G. B. (1979). The measurement of marital quality. *Journal of Sex and Marital Therapy, 5,* 288–300.

Tiefer, L., Pedersen, B., & Melman, A. (1988). Psychosocial follow-up of penile prosthesis implant patients and partners. *Journal of Sex and Marital Therapy, 14,* 184–201.

Turner, L. A., Althof, S. E., Levine, S. B., Bodner, D. R., Kursh, E. D., & Resnick, M. I. (1991). External vacuum devices in the treatment of erectile dysfunction: A one-year study of sexual and psychosocial impact. *Journal of Sex and Marital Therapy, 17,* 81–93.

Walsh, P. C., Lepor, H., & Eggleston, J. C. (1983). Radical prostatectomy with preservation of sexual function: Anatomical and pathological considerations. *Prostate, 4,* 473–485.

Witherington, R. (1991). Vacuum devices for the impotent. *Journal of Sex and Marital Therapy, 17,* 69–80.

Zorgniotti, A. W., & LeFleur, R. S. (1985). Auto-injection of the corpus cavernosum with a vasoactive drug combination for vasculogenic impotence. *Journal of Urology, 133,* 39–41.

12

Genital Pain in the Context of Chronic Pain and an Incest History

JULIA R. HEIMAN

INTRODUCTION

Numerous studies have found a higher incidence of adult physical and psychological complaints associated with a history of childhood incest (Russell, 1986; Wyatt & Powell, 1988). These results have not necessarily led to more clearly articulated treatment approaches, often because the clinical picture is complex and treatment more protracted. In the therapy outcome literature for incest survivors, there has been only one controlled study demonstrating effectiveness (Alexander, Neimeyer, Follette, Moore, & Harter, 1989), although there are numerous self-help books available to treat sexual abuse (Bass & Davis, 1988; Blume, 1990; Lew, 1990). In addition, a set of self-help texts has appeared that focus on sexuality issues in the lives of adults who have experienced incest (Graber, 1990; Maltz, 1991; Maltz & Holman, 1987; Westerlund, 1992).

At this point in our work on the sexual ramifications of incest, most clinicians are struggling to find an integrated, multifaceted approach that addresses the long-term sequellae of incest. Exactly what was caused by the incest always remains a question. In an attempt to understand current suffering, there may be a tendency to overattribute specific problems to the effects of sexual trauma. Exposing and addressing the trauma may then take on disproportionate importance in the healing process, as these activities may mark only the beginning stages of complete recovery.

209

Sexual issues can be particularly vexing to address for clients and therapists alike. The heart of the incest experience is sexual activity and the problems of differentiating sexual abuse from sexuality can be discouragingly incomplete. In addition, sexuality is usually not the only problem, as in the case I discuss here, where chronic pain and depressive symptoms were also present throughout the therapy.

Developmental, systemic, and cognitive-behavioral frameworks are valuable theoretical bases to draw from in treating these conditions. The key developmental issue is the child's age at which the incest occurred, reflecting the availability of language and degree of physical maturation. The systemic issues include the family of origin and the patient's past and current patterns of relating around territoriality, ranking order, and attachment interactions (Verhulst & Heiman, 1988). The cognitive-behavioral perspective is used to reformulate ways of thinking about self and sex (Westerlund, 1992). In addition, trance work can be employed in solving the problems that seem most recalcitrant (Dolan, 1991).

The case presented, Mary and Paul, was chosen because it was challenging, rather complex, yet had a positive though imperfect outcome, both by the therapist's and the couple's account. The case also illustrated the limits of our principles for working with trauma individuals and couples. Little has been written about couple therapy with survivors and their husbands, though Bolen's (1993) recent work is an interesting exception. It is hoped that the present case will further expand the approaches one might take within this therapeutic context.

An important ingredient in this chapter is that I have asked the couple to review it and to check for the adequacy of the confidentiality protection, errors in content, and any misrepresentation of their perspective. Their willingness and interest in doing this are greatly appreciated. I originally asked their permission to discuss their case as part of an increasing belief that this collaborative effort is important for clients, especially sexually abused clients, and because I planned to include specific details of the treatment rather than just a summary. Consent for using written treatment material is not new, of course. Inviting additional editorial input is less common, however, and has been most vocally promoted in recent years by feminist clinicians and researchers.

BACKGROUND

Mary was referred to the Reproductive and Sexual Medicine Clinic by a colleague at the Pain Clinic; both clinics were within the University of Washington's Medical School. At the time of her referral in 1990, Mary was 44, married to her second husband Paul, 63, for 10 years. Mary had no children. Trained as a lawyer, she stopped working due to pain about 2 years prior to entering treatment and was on long-term disability. She was interested and usually able to be involved in church activities, as well as limited activities around the house, some writing, and fishing with her husband.

Paul had also been married once before and had two children. His daughter developed brain cancer and died in her 20s after years of illness. His wife committed suicide 6 years after their daughter's death, in large part, according to Paul, because she never recovered from this loss. Paul retired from his profession about 1 year after Mary stopped working. He took early retirement to be able to spend more time in personal interests and outside activities with his wife.

Medical and Psychiatric History

Mary had an extensive history of pain and depression. She reported being depressed for much of her life, with a prolonged adolescent depression and suicide attempt at age 18. In addition, she had a history of irritable bowel syndrome, ulcers, and migraine headaches. She had a hysterectomy at 35, due to painful menstrual periods. She also suffered from chronic interscapular, neck, and myofacial pain and was diagnosed by her physician with fibromyalgia during the course of our treatment. The head, neck, and facial pain had begun shortly after the separation (initiated by her) from her first husband. Eight years later, an MRI (magnetic resonance imaging) revealed C_5–C_6 herniation and she underwent C_5–C_6 fusion 2 years prior to our therapy. The surgery did not improve her pain and, in fact, when I first saw her, interventions with her pain symptoms had failed or only temporarily been helpful. These interventions included several different antidepressant medications, trigger-point needling, relaxation, and biofeedback. In addition, physical therapy, transcutaneous electrical nerve stimulation (TENS; to stimulate acupuncture points), ultrasound, massage, traction, chiropractic treatment, and certain antidepressants (e.g., amytriptyline and Prozac) had made her symptoms worse. At one point, the Pain Clinic had recommended inpatient treatment, but Mary's insurance would not cover it. She continued in treatment with the outpatient team, however, trying different interventions and seeing a psychologist for individual therapy to better manage her pain. This therapy continued for 2 years with an increased focus on Mary's sexual abuse history. Periods of improvement in the pain symptoms were noted when Mary was less stressed (less pressured to be or to perform in a certain way), was less perfectionistic, used relaxation imaging, engaged in exercise, and was in the initial phase of taking certain antidepressant medications.

Paul, by contrast, was quite healthy. He had experienced hernia and hemorrhoid surgeries plus kidney stone attacks in the 10 years prior to therapy. He had no history of psychiatric symptoms. He had occasional backaches and rheumatoid symptoms. He tended to cope by not focusing on the negative and minimizing his own psychological discomfort. He was troubled by Mary's pain and had a special sensitivity, certainly augmented if not created during the dying of his daughter and misery of his wife, to feeling helpless to soothe Mary's pain.

Sexual Issues

Mary reported clitoral pain upon sexual arousal as well as dyspareunia, occurring with penile entry but not with her husband's digital penetration of an equivalent diameter. Hip pain continued "in waves" up to 24 hours after having coitus. These complaints had been present since the beginning of their relationship but had worsened, as had the sexual desire discrepancy between them. Mary's manifest response to the sexual problems was guilt; Paul's was intermittent irritation.

Important historical sexual issues included Mary's incest history. Over her adult life, Mary had pushed out of her awareness the extensiveness, severity, fear, and anger over her incestual experience. These details became clearer as we attempted to address the sexual problems. To summarize her history of incest, she reported that it began when she was about 6 years old and continued until she was 14. Sexual activities included her father fondling her breasts and genitals, as well as fellatio and vaginal and anal intercourse. She recalled much fear, tension, and pain surrounding these experiences, which occurred when her mother was out of the house. She could not remember the frequency but was sure it was more than two times per month and less than once per week. Mary's recollection of the termination of the abuse was when she was 14 and her mother walked into the bedroom when Mary's father was having anal intercourse with her. Mary recalled saying, "It isn't my fault," and running out of the room. It was subsequently never discussed, and Mary felt that her mother and she had a difficult relationship throughout her adolescence no matter how well Mary did in school or how hard she tried to please at home. She felt her mother liked her sister but not Mary.

Between age 14, when the abuse was witnessed by her mother and immediately terminated, and age 19, Mary was unaware of any memories of sexual abuse. However, it is not certain that they were truly repressed at that time because the context—family members who refused ever to speak of it—itself communicated rejection of the reality of the incest. At

19, away from her father and attending college for 1 year, she recalled a few brief encounters, less invasive than she eventually remembered in her work at the Pain Clinic. When she was 20, among her father's last words to her as he was hospitalized and dying of cancer was a proposition to have sex with her since her mother was not present.

Two other family features are pertinent to Mary and her sexuality. One was that, as a preteen and teen, her father, with her mother's support, paid her $1 per pound to gain weight (her mother incidentally was quite overweight) and her father called her a nickname, "Rolly," which referred to her roundness in a way that Mary found embarrassing and humiliating. From photos she has shown, Mary was not overweight but had the typical shape of a developing 10–14-year-old pubescent. His comments about her body were far more intrusive and shameful for the patient given his secret and private knowledge of and access to it.

The other issue Mary recalled was that her parents did not tolerate complaints about pain. Their attitude was stoical acceptance. Complaints about pain would be met with minimization or indifference. She reported spending allowance money on aspirin for her headaches because she was afraid to ask for or take it from her parents.

Mary's first marriage, which lasted 14 years, replicated her being controlled in the sexual and physical appearance domains. Her first husband was verbally demeaning about her physical attractiveness and value as a sexual partner. Her poor self-esteem and interactional pattern of trying to please those who refused to be pleased was reinforced in this marriage. Her sexual relationship consisted of servicing her husband's needs. She experienced dyspareunia throughout their sexual relationship. She did earn her law degree, however, and managed eventually to exit from the marriage.

Formal Assessment

Both individuals completed a Medical History Form, Spanier's Dyadic Adjustment Scale (DAS), Brief Symptom Inventory (BSI), and Recent Life Stress Events Scale before and after therapy. At intake, Mary was slightly elevated, 55th percentile, on the BSI's Somatization Scale using outpatient norms. No other BSI scales were elevated at intake for either Paul or Mary. On the DAS both scored above the total score mean for married couples (Mary 126; Paul 132), with only the Consensus subscale score being slightly below the mean but still within one standard deviation of the mean of married couples. Cohesion, Satisfaction, and Affectional Expression were, respectively, the most positively rated areas of the relationship for both individuals.

CHARACTERISTICS OF CLIENTS AND TREATMENT CONTEXT

The setting for this work was a university medical school psychiatry center in an urban location. The center has a "medical" atmosphere to it, with a large, nonprivate waiting room, physical exam rooms, and private psychotherapy offices.

In presenting for treatment, these clients were referred to the director of a specialty clinic on sexual disorders, a clinic where treatment, teaching, and research (with client permission) occurs. Some commitment to addressing sexual issues was thus built into acceptance of the referral. In addition, at this site, clients are expected to pay for treatment at the usual, or somewhat higher than private practice rates. This couple had insurance that provided them some discount, but the financial commitment was still substantial.

Mary was of average height and weight with a sense of carefulness and neatness about her appearance. She was also measured and careful about her words. She appeared tense frequently and also needed more time than most people to walk. Both the tension and slow movements were related to the chronic pain she experienced.

Paul was rather tall, average weight, and casually dressed. He appeared relatively relaxed and attentive. Although cooperative, he did not find it easy to discuss his past, except briefly. I found it more difficult to ask him about it and, therefore, still have a sketchier picture of his family of origin than of Mary's. He assisted Mary a great deal by carrying heavy objects for her, driving longer distances, grocery shopping, and other tasks. Her pain was of great concern to him. He was fearful that she might become more disabled. He also felt both frustrated about their sex life and terrible if she experienced pain during or after a sexual interaction.

As a couple, there was obvious mutual respect of one another. They consulted one another and shared a sense of humor, though in sessions Paul was more often the instigator of an aside. Paul was more able to express negative feelings to Mary than the reverse, and more quick to express and let go of his anger. Both were thoughtful and verbal, paid careful attention to the other, and were openly appreciative of each other.

COURSE OF TREATMENT

We met for a total of 55 sessions, spread over 3 years, all but five of them including both Paul and Mary. They were always early to their sessions and only canceled one session due to Mary's pain. They drove 30 to 40 minutes each way to attend treatment. They saw me approximately every 2 weeks, with vacation breaks for them about twice a year.

When we began therapy, Mary had been in treatment for a total of 3 years. The sexual abuse had begun to be addressed over the prior year. Thus, it appeared reasonable to address the sexual relationship between Mary and Paul, while recognizing the likelihood of revisiting sexual abuse issues. Thus, the overt contract was to improve the sexual functioning. Mary also hoped to experience more healing regarding the sexual abuse than she had previously found. For the first 10 months of treatment, she continued to see the psychologist at the Pain Clinic on alternate weeks.

Early in Treatment

We began to address the sexual issues almost immediately, with agreement to explore various ideas and exercises outside the therapy session. An early suggestion was to associate to the word "penis" (recall her dyspareunia was limited to penile, not digital, stimulation). It was helpful for me and her husband to hear the extent of her negativity regarding the word "penis": "hairy, ugly, disgust, rage, purple, hard, betrayal, invasive, snake, demand, guilt, need, insatiable, hose, alien, fear." She also stated that she had negative feelings (related to this exercise and the incest) that "I don't have words for."

Simultaneously, Mary and Paul were sent to a middle-class sex accessory shop to buy a latex penis which she would, at home, try to partially insert with a lubricant, preceded by finger insertion. I usually tell clients that whatever their response to an assignment, it would be helpful to our work. For example, this exercise had several possible outcomes. Not being able to do it would not have been a failure but material for discussion. Doing it might help answer how critical issues of control are and might begin to address the meaning of a penis, differentiating her father's from her partner's penis and separating sexual abuse from healthy sexuality. While Mary was reluctant, she did attempt to use the penis both in individual and couple work for about four sessions but decided that she "hated it," and it only reminded her of her father's penis. Several months later, the penis met its fate by being buried in a Canadian lake, along with several other mementos from Mary's childhood, as part of a small "cleansing ritual." This was interpreted as an unexpected but therapeutic outcome in Mary's ability to say no to me and be respected in her willingness to collaborate rather than to just cooperate with treatment, and in the meaning of "cleansing" that she gave to the "burial" of the penis. In fact, the latter point was symbolically layered, and I had some concern that this act might be one of banishment of any penis. On the other hand, the exercise may have been too much too soon for a client who needed to have considerable control over the therapeutic tempo.

Other recommendations for sexuality during this period included Kegel exercises, sensate focus, vaginal containment, and masturbation using the fantasy of penile containment at the point of orgasm. Although most of these exercises were attempted, the only consistently satisfactory activities involved the couple and mutual touching assignments. Intercourse, if attempted, remained painful.

Early in therapy it became clear that Mary's sexual abuse issues were far from resolved. Within the first four sessions, she recalled additional memories of the incest, including more specific acts and sensations. She began to realize that the abuse began earlier, was more extensive, and ended later than she previously believed. During this time, the psychologist at the Pain Clinic was helping Mary to pursue these memories directly while I dealt with those sparked by our focus on sexuality. I worried about there being either too much or too little focus on the memories of sexual abuse. Too little attention to the memories might not be respectful of Mary's suffering and reenacted desire to be (finally) heard. Too much attention to the memories might put excessive focus on the power of the past, making change feel more impossible, or at least slowing down the process.

We elected to (1) review the past memories until Mary felt it was sufficient and I agreed and (2) deal with the ways in which past memories appeared to contribute to feeling currently blocked in terms of sexuality. Meanwhile, Mary still saw the other psychologist approximately every 2 to 4 weeks. Although there were disadvantages to this arrangement, overall it was useful in giving Mary control over termination and making explicit the fact that therapy was not to be focused entirely on issues relating to pain but on those relating to sexuality and relationship satisfaction as well.

Pain entered into the therapy process in an interesting and meaningful way. About five sessions after we began, Mary reported that the night before sessions, she would be in tremendous shoulder, neck, and headache pain. On one occasion she went to an emergency room for treatment of her migraine. She also reported that some sessions were physically painful for her. We dealt with this on two levels. One was to reiterate that this topic was painful, perhaps more than she was able to put into words, and that therapy should gradually assist her by putting pain into words. Also, her body had suffered in the abuse. On a related level, I acknowledged that she might at times be angry at me or the process but not able to say so, thus increasing her tension. I invited her to say no or report when she did feel increasing tension or pain and we would deal with it. Her husband noted that she often suffered without admitting to others that she was in pain or even consciously acknowledging it to herself. I encouraged her not to reiterate this pattern in our sessions. In part, this was intended to increase her sense of control; in part it was to allow her pain to be heard, which was not permitted during her years growing up.

Six months into therapy, the patient's mother died of cancer complications. The illness preceding her death allowed Mary to review several emotional issues regarding her mother. Of particular importance was Mary's increased awareness that her mother knew about the abuse, and her recollection that her mother had walked in on her father having anal sex with Mary and had never subsequently discussed it with Mary. The abuse did, however, terminate at that point. Mary's conceptualization of this was that her mother had seen the abuse, but forgotten it. We discussed in therapy the idea of reviewing this aspect of the past with her mother, although she believed her mother would deny it (she would "disown" Mary's memories) and the consequence would be mutual hurt. Mary felt it was not worth the effort it would take to go through the experience. My own reaction was ambivalent. I wondered whether Mary's response was simply recapitulating the earlier powerlessness she felt as a child and adolescent, and that she was missing an opportunity (albeit somewhat risky) to engage one of the key figures from her history in a reexamination and perhaps reconceptualization of the event. After all, her mother knew she was dying and might just want to set things right. However, Mary was quite resolved about not discussing this issue with her mother. Her vulnerability to rejection and fears of it might have been amplified by the experience of so recently becoming aware of the extensiveness of her sexual abuse. Ultimately, Mary would have to live with the consequences of her decision to face or not to face her mother on this issue. Paul was in agreement with her decision. Thus, upon some joint reflection, I stood by her as she let her mother die unconfronted. She has not regretted this decision over the subsequent 3 years.

Therapy was able to utilize the passing of Mary's mother as an opportunity to cleanse some aspects of the past. This metaphor materialized in the cleaning out of her mother's house, which included photos, trinkets, and some of her father's belongings. Sorting, throwing away, and letting go became physical expressions of the emotional work.

Her mother's death was a meaningful marker for the end of the initial phase of this therapy. The major *content themes* of these first 7 months were (1) the revelation of the extent of her sexual abuse; (2) the importance and value of Mary's relationship with Paul in contrast to her prior marriage, but her fear of its loss if sex did not improve; and (3) past intimate relationships with men and women as ones of, at best, distance and dislike and, at worst, betrayal, confusion, and abuse. The major *process themes* included establishing the ground rules that (1) the patient had power and collaborative control over the therapy and could say no to interventions (e.g., the latex penis), (2) experiences of abuse would be listened to, (3) an exploratory attitude toward solutions would be used, (4) therapy via assignments goes on inside and outside the session, and (5) pain, both physical and psychological, would be addressed in therapy.

Midtherapy

The next phase of therapy focused on sexual issues. The patient stated that she was frightened of sex. "I'm scared before it begins." Two issues were related to this, the first being that the anticipation of sex was more frightening than the actual sex itself. The other meaning had to do with a generalized response to her interactions with men. "Sex is such a powerful thing in the lives of men I have known. Men have done terrible things to me and all said they cared about me." It was like "being around a poisonous snake." Certainly these fears made sense given her past experience with abuse by her father and first husband.

The presence of Paul, though he was a less verbal participant in most of the sessions, became increasingly important. His capacity to listen and his willingness to understand and be affected by Mary's struggle were critical to her effort. In addition, Paul would challenge Mary if he disagreed but not in a hostile way, and he could get angry but not be embittered. He did not conduct himself "like a poisonous snake," which was helpful on one level of dealing with Mary's suspicious mistrust of men by discriminating him from other men in his overall treatment of her. The problem was that he still wanted to have intercourse with her, which automatically raised Mary's fear and mistrust.

Several strategies were used to deal with Mary's fearful imagery. With respect to the metaphorical fear, encompassed by the snake imagery, I asked her to search for an image that would neutralize or transform the snake into a less threatening image. This was a request to both her conscious and unconscious states because she was having relatively frequent dreams about snakes and was also aware of how they encapsulated her reaction to the sexuality of men. Her dreams consisted of scenes such as a chasm of snapping snakes, experiencing fear that they would hurt her if they touched her; seeing snakes that only she thought were dangerous; and trying to "be good in a balancing act," which would keep them from touching her. Although Mary was unable consciously to develop a transformational image, she did report a dream in which a caricature of a snake scooted up a ramp into her arms and became a cat. Cats were her favorite creatures. While not a formal conscious transformation, it was integrated as one that fit rather well. Her snake dreams were very infrequent after this session, until the termination phase of therapy, which will be discussed separately.

Regarding the actual fear of sex, there were three approaches that were used at this point. One was to openly tell Paul and Mary that I thought the fear had a reasonable basis in the past and perhaps was more intense and entrenched because it began when Mary could not protect herself or expect to be helped. Although this is an obvious point, I believe it is important to acknowledge with trauma victims and their partners in order to make sense of their feelings while also emphasizing that the present is different from the past. The differentiation of past identities and relationships from the present realities of the patient with her adult capacities and her current partner requires repeated and varied efforts from the therapist. Drawing attention to the patient's current adult ability to say no, protect self, identify danger, and so on., is one avenue. Another is to have the patient, with her partner present, draw direct distinctions between personality, appearance, and even genitals of the good and bad men in her life. One session and an assignment is not sufficient; repeated opportunities to have the patient look for and believe these differences are the more likely path.

The second direction we took was to introduce sensate focus exercises with the couple to decrease fears of intercourse. They had already initiated this on their own, but we made it explicit to exclude intercourse. Mary said she would like to try intercourse again sometime later, and Paul definitely wanted eventually to include it in their sexual script because of what he perceived as a special closeness it provided for him.

Third, we utilized a systematic desensitization approach for the activities around sex that made Mary more or less afraid. My own thinking was that she would prefer this over another alternative, trance work, because it would appear to allow her more control. The least stressful/fearful items on her list were:

1. Holding hands with Paul while going shopping/to a restaurant.
2. Paul and I are in the kitchen. We hug each other; he touches my hair.

The most fearful/stressful items on her list were:

13. Paul's penis penetrates me fully. It is very painful.
14. Paul touches my breasts when we don't intend to make love.

I mention these items to show that there was some fairly comfortable touching that could occur, and also to point out item 14, which is not in a typical position with respect to item 13.

Three sessions of desensitization were conducted, with Mary using a relaxing visual image to pair with stressful images (she could not do deep muscle relaxation because it exacerbated her chronic pain). At the

third session she stated that she did not want to continue the desensitization due to increasing shoulder and neck pain. Psychologically, she
found the exercise made things worse because she could anticipate what
was coming next. I decided not to pursue the desensitization, mindful of
the fact that therapy was again being intruded on by Mary's pain. However, given Mary's overt message, it was also possible that this approach
was too stressful for her at this point. At the end of therapy she still felt
this had not been helpful. There were several indirect and useful consequences of our attempt with this technique. One was a clearer understanding for me about how upsetting the anticipation of sex, even in
imagery, was for Mary. Another was the management of item 14 by
bringing Paul in and having Mary explain why it bothered her. It was
hard for her to ask him not to do something in the sexual realm because
of feeling guilty about the larger sexual problems. A third consequence
was the opportunity for Mary to refuse an activity having sexual content, to be heard, and to have the relationship continue—a partially corrective emotional experience.

At this point in therapy (and 6 months after her mother's death)
Mary's sister was diagnosed as terminally ill with Hodgkin's disease. Her
sister's house was 2 hours by car from Mary's. This relationship was
complicated because Mary saw her sister as having been favored by their
mother, and Mary and Paul both viewed the sister as very self-centered,
a particularly unacceptable quality in both their value systems. We discussed a reasonable role for Mary as she waited for her sister's death
and again the possibility of discussing the sexual abuse with her sister
and seeing whether it might have happened to her as well. Mary decided
not to discuss the abuse with her sister.

We did, however, continue to deal with sex in the final 2 months of
her sister's illness. Mary mentioned Paul's restlessness if he did not have
sex every 2 to 3 weeks. Paul clarified what he saw as his response, which
was less a reaction to Mary than part of an earlier pattern where his first
wife would withhold sex to "get even." His usual response to infrequent
sex was more often a sense of missing something than of being manipulated. This was a different emphasis than Mary was picking up and I
suggested that Paul had a right to feel disappointed and Mary needed to
know and accept Paul's feelings without feeling she had to solve them
by giving in to sex when she did not want to do so. Both accepted this
formulation and decided together that their lovemaking, while not perfect, was satisfactory with partial entry rather than full entry for intercourse.

Still, the anticipatory fears and low desire remained distressing for
the patient, who wanted sex to feel like a more loving, intimate activity
and with less pain. We had talked about the clitoral pain. This pain

occurred only on arousal and then went away. I labeled this as probably the experience of her clitoris becoming erect and more exposed to sensitive contact and also a signal that she was aroused. Being sexually aroused was historically a very upsetting experience for Mary. She felt humiliated and betrayed by her body, which as a child, in response to her father's touching, had been aroused and orgasmic. The consequences of this went far beyond clitoral pain and formed the core of her sexual despair: She hated her body as a child, she blamed it for betraying her, and she hated and objectified "that pathetic, whining, ugly little girl." She never referred to herself as a child as "I," "me," or "mine."

My first approach to this issue was direct. I asked Mary if she could come up with a way to explain to and comfort herself as a young child regarding why she had become aroused during incest. I did not force the integration of childhood and current selves as she was not willing to accept it. I did ask her to think about her own sexuality, at least to acknowledge the fact that she was able to respond sexually as an adult, as a first step toward accepting the adult sexuality that already was part of her.

In retrospect, this direct approach was too provocative as a change intervention but quite useful in unearthing the underlying issues Mary encountered in recalling her past, her body, and her sexuality. Among the issues we dealt with, in the approximate order they appeared in treatment were the following:

• Her response to finding a way to comfort the child was that she could *not* forgive the child for having a body. She felt the child's body should not have responded to her father's sexual touch. "Why did her body do that? Her body is bad. Her body betrayed her." She tried repeatedly to approach this issue but was unable to move forward. Instead, issues connected to religion, her former husband, and pain were stimulated.

• Mary's faith in God, adopted early in her life as a comfort and escape (and a rebellion against her family's professed atheism), was revealed to be intimately interwoven with therapy. For example, she mentioned that as a teenager she had a sense of her self as a "spirit only." What she began to recognize during therapy is that the Christian faith values people as both spirit *and* body. In between our sessions she would often use prayer. After one of these prayers, she observed that God's "greatest gift" was a body. Jesus, after all, had a body. This raised other issues with respect to Jesus's physical suffering, which Mary also identified with, presenting complications for the pain and its resolution because Jesus's pain was not resolved. It also allowed a strong source of meaning for her pain. After another prayer specifically about her pain, she recalled an answer of "receiving something golden from it." When

Mary read through this section, she commented that identifying with Jesus's pain encourages her to "find in or through the pain the healing that allows me to go on living in a valuable way to myself and others."

• Paul was observant of Mary's inability to like or love her body and offered to discuss this with her.

• She looked at photos of her childhood and brought some in to therapy. My hope was to stimulate her empathy for "the little girl." Her response was detachment: "It doesn't seem like me." What did happen was a surge in my own empathy for Mary as a child. I was especially moved by one family photo in which members were arranged by alliances: mother cuddling the new baby sister, boys standing a bit off to themselves, and Mary holding one of her beloved cats while her father's hands were placed firmly on her shoulder and arm. Her innocent (she was about 9), wholesome beauty and natural affection so apparent in the photo made her story of incest even more bleak. I expressed my responses to the photo, focusing on her in them and how she seemed to me. She continued to work with the photos afterwards, with some modest improvement and connection to herself as that child. She saw that the child did not appear in the photo the way she remembered her ("ugly, sniveling"). That paradox was too difficult for her to resolve directly but was a positive contribution nonetheless.

• We discussed her father's background and what might have contributed to his incestual treatment of her. There were no unique revelations here, and there was no expectation from me that she was required to forgive him. She also experienced many dreams about her father, some showing progression (dreams in which she experienced getting away from her father or, as an adult, saying no to him) and other dreams that showed no progression (those in which she was pursued sexually by her father until she woke). The dreams stimulated other associations which were useful. In particular, one dream reminded her that "the worst part about the abuse is that I had to tell him [her father] how it felt."

• Her desire for sex, expectedly, had not yet changed. Her clitoral pain, unexpectedly, was much improved—less intense and less frequent. Part of her never wanted sex again. Sex was connected to pain. It was a cause for rejection directly (her mother) or indirectly (her father telling her how unattractive she was and her first husband telling her that she was not lovable and there was nothing she could do about it). Her anger over these rejections was only minimally expressed and, after one session of discussing it (in particular her experiences with her first husband), she ended up going to the hospital with a migraine. Though her manifest anger was at her first husband, I asked about her anger, realistic or not, at Paul. She denied it but during the next session reported a dream of her first husband invading Paul's body. She also dreamt of Paul dying of tuberculosis. Both dreams had a feeling tone of panic and fear. Given what I had witnessed of their interaction and of Paul's treatment of Mary (by both accounts), her core anger was toward the prior male figures in her life and Paul was primarily the recipient of unresolved and over-generalized feelings.

Her sense was that these earlier men were "locked inside of me." We discussed ideas around removing them or finding a less pervasive place for them. These included joining a women's group of incest survivors (for emotional validation and for exposure to women who have used different approaches), talking to other family members (only her aunt and uncle knew and had been supportive; she did not want to tell her brothers for fear of losing the relationships), and continuing to write down memories of the abuse, as they surfaced, and her feelings about them which she would put on a floppy disk, appropriately labeled and compartmentalized (she enjoyed word processing and was proficient at it). She did continue to record her memories, but none of the other suggestions proved helpful and she expressed some discouragement about the lack of progress in therapy.

• The dilemma that Mary was in with regard to resolving the sexual issues and her sexual pain, given the background of somatic disorders, was much clearer. Her physical discomfort was continually present via fibromyalgia. Thus, as she mentioned several times, she wanted to ignore her body and sex was again putting attention on the acceptance of herself, including her sexual body as a child and an adult. During this period she had an exacerbation of pain symptoms, sought additional medical consultation for sleep disturbance, changed physicians to a local specialist in fibromyalgia, and was switched to Prozac (fluoxetine) to manage her pain and depressive symptoms. The relationship between facing her sexual issues and her increased pain was circular, not linear.

• It was likely that Paul, being a nonabusive and loving man, made it *more* difficult for Mary to say no to him if she did not want sex. This dilemma may have unintentionally played into the continuation of coital and postcoital pain.

Given the latter two points, one can appreciate the importance of Paul giving a clear message that he chose to give up full intercourse rather than for Mary to suffer pain. This was not martyrdom, nor did he promise not to be disappointed at times, which Mary, in turn, needed to deal with, but that "in the broad scheme, some things are more important than others." If we examine Mary's interactional history around pain and sexuality in the context of "love," we can see the power that this message had for her as a corrective emotional experience.

Later in Therapy

Nearly 2 years (34 sessions) into treatment, Mary and Paul came in very discouraged and concerned over their lack of progress. "The [fibromyalgia] pain is worse, Mary's decreased energy is the same, and the past is still not in the past." Paul stated this; Mary and I agreed. Notice that sex was not mentioned. For Paul this situation raised memories of his first wife whose "energy was drained from her" in the course of their daughter's dying and trying to adjust to the loss. Feeling helpless, as he did at this point in our work, was very difficult for Paul.

Their discouragement and my response to it revitalized and refocused therapy and allowed it to enter a final phase with the goals of putting the past in its place and briefly exploring the connection between sexual abuse and pain. What may be important to recognize is that the course of treatment had slipped away from the sexual complaint to a broader hope that dealing with the sexual abuse would impact Mary's overall pain.

I will briefly summarize this phase as it is less directly related to ongoing sexual issues though it was very meaningful for the patient in other areas.

Several sessions of trance work were employed for the purpose of understanding the pain–sexual abuse connection and exploring a means for incorporating Mary's past experiences into her present adult self. The theory was that by blaming the child via her body and gender, she was keeping the past alive and continuing to punish herself.

Mary found trance work easy. Through it, she revealed that there were some moments when she felt safe in her parents' house. When she visualized an abuse experience as a child, she realized that her body, when she was a child, became extremely rigid and tensed in anticipation of the intercourse and her inability to escape, a tension not unlike what she currently experienced, and which clearly increased her pain. In trance, when asked (as an adult) to comfort the child, she felt the child could not be comforted. In fact, the child did not trust others to comfort her, especially by physical touch, except for a touch on the hand. In a later trance session, she was, as an adult, able to take the little girl back to the present with her, but with some trepidation, "I'll try to love you, to protect you. I don't know what we will do with the memories." When I asked what the girl's idea was to deal with the memories, she said, "Play with them."

Overall the effect of our trance work and subsequent discussions was quite powerful. It allowed Mary to fully appreciate herself as a child. She began to see her child self as a "pretty, courageous, and graceful" girl. This revision of her images allowed Mary to begin to incorporate

her child self in a more empathic way. The question of what to do with
the memories of the abuse remained important. She could not tell the
child not to remember as that is what she felt she had been told by her
parents. The goal was to find a way to remember that was less invasive
and allowed Mary to live her life.

Her solution was to put the memories more on the periphery through
prayer and through occasional writing. In response to a suggestion that
she set up a museum box or a special section on her computer, she came
in with a poem she read and gave to me:

REMEMBERING

He slinks toward her, sniffing
for her in the darkness.
No, for me, my pain, my memories.
His thick animal hands touch
her small curveless body.
No, they paw at me.
The little girl is me,
She, no I, rigid, retreating
against a prison of sofa cushions.
He blots out her light,
smothers her breath and enters her.
Pain! Escape. Forget.

No, it is my darkness.
It is I who cannot breathe.
I will remember.
When I was that little girl
my father raped me, over and over.
My pain, my memories.

This was a moving moment and in some ways a crystallization of
therapy issues and a new direction toward resolution. Indeed, in this same
session Mary began to talk about still needing to know the memories
would not engulf her. During a trance, I asked her to consult her "strong
and competent part" regarding ideas for solutions to this issue. Many
ideas were mentioned, but one recurring theme that united most of the
others was the idea of a ritual. She ordered and read specific books on
the topic (Flaherty, 1992; Pellaver, Chester, & Boyajian, 1987) and eventually decided to create for herself a healing ritual. She did this while we
continued to work in therapy on managing memories and incorporating an appreciation of herself as a child. Also, through the religious education groups she and Paul conducted, she listened to several women's
stories about their abuse. This experience helped her to see her own

progress in working through her past. She was able to tell the women she worked with about her abuse. We observed that telling others helped the memory to become less burdensome because it is then also held by someone else.

The subsequent sessions continued to be fruitful, with Mary and Paul both sensing significant gains. They both felt healing taking place. Mary began to see her abuse as both a strength and a weakness. She became less perfectionistic and more relaxed. She became more accepting of her body and found a somewhat greater interest in sex.

She planned the ritual to take place at her house and asked if I would be present with her and Paul, along with five friends. She felt my presence was important given my role in her therapy to this point. We discussed several issues. My main concern was whether I could participate and still be able to maintain a therapeutic role with her. I explained that I would not be able to interact as a friend but as a therapist, which might feel awkward at times for everyone. They accepted this.

Overall, the ritual was important for it marked the recognition that much work had been done and some issues were resolved and others redefined. It lasted for 45 minutes and included candles, a display of pictures of Mary as a child and an adult, spiritual readings, and a carefully thought through litany written by Mary using the words, "Woman, why do you weep?" (inspired by the title of the book by Flaherty) and turning it into a very personal response prayer by also asking, "Woman, why do you rejoice?" The couple informed me that they very much valued my presence there, and I also thought it was important that I took part.

The next 7 months were spent consolidating therapeutic gains and finally terminating. One other somewhat difficult period arose after a 2-month vacation Paul and Mary had planned. Mary's dreams of snakes reappeared two to three times per week. It was clear that this was related to her hope, although she realistically knew otherwise, that all sexual abuse issues had been eliminated and that she would thus not *ever* have to think about them again. This was too much like forcing herself to forget, which was breaking a promise to herself. Also, it turned out that a snake does not equal a snake, even in her dreams, which was helpful; for example, in some cases they were inescapable and invasive and at other times she could walk away from them without being touched. Ways to compartmentalize attention to these themes were discussed.

OVERALL OUTCOME OF TREATMENT

With respect to the formal assessment, no significant changes occurred on the BSI or the SDAS. Somatization on the BSI was still slightly elevated

(58th percentile) for Mary. Marital adjustment had increased somewhat to 130 (Mary) and 138 (Paul). Most of the increase from intake to posttherapy marital adjustment scores occurred because of an improvement in the Consensus subscale.

Regarding sexuality, Mary and Paul completed independently a sexual activity form at the end of therapy. Their sexual intercourse frequency was once every 2 weeks, at her current desire level but different from Paul's desired level, which was once per week. Mary was always orgasmic during manual stimulation by her partner and orgasmic during intercourse alone about 25% of the time. If accompanied by manual stimulation, she experienced orgasm on about 90% of coital occasions. She reported genital pain during intercourse about 55–75% of the time. She reported being sexually aroused during sex over 90% of the time, and seldom (less than 25% of the time) having negative emotional reactions during sex. Her general sexual desire level was one time per month. Paul also reported difficulty in achieving and maintaining erections about 50% of the time. However, he felt very aroused during sex with Mary (90% of the time). He reported his general sexual desire level to be two times per week. Both reported feeling moderately satisfied overall with their sexual relationship (5 on a 6-point scale from extremely dissatisfied to extremely satisfied).

I was surprised by the fact that sex was still painful for Mary and asked her to elaborate. She said that she first has an orgasm with manual stimulation by Paul, so that any discomfort of intercourse is not associated with orgasm. Also, this pattern "allows me to control the length of time of my orgasm. I do this because I know that the muscle contractions of orgasm will cause subsequent fibromyalgia pain" in her hips and shoulders. "The longer the orgasm, the greater the subsequent pain." In response to my question as to why she can enjoy sex if it still is often painful (and why not give up sex), she replied, "Virtually nothing doesn't hurt. If I lived my life avoiding pain, I would do nothing. This pain is comparable to that I feel doing other positive activities, such as computer work and teaching my church group."

The formal assessment was consistent with the clinical picture. The marriage was extremely satisfying to both individuals. Sexuality had improved somewhat, as there was no clitoral pain (although occasionally still "tightness") and the intercourse pain was slightly less frequent and considerably less intense than at the onset of treatment. Of note, they no longer attempted to have full vaginal intercourse but rather partial entry, which both felt was adequate.

Mary's chronic pain was, however, still very much present and at times worse. When we ended treatment, she was still searching and hoping for a medical solution. She commented that 12 different antidepressants and antimigraine medications had not been effective and felt quite discouraged about the medication route. As it was, her daily medication regimen included Desyrel (trazodone), Xanax (alprazolam), Tagamet (cimetidine), Estinyl, Ergotrate (ergonovine), Tylenol (acetaminophen), Darvocet (propoxyphene napsylate and acetaminophen), and DHE (dihydroergotamine mesylate) inhalant, approximately the same list with some antidepressant and antimigraine medication shifts since the beginning of treatment. Soon after therapy ended, she discontinued the Ergotrate and Xanax; the latter had worsened the pain. Although our work was not directed at the chronic pain, we had all hoped it would improve with more complete resolution of the sex abuse. It did not.

In session, Mary felt satisfied with her progress in treatment: She noted that she liked herself better and had made progress on the sexual abuse. Paul agreed, noting the extent to which Mary accepted all of herself, including the childhood she had experienced. We critiqued the therapy. Mary noted the plastic penis and systematic desensitization as not being helpful. They felt the most important aspect of this therapy was that I listened and reacted, meaning that I acknowledged that what happened to Mary in the past was a terrible experience and that she did nothing to deserve it. It was also essential to Paul that someone see and believe Mary's suffering, and he "would have walked out" if I had sat and said nothing or been too passive. Mary also mentioned repeatedly that I "allowed and encouraged" her to include her faith in the therapy. She perceived me as open to this expression of herself and to welcome hearing about her insights inspired by her faith. I believe I was able to accomplish this because her religion was a core authentic part of her identity, and indeed had been an instrument of her differentiation from her family. Thus, my acceptance of this aspect of Mary (and Paul) also differentiated *me* from her parents.

Perhaps it is important to be reminded of the power of different styles of reacting to clients, and certainly Mary, whose father would not hear her and whose mother would not speak with her about her incest, would find a therapeutic experience in being heard. It is probably useful to be permitted to say it repeatedly and be reacted to in a way that recognized her past misery while drawing on her present courage. As seen in this couple, finding an appropriate place for the past, so that it is not again stifled and ignored, is one of the creative challenges of treatment. Especially when one of the major goals of treatment is to improve the sexual relationship, retiring the past proves difficult. My approach to resolving this dilemma has been to work out ideas collaboratively with clients and ultimately to permit them to come up with their own solution in an atmosphere of attentive exploration.

A final set of outcome remarks follow. They are selected from Mary's written response to reading and commenting on this chapter. They were useful to me in understanding the experience of being written about as a patient and in terms of another aspect of therapy, termination.

"It was strange, seeing myself in print through your eyes. I don't think I have ever before read anything written about me. It was like a view through a slightly somehow different mirror. While you were, we thought, quite open in expressing your reactions to us during therapy, still this manuscript contains some thoughts and assessments I don't remember you mentioning. It was not, though, an uncomfortable experience. (In fact, it was a good experience.) I think that is because I have come to know and trust you. At its most basic but very important level, given my past, that means that I know that you will not hurt me.

"For me this was a helpful concluding experience to the therapy. I spent time reflecting on my conclusions about our three years together and then could assess how closely they resemble yours.

"In reading and reflecting on this chapter, I found some revelations. I realized that I am quite a bit happier with Paul's and my sex life now than when we began therapy. I can now talk quite openly with Paul about it, even about my still sometimes negative reactions. (We recently had a long conversation about why he experiences sex as more romantic and expressive of love than I do.) And I feel much less guilt (but not none) about our sexual frequency being less than Paul would like. This lessening of my guilt feelings results mainly from our being able to talk now about the frequency of our sexual relations and also Paul's loving way of not blaming me. Paul has asked me to tell him that I am concerned about the infrequency of our lovemaking which will allow him to also express his feelings about that and will let him know that I do think about it, which I do. I have been comfortable with doing that.

"Reading this chapter has also created a good occasion for me to reacknowledge that, while much healing has occurred, my abusive past will always be with me, part of who I am. And I expect that the pain it causes me, palpably physically (for I am convinced that there is a connection) and also, but diminished, psychological and emotional, will always be with me. I can also acknowledge that, in dealing with the abuse, I have become stronger and (very important to me) able to use my experience as a survivor to help others.

"Seeing my name as 'Mary' really stopped me. I couldn't read on. I thought about what name other than mine I would choose for myself. None felt comforable. I realized that I like my name. It is me. And I pretty much like who I am. I thought, 'What a surprise! I wonder when this happened?' I used to hate my name, especially when I was a child and teenager. I associated it with all the other ugly things I thought about myself. I am glad that I like it now, a sign of healing, I think."

CLOSING COMMENTS

Mary is not every incest survivor. Both she and Paul have unique strengths and specific problems. Their educational and socioeconomic level provided them with resources and experiences that they could draw from in responding to therapy. Religion was a valuable source of inspiration and coping for them. Mary's poem and ritual, while making excellent sense for her, may be wholly inappropriate for an incest victim with different sensitivities. Age may also play a role in the extent to which this couple was willing to adapt to the sexual imperfections. These factors, combined with the particular parameters of incest in Mary's case and loss and caretaking in Paul's, contributed to their unique capacities to address different issues in treatment and in their lives.

It is clearly up to the therapist to recognize commonalities and uniqueness across individuals. An "experimental attitude" toward therapeutic interventions and techniques was a key feature in the present case and, in my opinion, is more broadly useful. This attitude requires a firm commitment to therapeutic flexibility, as well as valuing the client's right to reject, change, or invent interventions. The opportunity to improve on the therapist's ideas should be available, as that ultimately allows the client a more personally owned solution and increased sense of mastery.

REFERENCES

Alexander, P. C., Neimeyer, R .A., Follette, V. M., Moore, M. K., & Harter, S. (1989). A comparison of group treatments of women sexually abused as children. *Journal of Consulting and Clinical Psychology, 57,* 479–483.

Bass, E., & Davis, L. (1988). *The courage to heal.* New York: Harper & Row.

Blume, E. (1990). *Secret survivors.* New York: Wiley.

Bolen, J. (1993). Sexuality-focused treatment with survivors and their partners. In P. Paddison (Ed.), *Treatment of adult survivors of incest* (pp. 55–75). Washington, DC: American Psychiatric Press.

Dolan, Y. M. (1991). *Resolving sexual abuse.* New York: W. W. Norton.

Flaherty, S. M. (1992). *Woman, why do you weep? Spirituality for survivors of childhood sexual abuse.* Mahwah, NJ: Paulist Press.

Graber, K. (1990). *Ghosts in the bedroom: A guide for partners of incest survivors.* Deerfield Beach, FL: Health Communications.

Lew, M. (1990). *Victims no longer: Men recovering from incest and other sexual child abuse.* New York: HarperCollins.

Maltz, W. (1991). *The sexual healing journey.* New York: HarperCollins.

Maltz, W., & Holman, B. (1987). *Incest and sexuality: A guide to understanding and healing.* Lexington, MA: Lexington Books.

Pellaver, M. D., Chester, B., & Boyajian, J. (1987). *Sexual assault and abuse: A* handbook for clergy and religious professionals. San Francisco: Harper Collins.

Russell, D. E. H. (1986). *The secret trauma: Incest in the lives of girls and women.* New York: Basic Books.

Verhulst, J., & Heiman, J. (1988). A systems perspective on sexual desire. In S. R. Leiblum & R. C. Rosen (Eds.), *Sexual desire disorders* (pp. 243–270). New York: Guilford Press.

Westerlund, E. (1992). *Women's sexuality after childhood incest.* New York: W. W. Norton.

Wyatt, G. E., & Powell, G. J. (Eds.). (1988). *Lasting effects of child sexual abuse.* New York: Sage.

13

Resistance versus Motivation:
Tipping the Balance

CAROL L. LASSEN

INTRODUCTION

The issue of patient motivation, or, conversely, resistance to change, is a key factor in sex therapy. While some authors have specifically discussed the concept of therapeutic resistance (Althof et al., 1989; Hartman, 1983; Kaplan, 1974, 1979, 1990; LoPiccolo & Friedman, 1988; Radin, 1989), the topic is frequently ignored. Even though not explicit, it is an implicit consideration in all case formulation and treatment planning. In the formative years of sex therapy, the approach of "bypassing" the resistance tended to dominate the field (Kaplan, 1974; Masters & Johnson, 1970). More recently, however, the term "complex case" has come to be synonymous with formidable resistance. Typically, new innovations in treatment have been devised to deal with resistance to previous forms of therapy (Kaplan, 1974, 1979; Lazarus, 1988; Masters & Johnson, 1970; Zilbergeld & Hammond, 1988).

The concept of resistance came originally from psychoanalysis, where it is considered to be both ubiquitous and the focus of the treatment (Wachtel, 1982). Behavior therapists originally took issue with the concept of resistance, but in the era of cognitive behaviorism, resistance has reestablished itself in the form of noncompliance (Lazarus, 1982) or automatic thoughts (Beck, 1976; Meichenbaum & Gilmore, 1982). Currently, practitioners of all schools tend to acknowledge the role of therapeutic resistance, which is usually assumed to be nondeliberate but can be conscious, preconscious, or unconscious (Hartman, 1983; Meichenbaum & Gilmore, 1982). Within the field of sex therapy, Kaplan has written extensively about differing levels of resistance (Kaplan, 1974, 1990). She places considerable emphasis on resistance as an unconscious process and in this regard views sex therapy as one variant of all psychotherapy, to which resistance is ubiquitous.

If resistance is resistance to *change* (Hartman, 1983), the components of that resistance, and the mechanisms of intervening to modify resistance, are far from agreement (Wachtel, 1982). In the wider psychotherapy literature, resistance has been viewed as the conflict of impulses versus defenses, unconscious versus conscious motivations, reinforcement history, the maintenance of a sense of self, the avoidance of anxiety, an individual's schemas and beliefs about how the world operates, noncompliance with homework assignments, and plain reluctance to do the necessary work. When the resistance of *couples* in therapy is reviewed, one speaks of interpersonal systems in balance, couple collusion, miscommunication, and shared anxiety about the impact of change on the partnership. But the theme in all of this, whether intrapsychic or interactive, is *equilibrium,* and it implies both stability and an economy of psychological effort. Looked at in this light, resistance can be seen as a biological organizing principle of living matter that aids survival. But in psychotherapy, where the purpose is planned change, it can play havoc.

Typically, the motivation *for* change is considered the key factor on the other side of the scales. In both individual and couple psychotherapy, motivation is a major variable in psychotherapy outcome. Change, like resistance, is also a biological and psychological quality in the human species. Motivation to change provides the energizing force to move resistance and inertia.

In the initial assessment for sex therapy, our clinical assessment of treatment motivation may or may not be accurate. Most clinicians have had the experience of believing a couple will do well in therapy, based on a positive relationship, good mutual communication, personal insight, etc., only to encounter a major therapeutic impasse. Or the reverse— occasionally a couple is seen on the verge of divorce, with the subsequent surprising development of a rebuilt relationship and a satisfying sexual life.

In couple therapy the clinician needs to assess the motivation of each partner as well the couple dynamics. Most therapists attempt to increase motivation for change through a wide variety of therapeutic interventions (Leiblum & Rosen, 1989). Sex therapy has been a prime example of the integrated use of diverse therapeutic approaches to the presenting problem (Heiman, 1986; Kaplan, 1974; LoPiccolo & Friedman, 1988). It is common for sex therapists to formulate cases from a psychodynamic, cognitive-behavioral, and systems approach simultaneously. There is also a strong emphasis on working with couples, although individual treatment is also employed in many instances. It is my contention, however, that no matter how well we may have formulated a case, no matter which panoply of treatment approaches we have chosen to utilize, we are flying blind much of the time. Our approach to treatment is inevitably refined and redirected on the basis of the response of the couple or individual. In this regard, Heiman (1986) has said, "the process of changing may be one of recognizing a change already occurring, permitting a change to occur, working for a change, or trying to direct the course of the change process. The processes of change are complex and at times difficult to predict" (p. 365).

The following case is one in which both the process of change and the outcome were difficult to predict. It is presented sequentially in order to provide a picture of changing motivation, change in the role of the therapist, and the way in which treatment may take on a life of its own.

CASE EXAMPLE

Michael and Nancy B were an attractive couple in their early 50s. They had been married for 15 years. They came to therapy in a state of crisis and total frustration—particularly Michael's frustration. He had a carefully scripted story to tell, simultaneously to both his wife and the therapist:

"Several years ago we came back from a wonderful sabbatical in Japan, where for three months, we never made love. I asked, 'Why aren't you interested in making love?'" Then to his wife: "You sobbed. But nothing changed." He recounted repeated similar episodes of blocked communication attempts over the last decade. If Nancy asked him what he desired for his birthday, he'd say, "Guess." Usually she did not respond. He concluded by saying with great affect, "I'm angry, I'm hurt and confused. I don't understand."

Nancy replied that she did not understand either. She loved Michael very much. "It hurts me to see Michael angry and upset—and I'm at the root of his anger. When we make love I'm orgasmic, but I have no interest." Her lack of interest was defined not as rejection of sex, not as avoidance or apathy, but simply as the absence of any thought about sex. Intercourse had started to hurt. She wondered whether it was her age and changing hormones. Estrogen cream helped but did not resolve it. And Nancy was not yet menopausal.

In the middle years of their marriage this couple had been through a period of intense distress related to infertility. They had attempted artificial insemination without success. Nancy was impregnated twice but miscarried both times. Both agreed that she had gone through an intense period of depression and self-deprecation, even asking Michael at one point if he wanted a divorce so he could marry someone who was fertile. Ultimately, the couple adopted a school-age child. Sexual problems following an intensive course of treatment for infertility are well-known (Dunkel-Schetter & Lobel, 1991; Leiblum, 1994). However, in this instance the couple wondered whether the problem had predated the infertility crisis.

Their description of the history of their relationship was remarkably consistent. Both had been married previously, Michael for a short time, Nancy for a longer period. Their previous marriages dissolved for similar reasons: They and their former spouses developed different values and lifestyles, and each had simply drifted away. Both had deliberately cultivated a variety of relationship experiences when single, and each felt that he/she had succeeded in accomplishing that goal.

When first introduced by colleagues, Nancy and Michael fell madly in love, were passionately attracted to each other, were engaged very quickly, and married within a few months. Neither one felt he/she had made the decision precipitously. Both had conscientiously developed a self-awareness during their single years and an understanding of their individual needs in a relationship. They were ideally suited to each other in terms of background, values, lifestyle, and families. On both sides, families and friends felt they were a perfect match. They had a strong sexual relationship, which was especially important to Michael. They were both bright and fun loving. Their communication was positive. There had been only one near hitch to their prospective marriage. Michael wanted children whereas Nancy had no desire for children. He almost called the marriage off but decided he did not want to give up Nancy, with or without children. To this day both felt they were indeed an ideal match. They were enormously supportive of each other through family crises, work stresses, and mutual advanced degrees. Both were enormously productive in their individual careers, and each of them had independent friendships and community involvements. They had successfully negotiated family and social activities, finances, household tasks, in-laws, a further decision about having children, parental responsibilities—everything but sex. At this point what had been a joyful and fun-filled relationship was no longer playful or satisfying. Michael was resentful and Nancy was increasingly withdrawn.

At the end of the initial session a number of possible contributing factors were tentatively identified to the couple: the role of vaginal pain, possibly related to a hormone deficiency (though she was still cycling regularly); their busy lifestyles; the contribution of the earlier infertility crisis; and possible depression at the time of Nancy's miscarriages.

During the individual evaluation sessions a number of themes became more prominent: Both agreed the first 3 or 4 years of their relationship had been marked by satisfying, invigorating, and mutually initiated sex. For Michael the sexual problem seemed to develop with no warning signs. Currently Nancy was quite disturbed about her ability to leave all thoughts of sex out of her consciousness. She wondered whether sex played a larger role in her life up until she felt emotionally secure and then became secondary to other activities. And she was very involved in both work and community activities. She remembered the attempt to get pregnant, with all the mechanics of the process, as a very stressful time. Two years into the marriage Michael still wanted children, and they spent hours discussing the matter with each other and sometimes with their minister. Nancy recalled: "Finally, I came around." She knew how important children were to Michael and she agreed.

After the miscarriages, which were devastating to Nancy's self-esteem as a woman, they compromised on adopting an older child. Given their stage in life, Nancy was not willing to deal with the needs and dependencies of an adopted infant. However, the little girl they adopted had a history of insecurity, emotional abuse, and neglect and, in addition, a diagnosis of attention deficit disorder and hyperactivity. She was an enormous emotional strain on them both, requiring the resources of both parents for effective parenting. Like many conscientious parents of an emotionally handicapped child, Nancy and Michael questioned their ability to succeed. They recalled the early months of the adoption, when after hours of their daughter's screaming and attention-demanding behavior, Nancy exploded, "This kid is ruining our marriage!" His internal response was "What marriage?" as he considered their passionless existence.

In addition, Nancy reported that she had experienced pain on intercourse with earlier partners. Her only really comfortable sexual relationship had been with a man who apparently did not have a fully rigid erection, and, most important, had had a vasectomy. Nancy had always feared pregnancy. Further exploration revealed *two* forms of dyspareunia. During the last few years she felt pain at the entrance to the vagina, with significant burning. All her life she had experienced pain with hard thrusting, which sometimes caused significant cramping the following day as well. She did not think she lacked lubrication but stated that she dried up rapidly after orgasm, which occurred through manual stimulation. She was urged to see her gynecologist for a thorough assessment, although Nancy said she had been told in the past that there was no physical basis for her pain. Her visits to the gynecologist had been only sporadic since the days of the fertility workups, but she agreed to see a physician in the near future.

Her husband described her as an overachiever and a workaholic. Nancy admitted to such tendencies but felt she had learned to limit her workload, not to bring her work home despite a responsible position, and to leave sufficient time for family activities. However, there were few opportunities for intimate time with Michael or, for that matter, for time to herself, and the latter was critical to her own sense of well-being.

Nancy was the second and late child born into a warm and affectionate environment. Her older sibling was already out of the home by the time she could walk, so she was raised essentially as an only child. She had learned to prize "alone" time, and her fears about raising an infant derived partially from her having no childhood contact with young children, including almost no baby-sitting experience. Nevertheless, she was popular at school and had a steady boyfriend throughout high school. Her sexual development was fairly typical and not particularly inhibited, with one exception. Her family, church, and community maintained a strong taboo with regard to premarital pregnancy, and she had seen a close adolescent friend totally ostracized because of pregnancy. Though she had a variety of positive sexual experiences throughout her development, fear of pregnancy was never far from her mind.

What troubled Nancy the most was the way she had neglected her husband's complaints about the lack of intimacy in their marriage. Her neglect was not deliberate; she just did not think about it. She did not want to lose Michael. "It boggles my mind, when I think what a prize I have. I just don't think about sex."

For his part Michael was furious with himself for letting the problem continue for so long without "making a bigger issue of it." He was extremely hurt and made no bones about it. Michael was a personable and engaging man, affectionate and supportive of his wife, and well liked by friends and colleagues. He had adapted easily to a "modern" two-career marriage with shared responsibilities. He had thought of having an affair, but felt that was only a good way to destroy a marriage. Michael did wonder whether *Nancy* had had one. He maintained that he was totally satisfied with everything in their relationship *except* for the sexual problem. He appeared to be somewhat clinically depressed. His childhood history was marked by family and personal losses. Michael's father died when he was 12, and his best friend was killed in an auto accident when he was in college. Clearly this rift in their marital relationship felt like another loss.

Most therapists in this field utilize a modified version of the Round Table, a feedback approach originally developed by Masters and Johnson

(1970), which incorporates the information developed from the early interviews and presents a model of causation and an initial treatment rationale to the couple. Typically this step is received positively, with hopefulness and relief and a feeling of being understood. The feedback usually engenders a stronger alliance between the partners and between the couple and the therapist.

Feedback in this case focused on five areas: (1) the strengths in their relationship, particularly their earlier satisfaction with sex; (2) the role of pain in developing an avoidance response to sexual intercourse; (3) life-style issues that focused more on work than on pleasure and included very little "recharge" time, either with each other or alone; (4) Michael's current resentment, diminished communication, and anger at the neglect of his needs and the ignoring of his complaints; and (5) several possible dynamic issues relating specifically to Nancy that required further exploration. These included the impact of the infertility procedures, her depression at the time of the lost pregnancies, the possibility that the "chase" or the time when the relationship was her entire focus was the time of intense sexual excitement for her, and the possibility that fear of pregnancy may have played a role in Nancy's reaction to lovemaking.

Nancy was responsive to this feedback, but much to my surprise, Michael responded with anger and resentment. He was particularly resentful that Nancy had not said much to him about the physical pain, though clearly this was not a surprise to him. Even before the feedback session Nancy had been trying to reach out to him, both physically and emotionally, and he had rejected her approaches. She asked him, "How long before we can do something?" I raised the question of what each could commit to. Michael said he would not stay angry forever but implied that he would not give up his anger in a hurry. This was a psychologically sophisticated man. Trying to engage him, I said, "I know you won't stay angry forever. But tell me this, how long do you think you'll need to sulk before you can feel better?" He smiled. He said he felt they could talk. The "sulking" he said would continue but decrease over time. For the upcoming week they agreed to Nancy touching and being affectionate to him and attempting to tolerate his rejection if that occurred. She felt she could do that at some times and not others. He agreed to deal with his anger by walking and probably some talking. As they left, he put his arm around her.

In the meantime, Nancy saw her gynecologist again, who by her report had discovered a cyst in the vulvar area, whose location she was totally uncertain of, and she required laser surgery. She had some fear about the discomfort this would entail.

They were more connected and affectionate during the next session. Michael said he was past his sulking but now implied that "sulking" was

Nancy's word. I did not let that go by, and I took responsibility for using that word. I never knew whether Michael attributed it to Nancy in an attempt to spare my feelings or to give me an indirect message about his hurt feelings or whether he truly had sufficient memory distortion as to believe that she had been the one to say it. I chose not to go into a transference exploration but to take the onus off his wife.

During the previous week Nancy had been *very* tentative about initiating physical contact. She was afraid of an angry outburst from Michael. She also found that any noise from their daughter was very distracting. Nancy felt she needed to be "cocooned" to get into the mood. Michael was willing to participate at her pace. She was worried about the surgery but felt she could handle kissing and massage. She was eager to try Kegel exercises and dilators if her doctor agreed. It is important to note that I had tried to reach her gynecologist several times without success.

When they returned, Michael was in a funk. Nancy had been out of the home for three evenings; in addition, she had not followed through on a planned walk together. *She* had been waiting for *him* to suggest the walk. She commented that she was assertive with everyone else but not with Michael. For his part, Michael acknowledged that he was being half-hearted about this process and was "testing" her. He promised not to "hit" Nancy emotionally anymore but would speak up to clarify situations when he felt ignored.

For the next month the couple were away on vacation. Upon their return, Michael was still angry, said he did not trust Nancy's attempts to be close, and that it was "like something for school." We spent considerable time on the issue of his willingness to participate. Nancy assured him that she was committed to change but that it was easier to approach him when he was not so angry. He was still testing her to take the initiative in sexual contact. She reminded him that she had, in fact, done so. He was surprisingly nondefensive in acknowledging that reality and thanked her for reminding him. This example was a good demonstration of the observation that spouses hold on to their assumptions about their mates even in the face of opposing evidence (Fincham, Bradbury, & Scott, 1990). They had, in fact, walked, spent time together, fondled each other, and become sexually aroused. Nevertheless, Michael continued to have suspicions about whether Nancy was really sincere. They established a regular date for caressing, but she set a limit on touching genitals. He said that was fine as long as they were working on it. For the first time, they made a specific plan to keep their daughter from intruding on their privacy and disrupting their mood. This appeared to be a positive sign of renewed emphasis on their intimate relationship. Michael continued to vacillate between being supportive and being sarcastic and angry.

It was several weeks before I saw this couple again. This case, like too many others, demonstrates the difficulty of maintaining regular therapy appointments in the face of pressured schedules. One can certainly interpret it as resistance (Kaplan, 1990), or as yet another enactment of the lower priority that people put on their relationship. It often disrupts the momentum of therapy. Nevertheless, this couple continued to improve emotionally. They had had two sessions of intense physical involvement, and Michael was ecstatic about one of those episodes.

I used this opportunity to ask what they had done *right*. This is a useful intervention for most couples. It requires their active observation and participation, renews optimism, and reinforces the idea that there is a rationale and a solution to their problems; it is not magical. Nancy and Michael could easily identify the important contributing factors: (1) She had had a lot of sleep, (2) they had time to get in the mood, (3) they kept their daughter occupied and out of the way, and (4) once they had established a planned time for intimacy, Nancy started thinking about it with anticipation and desire. They had gone on to genital play, she had been well lubricated, and both were more confident that they could work out their sexual problems. Nancy had also been diligent in doing the Kegel exercises.

She had not, however, followed up with her gynecologist. She had yet to schedule the laser procedure. There had also been some mixup about ordering the dilators, although in his eventual telephone discussion with me, her doctor supported the idea. However, he was not terribly concerned about a physical basis for her pain.

The next few sessions were spaced out as Nancy was very pressured at work. As a highly productive attorney in a busy law firm she could easily keep two paralegals and two secretaries busy full time. She still maintained time for their intimate sessions, but she was regularly preoccupied. Michael continued to wait for her to initiate, although they had specifically been asked to alternate initiating intimacy. He also continued to play Devil's advocate. If Nancy suggested tomorrow night, he would say, "Why not tonight?" She also began to have what she believed were hot flashes, which subsequently turned out to be a high fever. But the biggest change in our sessions was the difficulty in getting them to respond or to provide information. Each session felt like pulling teeth. Eventually it became apparent that their physical involvement had decreased, although they remained affectionate with each other. Hendrix (1988/1990) observes that couples frequently will make significant improvement in a specific area of their relationship, only to revert to previous patterns as therapy continues. He and other authors analyze this development in object relations terms, as an unmet need left from the unfinished business of childhood that creates a hidden agenda in the relationship.

It was apparent that it was time to focus on the resistance. They were asked to explore what might be the downside of their continuing progress (LoPiccolo & Friedman, 1988). They reviewed several aspects of the relationship that were going well and not so well: Time together and time alone were good, their daughter was under control, the dilators were now available, but Nancy had not seen her doctor, and she was worried about pain after laser treatment. Nancy was encouraged to ask her doctor to reproduce the pain that she was worried about. We reviewed the whole sequence of events: pain, anxiety, flinching, contraction, and more pain. Michael asked for more explanation. It became clear that he never saw Nancy as anxious, only as withholding. It was also clear that I still did not have a good understanding of the negative change in their progress.

The couple were away for several weeks and when they returned, Michael had totally withdrawn. He told Nancy in no uncertain terms that he was no longer interested in sex or in working on their sexual relationship. Emotionally, he had resigned from the relationship. She had finally scheduled an appointment with her gynecologist and was confused about why she had avoided it for so long. Michael maintained that there was no particular reason why he had reached the end of his rope, but in fact, in a moment of total frustration, when Nancy could no longer stand the unending stress from their daughter, she told Michael privately that she wished they had never adopted. He took this comment very personally and said that maybe she did not want *him* either. The therapist was struck by how little Nancy seemed to empathize with his pain. But she felt desperate and asked to see me alone. I was also concerned about him. He was clearly angry and depressed. I agreed to see each of them separately to consider our options.

Nancy talked more easily alone. She was now afraid of Michael's anger and would not approach him even when she wanted to. She was also totally confused about why she had not followed through. She had obviously given a lot of thought to the issue. She realized that although she had very solid friendships, she always let others come to her. It was much easier if Michael approached her. And when he got angry she became totally paralyzed. I tried repeatedly to arrange an appointment with Michael, but although he did return some of my calls, we were never able to connect. Then I stopped hearing from Nancy as well. When the decision is made to see a couple separately, it is both a clinical and an ethical decision. The decision is not made lightly, and I take personal responsibility for carefully weighing the consequences, both the potential hazards and the benefits. This was one of those times that I was concerned that I had made a mistake. But the alternative of not meeting at all was not very attractive either.

Six months later Nancy returned to therapy, but this time she was insistent that she had to understand why she had stopped initiating sexual intimacy. She loved Michael deeply, but she experienced neither the thought nor the spontaneous physical desire for intimacy. He had become hostile again and had withdrawn all support and comfort. Nancy hated conflict but finally got up her nerve to ask him about it. He pointed out to her that although she had completed the laser procedure, she never returned to her doctor to learn to use the dilators, and she had completely stopped approaching him. Nancy's version was that she naively believed that Michael had meant it when he had said he was no longer interested in sex. That seemed very hard to believe, given how upset he had been. While Michael agreed to Nancy seeing me individually, he was not inclined to be overly cooperative.

What followed was a much more intense period of individual therapy than had occurred with the couple. It was both insight oriented and problem focused. Several issues became much more salient, and Nancy was more emotionally involved. She explored her avoidance of conflict in depth. We began specific training in sensory awareness of physical signs of emotions (LoPiccolo & Friedman, 1988) to deal with her tendency to "go intellectual." This affective focus led to some pertinent history that she had not previously shared: She had been quite severely injured as a kid, with intense pain and multiple surgeries, and wondered whether she had learned to screen out all feelings in response to the pain. Other themes were as follows: the contrast between how others perceived her, as a leader, assertive and tough, and how she saw herself, as shy and fearful of disapproval; a heavy parental emphasis on responsibility and duty over pleasure; and her fear and anxieties, both present and historical, about intercourse and pregnancy.

Michael never asked her about her therapy sessions. She began to be concerned about his having an affair because he was getting careless about wearing his wedding ring. With her new insight about conflict avoidance she was able to question him. He told her there was no one else but also used it as an opportunity to comment sarcastically about what mattered to her. Her new focus on feelings led her to experience a variety of conflicting emotions, from anxiety to eroticism. She started approaching him for sex (without coitus) fairly frequently. Often both would reach orgasm, and then he would pull away from her, either emotionally or physically, sometimes for days. She began a period of intense grieving, feeling isolated from Michael and from others. She felt she could not talk to their friends about this, and she came to appreciate that this was how *he* usually felt—alone.

By this time Nancy had taken charge of her own therapy—much in contrast to the previous couple sessions. She became more open with me, and then with Michael. When she connected with him in a real way, this would often lead to a sexual encounter, though not necessarily intercourse. These encounters were often associated with intense closeness but were followed by a spike in his hostility. I came to realize that each time they made a real connection and Michael actually felt heard by her, he would unload more of his anger. I tried to prepare Nancy for this pattern. On one occasion when Michael was venting his anger, she asked him whether he loved her at all. "I don't know," he replied. She was devastated. He told her he felt abandoned by her and was still very angry. This time *her* anger spilled over and she accused him of retaliating. He agreed. Nancy connected this with his background of losses, and he angrily agreed.

By this time Nancy was feeling very guilty about the relationship. I urged her to take her share of responsibility but not his. I stressed that he too had a share in this problem. This led to an expression of anger about her constantly taking on unwanted responsibilities. She had not wanted kids, she hated the fertility procedures, and she did not want to adopt but deferred to Michael. She truly had not thought she was resentful, but on reflection, she now thought their problems had begun when they started talking about having children.

The next session Nancy began, "Something amazing has happened." They had unexpectedly had a day to themselves, without their daughter. They had had a passionate and mutual sexual encounter, and *she* suggested that they try intercourse. He was not too erect, she was well lubricated, and penetration had not been painful. She asked him not to go too far, and he complied. Since then Michael had been more affectionate and attentive, even in public. Nancy was amazed. She now believed seriously that the "shutdown" had started with the issue of children. She also was convinced that she missed just how important sex was to Michael because she had been raised to avoid seeing vulnerability. Nancy had missed seeing this in him, and it was also what she missed seeing in herself.

But the next two attempts at intercourse were painful and unsatisfactory. Michael became very depressed. Nancy continued to initiate sexual encounters but not intercourse. She worked at staying emotionally present. She had returned to her gynecologist, who told her she did not need the dilators, that she should work on the problem psychologically. She experienced this response as patronizing and decided not to return to him. I referred her to a pelvic pain specialist—a referral she did not pursue, however. She did gather data on other doctors, and seriously considered seeing a woman physician. Six months later, however, she located a new male gynecologist.

She began to skip sessions with me because of her busy practice but continued to work on the marriage. She was more keenly alert to Michael's moods, particularly if she had been unavailable. In an intense and vulnerable moment she shared with him all her conflict about children and adoption. She was feeling close to Michael again.

I had been emphasizing maximizing the pleasure to deal with the pain, an approach I have used with some success with other couples (for whom there has, however, also been a thorough medical workup for pain). Combining that approach with the lecture I had given them months before on physiology, the couple tried intercourse *before* she reached orgasm and discovered they were quite successful. If intercourse occurred after orgasm she could not tolerate the pain of intromission. She was more convinced than ever that there were two sources of pain, on entry and with deep thrusting. She had still not seen a gynecologist for another opinion. Michael did not easily resolve his anger. He alternated between being loving and attentive and skeptical and angry. The last time I saw Nancy, intercourse was occurring once or twice a week. She had revamped her work schedule to reduce some of the pressure. Their daughter was doing well and seemed to have accepted her parents' new focus on their relationship, though family activities were still frequent and important. Nancy had not brought her calendar and intended to call me to reschedule, but for sporadic appointments to "stay on track." However, she never contacted me. Several months later I called her for a followup. She was very positive about their emotional and sexual relationship. Their gains seemed to have been maintained. She seemed happy to hear from me, but at this point saw no need to come in. She was happy with her new gynecologist and she never mentioned the pain.

COMMENTARY AND DISCUSSION

There is no question that Nancy's prime motivation for change was the preservation of her marriage and, most particularly, of her marriage as a nurturing and affectionate relationship. But this was true in both phases of treatment. Furthermore, it seemed that Michael's withdrawal and hostility, even given his typical caring and nurturing proclivities, did not augur well for resolving this couple's sexual deprivation. His anger could easily have escalated the conflict between them (Notarius, Benson, & Sloane, 1989; Notarius & Markman, 1993). However, in all probability Michael's sullen hostility led to Nancy's experiencing so much psychological distress that she was willing to take on the painful task of exploring her own resistances and dynamics. This entailed overcoming an intense fear of anger from the man she loved most. It took a great deal of courage for Nancy to approach the husband she correctly perceived to be hostile and rejecting when she still could not grasp his underlying pain of abandonment and neglect.

There are several aspects to this case that are known to be associated with sexual and marital distress: Infertility procedures are known to precipitate sexual problems (Leiblum, 1994). The parents of children with illnesses or disabilities are known to be at much higher risk for divorce (Belsky, 1990). Depression in one or both partners is correlated with marital distress (Gotlib & McCabe, 1990) and difficulty in treating sexual problems (LoPiccolo & Friedman, 1988). And obsessive traits, which correlate with hyperresponsibility and diminished affect, are often seen in resistant cases (LoPiccolo & Friedman, 1988).

There were some distinct differences between the period of couple treatment and the phase of individual psychotherapy. Most striking were Nancy's openness and her active direction of her own treatment. This may have occurred because she was less concerned with hurting Michael, or because individual therapy fit better with her attribution that she was the source of the problem.

There was also a striking difference between Phase 1 and Phase 2 in the affective tone expressed by the couple. The level of Nancy's awareness and atunement were different, the degree of playfulness and pleasure was different, and the degree of openness with each other was different. Horowitz (1987, 1991) makes a cogent case for the existence of contrasting affective and cognitive "states of mind" during which events, self-image, and coping strategies are remarkably different in the same individual. Most of us are familiar with the sense of disorientation that occurs in us when a patient "forgets" a highly significant session or statement or when the patient's whole tone, demeanor, and level of optimism change from one session to another. Often clients do not even realize the degree of change that has occurred since the last session. Instead of reflecting the recent powerful insight or newfound hope, the current state of mind represents a cluster of mood, thought, and motivation, which is linked directly with some prior *similar* (usually negative) affective state. But the alternate state can be out of awareness, and not just in individuals with severe pathology (Fincham et al., 1990). It is useful for the therapist to comment on the remarkable differences, and to help create an affective bridge between these differing states. Also, for a time the therapist can deliberately function as the patient's memory until his/hers develops sufficiently. I utilized this therapeutic strategy with Nancy, though she was probably not aware of it.

This brings up the importance of each client's relationship to the therapist, and the role of countertransference in this case. During the second phase of therapy Nancy seemed more accessible and open, but it would be difficult to conclude that she developed a strong therapeutic attachment to me. I attempted to be very supportive but also sensed her need to remain independent. My interventions had decidedly more influence in our individual work, and there was more sense of collaboration, but the lack of a termination session would suggest little need for "good-byes." It could also be argued that I may have alienated Michael, particularly with my "sulking" comment, but there is some evidence to suggest otherwise. At the time that he stopped therapy it seemed part and parcel of his stonewalling behavior toward Nancy. In hindsight, it seems likely that we repeated his dynamics of abandonment by our not succeeding in connecting for an individual session at the point that he went "on strike" in his marriage.

My countertransference was marked by some ambivalence. Initially I found Michael to be warm, psychologically minded, and caring, and that facilitated my ability to support Nancy through the most difficult phase of the treatment, despite his hostility. There was also a lot to admire about Nancy. She was less spontaneous in relationships than Michael, but her relationships were long and loyal. As I got to know her I came to realize that her reserve was a combination of shyness, independence, and competence. Her steadiness and persistence were quite remarkable. Furthermore, one could envy how much they had worked out between them as a couple. Despite the exacerbated stresses of childrearing, they worked well together as a team. Their decision to adopt a child was the issue that caused me the most difficulty, as it had for them, and my countertransference probably paralleled their dilemma. It is instinctive for us as therapists to empathize with the wife who desperately wants children and the husband who does not. But our cultural biases are apparent when the gender roles are reversed. It was easier, though not necessarily rational, to empathize with his position than with hers. And this was a situation where the husband had *agreed* to a childless marriage and then reversed himself. On the other hand, as Nancy explored the emotional dimensions of her acceding to his wishes, I could truly understand the unconscious bind that she was in. One could also raise the question about the level of bonding between Nancy and her difficult daughter. Would one automatically raise that question regarding a man? In fact, I believe she was very attached to her daughter, though ambivalently. And because of her proclivity to responsibility, she made every effort to be a consistent and effective mother. Furthermore, I think she interpreted her own dynamics correctly: She came to understand her defenses against vulnerability. Though not explored, the care of a vulnerable infant probably would have seriously threatened those defenses.

How does one account for her resistance to returning to her gynecologist? Without the availability of a team approach, individual sex therapists must rely on a patient's physician or preferred consultant. I had not worked much with this physician previously, but several of my colleagues had, and his reputation was sound. Clearly, her greatest concern was with pain, whether from intercourse or laser surgery, and in light of her past experience with surgery, that was understandable. In any case this was not a good match. Possibly because her gynecologist appointments were so far apart, my interaction with her doctor was not productive either, and she resolved this problem by eventually finding another physician. But that was 6 months after she discovered her own solution to the pain.

With respect to Michael, there was a repetitive pattern that could have destroyed their intimate relationship. Each time that Nancy successfully approached him sexually and they had some long-delayed satisfaction and closeness, he would follow up with further venting of his anger and hurt. It was as if her empathy released his rage and pain and the toxic feelings would dominate their interaction. This is a response to empathy that we might expect in individual therapy, but not one we anticipate well in marital therapy. It could easily have created a cycle of revenge and spite (Notarius & Markman, 1993), but in this case when Nancy reached her limit and became angry in response, the relationship began to move back into balance. This couple was able to tolerate the swings from closeness to anger and back again.

The curative factors here were probably the following: (1) Nancy's courage in dealing with the conflict with her spouse despite her fears; (2) a working and positive synchronization in most areas of the marriage (Heiman, 1986); (3) a systematic sensory awareness program to access and experience both positive and negative feelings (LoPiccolo & Friedman, 1988); (4) three major insights that Nancy developed in individual therapy—her avoidance of conflict, her defense against vulnerability, and her resentment about the decision to have children; (5) a workable solution to the pain problem in which both partners participated; (6) a conscious existential decision to be aware of vulnerability in herself and in her husband; and (7) the evolution of a joint plan to maintain a private intimate life despite the demands of their daughter.

But what was the critical difference between Phase 1 and Phase 2 of the therapy? What tipped the balance between resistance and motivation? Different therapists would, in all likelihood, focus on different factors in this case. In my judgment Nancy was characterologically competent, compulsive, rational, perfectionistic, and a peacemaker. Defenses that she took for granted were also valued as part of her sense of self. In classical terms, these characteristics were part of her ego ideal, and therefore ego syntonic. Most therapists will attest to the difficulty in changing behavior when that behavior conflicts with characteristics that an individual *values* about him/herself (Lassen, 1976). Only when Nancy's anxiety about losing Michael's support and love outweighed the anxiety created by changing long-held coping strategies was she able to expand her awareness and modify some aspects of her character. Cognitive therapists would argue that because Nancy exposed herself to the feared stimulus of her husband's anger, and there was a partial positive outcome, her anxiety was extinguished, or at least diminished, and a sense of self-efficacy reinforced. That was partly true, and to that extent the defense of avoidance or "nonthinking" about sex was less necessary.

However, the sophisticated reader will raise the question whether this represents a lasting solution. There are two major risk factors here: The first is whether, as comfort replaces distress, Nancy might revert to her old style of avoidance, distance, and disinterest. Clinically it appears that this threat is considerably reduced. The other risk is based on an object relations or systems model of marital relationships (Segraves, 1982). Given Michael's susceptibility to abandonment and rejection, he might recreate the sexual stress between them because he may not yet have mastered the challenge of his own dynamics in this evolving sexual dance.

REFERENCES

Althof, S. E., Turner, L. A., Levine, S. B., Risen, C., Kursh, E., Bodner, D., & Resnick, M. (1989). Why do so many people drop out from auto-injection therapy for impotence? *Journal of Sex and Marital Therapy, 15*, 121–129.

Beck, A. T. (1976). *Cognitive therapy and the emotional disorders.* New York: New American Library.

Belsky, J. (1990). Children and marriage. In F. D. Fincham & T. N. Bradbury (Eds.), *The psychology of marriage.* New York: Guilford Press.

Dunkel-Schetter, C., & Lobel, M. (1991). Psychological reactions to infertility. In A. L. Stanton & C. Dunkel-Schetter (Eds.), *Infertility: Perspectives from stress and coping research.* New York: Plenum.

Fincham, F. D., Bradbury, T. N., & Scott, C. K. (1990). Cognition in marriage. In F. D. Fincham & T. N. Bradbury (Eds.), *The psychology of marriage.* New York: Guilford Press.

Gotlib, I. H., & McCabe, S. B. (1990). Marriage and psychopathology. In F. D. Fincham & T. N. Bradbury (Eds.), *The psychology of marriage.* New York: Guilford Press.

Hartman, L. M. (1983). Resistance in directive sex therapy: Recognition and management. *Journal of Sex and marital therapy, 9*, 283–295.

Heiman, J. (1986). Treating sexually distressed marital relationships. In N. S. Jacobson & A. S. Gurman (Eds.), *Clinical handbook of marital therapy.* New York: Guilford Press.

Hendrix, H. (1990). *Getting the love you want. A guide for couples.* New York: Harper & Row. (Original work published 1988)

Horowitz, M. J. (1987). *States of mind: Configurational analysis of individual psychology* (2nd ed.). New York: Plenum Press.

Horowitz, M. J. (1991). States, schemas, and control: General theories for psychotherapy integration. *Journal of Psychotherapy Integration, 1*, 85–102.

Kaplan, H. S. (1974). *The new sex therapy.* New York: Brunner/Mazel.

Kaplan, H. S. (1979). *Disorders of sexual desire.* New York: Brunner/Mazel.

Kaplan, H. S. (1990). The combined use of sex therapy and intrapenile injections in the treatment of impotence. *Journal of Sex and Marital Therapy, 16*, 195–207.

Lassen, C. L. (1976). Issues and dilemmas in sexual treatment. *Journal of Sex and Marital Therapy, 2*, 32–39.

Lazarus, A. A. (1982). Resistance or rationalization? A cognitive-behavioral perspective. In P. Wachtel (Ed.), *Resistance.* New York: Plenum Press.

Lazarus, A. A. (1988). A multimodal perspective on problems of sexual desire. In S. R. Leiblum & R. C. Rosen (Eds.) *Sexual desire disorders.* New York: Guilford Press.

Leiblum, S. R. (1994). The impact of infertility on marital and sexual satisfaction. *Annual Review of Sex Research, 4*, 99–120.

Leiblum, S. R., & Rosen, R. C. (Eds.). (1989). *Principles and practice of sex therapy* (2nd ed.). New York: Guilford Press.

LoPiccolo, J., & Friedman, J. M. (1988). Broad-spectrum treatment of low sexual desire: Integration of cognitive, behavioral, and systemic therapy. In S. R. Leiblum & R. C. Rosen (Eds.), *Sexual desire disorders.* New York: Guilford Press.

Masters, W. H., & Johnson, V. E. (1970). *Human sexual inadequacy.* Boston: Little, Brown.

Meichenbaum, D., & Gilmore, J. B. (1982). Resistance from a cognitive-behavioral perspective. In P. Wachtel (Ed.), *Resistance.* New York: Plenum Press.

Notarius, C. I., Benson, P. R., & Sloane, D. (1989). Exploring the interface between perception and behavior: An analysis of marital interaction in distressed and nondistressed couples. *Behavioral Assessment, 11*, 39–64.

Notarius, C., & Markman, H. (1993). *We can work it out: Making sense of marital conflict.* New York: G. P. Putnam.

Radin, M. M. (1989). Preoedipal factors in relation to psychogenic inhibited sexual desire. *Journal of Sex and Marital Therapy, 15*, 255–268.

Segraves, R. T. (1982). *Marital therapy. A combined psychodynamic–behavioral approach.* New York: Plenum Press.

Wachtel, P. (Ed.). (1982). *Resistance.* New York: Plenum Press.

Zilbergeld, B., & Hammond, D. C. (1988). The use of hypnosis in treating desire disorders. In S. R. Leiblum & R. C. Rosen (Eds.), *Sexual desire disorders.* New York: Guilford Press.

14

Relinquishing Virginity: The Treatment of a Complex Case of Vaginismus

SANDRA R. LEIBLUM

INTRODUCTION

Vaginismus is a perplexing and challenging clinical problem. Women who experience the involuntary, spasmodic contraction of the pubococcygeal and related muscles controlling the vaginal introitus may be unable to tolerate vaginal penetration or to have intercourse but may be living in long and relatively happy marriages with regular sexual exchange. Often, they are orgasmic with manual or oral stimulation but display a striking phobic response to the anticipation of or attempt at vaginal entry. Over time, the sexual script shared with their partner or spouse becomes constricted, invariant, and, ultimately, unsatisfying. Usually, it is only when the pressure to overcome the problem becomes unbearable, because of either internal humiliation or external pressure, that the woman seeks sex therapy.

INCIDENCE OF VAGINISMUS

Although figures concerning the incidence of vaginismus vary widely, it is likely that it occurs with greater frequency than is typically acknowledged. Vaginismus rates have been reported as being between 12% and

17% of women presenting to sexual therapy clinics (Hawton, 1982; Spector and Carey, 1990). While primary vaginismus is not uncommon, many women experience partial or situational vaginismus; that is, they may be able to tolerate tampon insertion or gynecological examination, but panic at the anticipation or attempt of penile entry. During sexual encounters, the vaginal entrance is so constricted that it feels like an impenetrable "wall," lubrication is scant, and penetration, if it occurs at all, is experienced as quite painful. Not surprisingly, a woman with a long history of vaginismus often has a partner who has developed erectile difficulties or who displays sexual avoidance because of the expectation of frustration and failure.

ETIOLOGY OF VAGINISMUS

Unlike dyspareunia, where physical factors are commonly implicated and must be carefully ruled out before beginning psychotherapeutic treatment, primary vaginismus tends to be of psychological etiology. Often, but not always, a history of sexual abuse, gynecological trauma, religious orthodoxy, or extremely restricted sexual upbringing predates the vaginismus. Usually, a variety of factors contribute to creating vaginismus. Fear of intimacy and of loss of control, negative maternal modeling concerning vaginal penetration, poor self-esteem, sexual ignorance and misinformation, intrusive gynecological examinations, physical or sexual abuse during childhood, and clumsy male partners are just a few of the etiological contributors to vaginismus. Lazarus (1989) has suggested that three classes of factors are implicated in the development of dyspareunia, and these same factors are often associated with the etiology of vaginismus as well: (1) developmental factors (e.g., negative psychosexual upbringing, religious taboos that invest sex with shame and guilt, intrapsychic fears and conflicts), (2) traumatic factors (e.g., rape, violent first intercourse), and (3) relational factors (e.g., conflicted and antagonistic feelings toward men in general or one's sexual partner in particular, poor sexual technique).

Secondary vaginismus is common. If women have experienced vaginal pain due to infection, surgery, or chemical agents, they are often understandably apprehensive about vaginal penetration and may develop arousal problems. The lack of arousal, coupled with lack of lubrication, can create a tightening of the vaginal introitus when penetration is attempted.

Vaginismus was cited by Masters and Johnson (1970) as being among the sexual disorders most rapidly and successfully treated. Nevertheless, the reality is that cases of unconsummated marriage are often quite refractory to intervention. Treatment can be lengthy, with many obstacles and roadblocks to progress created by both the identified patient and her partner. Often, the motivation to overcome the problem is mixed and each step forward may be followed by periods of sexual inactivity or, at times, lapses into sexual avoidance. Even when success seems tantalizingly near, the couple may dally and linger, fearful of accomplishing the last but most critical step of intercourse. Then, having accomplished successful intercourse, they may or may not pursue future coital contact with enthusiasm and pleasure.

TREATMENT MOTIVATION: HIS? HERS?

The woman with vaginismus is oftentimes a reluctant patient. Typically, she has been plagued by fears of vaginal penetration for many years, beginning in early adolescence. While her peers have begun menstruating and have made the transition from sanitary pads to tampons without fanfare or difficulty, the vaginismic woman typically is unable to do so. In fact, attempts at vaginal penetration are often so fraught with anxiety and tension that fainting and nausea may accompany early efforts. She finally abandons such anxiety-laden attempts and keeps the shameful secret of her failure to herself.

Early dating is often associated with anxiety and ambivalence. Although the vaginismic woman may enjoy necking and petting, genital exploration arouses anxiety and avoidance. When other girls are at an age to lose their virginity, during adolescence or early adulthood, the vaginismic woman typically guards her vagina from being touched or entered. Thoughts of vaginal penetration often elicit overwhelming fears of being ripped apart and injured.

When she does find a sympathetic and nonintrusive partner, they often collude (consciously or unconsciously) in establishing a sexual script that precludes vaginal exploration. Manual and oral stimulation may occur readily, and satisfying orgasms may accompany sexual encounters. Nevertheless, any attempt at vaginal penetration usually results in frustration, failure, and feelings of fear and incompetence. The male partner may develop arousal or erectile problems of his own as a reaction to his partner's visible tension and anxiety during attempts at penetration. Over time, all such efforts typically diminish or disappear altogether and the couple's sexual life either withers away or is very narrowly scripted. There can be no spontaneity in the sexual script if each partner must guard against receiving or inflicting pain or discomfort.

This state of affairs may continue for many years until the male partner becomes so frustrated that he threatens separation and/or an affair, or, alternatively, the pressure and desire to start a family are compelling. Often, it is only when no alternative to the status quo is obvious that the woman is propelled into treatment.

The example that follows is a complex and extended, but in some respects characteristic, case of long-standing vaginismus. It illustrates the fact that "sex therapy" is seldom characterized by step-by-step "cookbook" approaches but rather a complex psychotherapeutic process that incorporates ongoing exploration of intrapsychic conflicts, couple dynamics and transference issues. Marital therapy is an intrinsic part of treatment, as is individual psychotherapy. Often, progress is slow and erratic and, at times, both patient and therapist may wonder whether successful intercourse will ever occur.

CASE EXAMPLE

Treatment in this case occurred over a period of 4 years. Because a session-by-session description of therapy is not feasible, the treatment is described as a sequence of five major phases.

Phase I: Building a Therapeutic Alliance

Gina, a 34-year-old lawyer, had been married for 13 years at the time treatment began. She entered therapy reluctantly after being referred for sex therapy following her discharge from an alcohol rehabilitation center where she had been an inpatient for the preceding 6 weeks. She had not sought help for her chronic alcoholism but rather had entered treatment following a planned confrontation by her husband, parents, and friends. She hated being an inpatient at the rehabilitation hospital and "felt like a prisoner there." She was deprived of her freedom to come and go at will and was subjected to an intense therapeutic regimen in which all aspects of her life and behavior were scrutinized. It was in the rehabilitation center that her sexual difficulties were identified and her unconsummated marriage became the subject of investigation. The psychiatrist at the center raised the possibility that her vaginismus was the result of her latent homosexuality and her fear and hatred of men. Although she had never considered herself "gay," the suggestion that she might be seemed plausible to her because she believed that homosexuality was partly inheritable and because her biological father was a closet homosexual who had "come out" shortly after she entered college. His disclosure resulted in the separation and subsequent divorce of her parents.

Gina was "confused" and extremely distressed by the suggestion that she might be homosexual without even realizing it; she denied feeling any sexual attraction to women. Upon discharge from the rehabilitation center, she was referred to a psychiatrist who referred her, in turn, for sex therapy.

At the first session, she was notably depressed, anxious, and tense. Talking about sexuality elicited considerable anxiety and she displayed a mixture of anger and guilt about her past history of alcoholism. Although she admitted that her drinking had "gotten out of hand" and was destroying her marriage, she was outraged and humiliated by the confrontation with her parents and friends.

She related to me in a tentative way, expressing uncertainty about all her comments. She looked for confirmation and watched my face closely for signs of approval or disapproval. Despite her evident discomfort, she was able to display flashes of wit and sarcasm, both at herself and at her predicament. Her face was mobile and expressive and she was easy to like. Her pain was palpable although disguised, at times, by her clever jibes at herself and others. She often elicited feelings of compassion and warmth from me.

The first 6 months of treatment were devoted to exploring her past history and reinforcing her abstinence from alcohol. Her husband was seen sporadically during this time. The major treatment goal in the early stages of therapy was on developing a relationship with Gina and establishing me as a nonjudgmental and supportive ally. This was deemed especially important because Gina's past relationships with "authority" figures were characterized by authoritarian overcontrol or servile obedience.

Over many sessions, the following history gradually emerged: Gina was the oldest of two siblings; her younger brother was 5 years her junior. Her mother was a homemaker; her father a salesman. She described a childhood filled with tension, physical abuse, and anxiety. Her father was an explosive and reactive tyrant who demanded absolute obedience. At any sign of misbehavior, he would physically strike out at his children, and the household was organized around placating and pacifying "Dad." If he came home from work in a bad mood, he would criticize his wife and beat his children, making them the scapegoats of his frustration and irritation. Trying to read his moods and ward off his anger were central features of everyday life.

Gina's mother played the role of a traditional wife who related to her husband in a passive, deferential way. When he had one of his "fits" in which he beat or pummeled her son or daughter, she would stand by helplessly. She never intervened to protect her children because she was fearful of becoming the next "victim." Gina recalls feeling indignant at her mother's failure to protect her.

Affection was virtually nonexistent in the household. Gina witnessed no instance of affectionate exchange between her parents or between her parents and herself. The only form of physical attention she remembers receiving was her mother brushing her long hair and spending hours setting and arranging it into fat curls around her face. In fact, Gina feels that her mother treated her like a "doll" to be played with and displayed rather than a flesh-and-blood youngster.

Sexuality was viewed as something dangerous and disgusting. Not only was there no evidence of any positive sexual feelings between her parents, but the whole topic was surrounded with prohibitions and shame. Gina recalls that her older cousin became pregnant out of wedlock and was held up to her as an object lesson. "If you ever get pregnant," she recalls her mother saying, "don't bother to come home!"

Gina learned the "facts of life" through information transmitted in a pamphlet provided by a manufacturer of sanitary pads. Her mother was clearly embarrassed at discussing sex and reproduction with her, and Gina responded by avoiding asking any questions that might embarrass her mother. She does remember complaining about menstrual discomfort and having her mother retort, "If you think this hurts, just wait till you go through childbirth!"

Gina had an intense but ambivalent relationship with her younger brother. Although he was subjected to the same paternal abuse that she was, Gina often made him the target of her own anguish and rage. Because she was physically bigger and stronger during the early years of their childhood, she would lash out at him whenever he "crossed her." Once he outdistanced her in height and weight, however, he would retaliate and physical brawls would result. Intermittently, however, they would join together as protective allies and privately express their impotent fury at their father. They both learned to use humor as a defense against their helplessness.

Gina was an excellent student at school and was a model of obedience and responsibility. She was popular and had many girlfriends. She never felt physically attractive, however, because she was tall, gangly, and awkward, with a large nose and mouth. She eventually had rhinoplasty during early adolescence, which improved her physical appearance and increased her self-confidence. Boys liked her for her outrageous wit and verbal quickness. She liked them as well but discouraged physical closeness.

When Gina entered college, she was ready to "break loose" and started to associate with a crowd that drank heavily. At the same time,

she became involved with a boyfriend who was domineering and physically abusive, not unlike her father. She was ultimatley "rescued" from
this relationship by the man who was to become her husband. He was
protective and kind, although rather passive and insecure. They quickly
formed an intense attachment, which was, however, dependent on alcohol and a rather symbiotic closeness.

In looking back at this significant part of her history, Gina realized
that three major events occurred within a single year of her life: She
started drinking, she moved in with her boyfriend, Paul (her current
husband), and she learned that her father was bisexual.

In retrospect, Gina speculated that living with Paul exacerbated her
sexual anxieties and she became increasingly dependent on alcohol to
"loosen" her up sexually. Paul was sexually naive and did not press Gina
to have intercourse, especially when she so visibly panicked at the approach of his penis. He, too, was sexually anxious and was afraid of
inflicting pain on her. Sexually, they depended on drinking to disinhibit
them, and they developed a sexual script that relied on manual stimulation and oral sex. Although sexual contact was relatively infrequent, both
were reasonably content.

This state of affairs continued for many years. It was not without
its costs, though. Gina felt inadequate and deficient as a woman and
avoided gynecological examinations. Paul would occasionally become
enraged at a seemingly small provocation and verbally attack Gina. Internally, he reported feeling humiliated, emasculated, and ashamed about
the nonconsummation of their marriage. When his coworkers teased and
joked about "getting it on" sexually, he felt alone in the private knowledge that he had never penetrated his wife despite 13 years of living and
sleeping together.

Eventually, as Gina's drinking escalated, the marital conflict grew
intolerable. When Gina was drunk, she would verbally berate and abuse
Paul. Her attacks and complaints about his passivity and lack of assistance with housework and her disparagement of his passion for sports
undermined the earlier closeness they had experienced. Although he
would usually tolerate her drunken tirades silently, he began to blow up
more readily and would verbally attack her. Thoughts of leaving the
marriage and/or having an affair occurred with greater frequency, although Paul was reluctant to do either.

Finally, he felt impelled to take action. Paul was depressed and dis-
enchanted with his life and increasingly worried about the possibility that
Gina's alcoholism would result in the loss of her job. He told Gina's
mother about her daughter's drinking and together with mutual friends
and his family's support arranged the confrontation that resulted in
Gina's admission to the rehabilitation center. It was only following her

inpatient hospitalization and commitment to sobriety that sex therapy could be initiated.

Phase 2: Sex Therapy Begins

After almost a year of individual and couple therapy, Gina was ready to seriously begin work on her sexual problems. Although I had encouraged Gina to engage in self-exploration and masturbation exercises earlier in treatment, Gina had avoided these suggestions. She would start each session with complaints about Paul, work, and her father and would skillfully distract me from focusing on her sexual conflicts. When this was pointed out, Gina would acknowledge that it was true but declared that as long as her relationship with Paul was so fraught with resentment and anger, she had no desire to be intimate with him. When I suggested that overcoming the vaginismus needed to be a personal goal rather than "something she did for Paul," Gina agreed but continued to behave as though intercourse would benefit Paul alone.

Nevertheless, through a combination of conjoint and individual sessions, the marital tensions ebbed and Gina became more tolerant of Paul's need to spend time away from her, primarily in sports activities. Gina also began to recognize that Paul would and did become more involved in sharing domestic responsibilities when she criticized him less for the way in which he performed them. For his part, Paul became more expressive and open as a reaction to Gina's greater acceptance. Over time, there were fewer and fewer explosive outbursts.

It was only when their relationship had become more stable and harmonious and Gina had maintained sobriety for 1 year that she finally began masturbation and self-dilation efforts. She was readily orgasmic with masturbation although she had difficulty inserting her fingers into her vagina despite adequate lubrication. I suggested purchasing a set of dilators, which would provide Gina with some measure of control and external confirmation of her therapeutic progress. Although Gina joked about their appearance, in sessions she would proudly announce her successful insertion of succeedingly larger ones and, in fact, at home she displayed them in a row across her nightstand.

Although progress was slow and periods of sexual inactivity were frequent, Gina was successful in graduated vaginal dilation and was encouraged to permit Paul to use his fingers to enter her vagina. This was a more difficult step for Gina and she had to be assured that she would remain in control and could "stop the action" whenever she needed to.

Paul was extremely gentle with Gina during these exercises. At times, he was overly cautious but supportive and involved. As the time for penile pentration approached, Gina became distracted by a host of family issues. Her anger at her father resurfaced when he reentered her life. His long-term lover had died of AIDS and he was responsible for the funeral arrangements. He called Gina and indicated that he wanted to live with her for 3 weeks while he attended to the affairs of his former lover. Gina was resentful at having to play "host" to him, especially as memories of his past abuse and selfishness returned. She felt trapped between wanting his love and approval and furious that he had never acknowledged his failures as a father. Rather, he felt entitled to be "taken care of," wanting his laundry done and his meals prepared. Gina's mother was not sympathetic to Gina's ambivalent feelings about her father and Gina felt alone and conflicted.

During this period, Gina remembered and relived many events from her childhood dealing with her father's physical abuse. She stopped doing her sexual "exercises," vented her feelings more readily against Paul, and was emotionally labile. It was only following her father's departure and further individual therapeutic work that she was ready to move forward.

Phase 3: Intercourse Accomplished!

As a result of Gina's success with vaginal dilation, she began to talk about the possibility of scheduling her first gynecological examination. She had never had a Pap smear taken and was cognizant of the importance of doing so, especially as she was approaching 40. Because she was successful at using tampons and was able to relax with dilator insertion, she was willing to consider a gynecological visit. Nevertheless, she delayed scheduling an appointment for some months and it required confrontation by me and a promise that I would speak to the gynecologist prior to her appointment to overcome her resistance. Although Gina was anxious during the 24 hours preceding the doctor's visit, the examination was a success and Gina felt triumphant about being able to tolerate what she had avoided for over 20 years. In fact, she was so proud of joining the ranks of "normal women" that she prominently displayed the follow-up card from the gynecologist informing her that her Pap smear was normal.

Shortly after this event, 2 years into treatment, Gina and Paul had successful coitus. Paul was ecstatic; Gina less so. In exploring their reactions to consummating their marriage and the implications of the "event," it was apparent they viewed it quite differently. Paul felt that his manhood was affirmed. He no longer needed to "fake" knowledge of intercourse and could join the ranks of effective lovers. Moreover, he was thrilled at the possibility that they could now attempt to start a family.

Gina was less enthusiastic. She stated that intercourse did not feel particularly good to her and that she remained "tight." Although she intellectually appreciated the fact that more frequent coital relations would increase her comfort and, possibly, her pleasure, she felt that she could no longer refuse to have intercourse with Paul since she was now capable of doing so. Moreover, she was terrified at the idea of childbirth.

Several sessions were devoted to exploring Gina's anxieties. Paul reassured her that intercourse was only an option, not a requisite part of their sexual encounters. Moreover, he assured her that she could refuse sex any time. To both Paul's and my chagrin, however, Gina took this permission literally, and avoided sexual intimacy whenever she could. It was only upon resolving her fear and ambivalence about motherhood that she was more receptive to engaging in additional attempts at intercourse.

Phase 4: Pregnancy and Parenthood

During the third year of treatment, Gina and Paul made two major life changes: They purchased their own home and they decided to try to have a baby.

Paul had always been clear about his wish to have a child: He loved children and was confident about his ability to be an effective and caring father. Paul was so eager to begin parenting that he told Gina that if she was unwilling or felt unable to tolerate a pregnancy, he would be happy to adopt a child instead.

Gina worried about her ability to be a good mother. She feared that she lacked patience and might abuse her child in the way that she had been abused. She recalled an incident at the beach when she had became so angry at Paul that she threw a book at him with the intent of hurting him. Moreover, she felt that she would be the one who would be "stuck" with all the childrearing responsibilities.

It took many months of therapy, working with Gina alone and with Paul and Gina together, to resolve these worries. She came to realize that it was unlikely that she would be physically abusive. As a result of her own therapy, she was extremely aware of the disastrous consequences of physical punishment on a child. Moreover, her brother had become a father and she was both observant and critical of how he treated his child. She was determined to be a gentle, consistent parent. In fact, I suggested that Gina would likely err on the side of under- rather than overcontrol, given her worries about abuse.

Gina was reassured as well by Paul's assertions that he was committed to sharing parenting responsibilities equally. They discussed various scenarios they might encounter (e.g., staying home with a sick infant, giving up recreational activities, dealing with overly intrusive grandparents). They eventually felt more confident about their ability to negotiate mutually agreeable solutions.

Gina then raised concerns about the gender of her prospective child. She said she really wanted to have a son rather than a daughter. "Girls were catty, hostile, and bitchy," declared Gina, and "I couldn't tolerate a coy, overly feminine, seductive child." We considered whether these fears were evidence of projections about herself and also explored whether she might be jealous of the possibility that Paul would prefer the company of a daughter to that of herself.

Finally, considerable time was spent dealing with her fears of pregnancy and childbirth. Gina was anxious about undergoing prenatal examinations, amniocentesis, and vaginal delivery. Each of these issues was discussed. The concern about having to deliver vaginally was discussed in depth as it was the issue that caused the greatest ambivalent feelings in Gina. She felt she "should" deliver vaginally in order to prove that "she wasn't a wimp," but she was terrified of being ripped apart and experiencing intolerable pain. I challenged Gina's belief that the only way to prove her worth as a woman and as a mother was through a vaginal birth. Evaluation of her success as a mother was contingent upon how she raised her child, not on how it was delivered, and, in fact, Caesarean section might be a more sensible birth option given Gina's long history of vaginismus.

Once these and other issues were worked through clinically, Gina became pregnant within 3 months. She and Paul were overjoyed. They displayed greater intimacy, humor, and compatibility during the pregnancy than ever before in their marriage. Gina threw herself into decorating the "nursery" and preparing for motherhood. Paul religiously attended all prenatal visits with Gina and radiated pride when teased about his impending fatherhood.

When Gina discovered she was going to have a daughter, she was psychologically "ready" and cried as she said that her daughter would never have to experience what she had undergone. Gina felt she now had a chance to "do it right" and could symbolically reparent herself through mothering her daughter.

As the time for childbirth drew near, Gina's anxiety increased and the issue of vaginal versus Caesarean delivery resurfaced. Gina's obstetrician was opposed to scheduling a Caesarean section if it was not medically indicated and Gina was increasingly conflicted about "chickening out" on vaginal delivery. Finally, with Gina and Paul's consent, I consulted with the obstetrician, explaining why a Caesarean section was psychologically important in this particular case. To run the risk of undoing all the therapeutic progress that had been accomplished over the preceding 4 years seemed senseless. The obstetrician concurred.

Soon thereafter, Gina gave birth to a healthy, beautiful 8-pound daughter without complication and I received a bouquet of roses and a heartfelt birth announcement.

Phase 5: Life after Birth

Gina and Paul did not live happily ever after. The first postpartum year was a time of conflict and anxiety. They argued, as do most new parents, about what to do, when to do it, and who was doing more. As might have been anticipated, Gina was an overly protective and devoted mother. In fact, she was so intent on doing things "right" that she only reluctantly permitted Paul to share infant care responsibilities. Despite these predictable "adjustment to parenthood" reactions, Gina and Paul were generally ecstatic with their role as parents and with their new daughter.

Nevertheless, the couple had a difficult time in recapturing the intimacy they had experienced during the pregnancy. Fatigue, disagreements, work responsibilities, and inertia/avoidance discouraged attempts at sexual intimacy. While they both acknowledged that "something needed to be done," neither took a particularly active role in reestablishing their sex life. In fact, because of Gina's involvement in full-time mothering and her satisfaction with this role, she decided to terminate therapy when her daughter was 3 months old, with the understanding that she could recontact me at any time in the future.

Pictures and notes arrived periodically, but Gina did not appear for a follow-up visit until her daughter was 1 year old. At that time, she called to discuss relations with her father, who had disappointed her yet again. When asked about her relationship with Paul, Gina replied that they were getting along well but had been coitally intimate only three times during the preceding year. Gina said that this state of affairs was agreeable to her and if it was a problem for Paul, it was his responsibility to "do something about it." With that comment and the announcement that she was thinking of having a second child, the session ended. At present, 4 years after termination, Gina contacts me only at holidays when she sends the latest picture of her daughter and an upbeat message about herself.

COMMENTARY

Was a successful outcome achieved in this case? The answer is not obvious and any judgment must consider both the patient's goals and those
of the therapist.

Gina entered therapy confused about her sexual orientation, phobic
about intercourse, and ambivalent about motherhood. Her marriage was
threatened and she had only recently come to grips with the fact that
she was an alcoholic. Her husband, Paul, was depressed, frustrated, and
uncertain about his marital commitment. The couple had been unable
to have intercourse during the 16 years they had been together. Each
felt signficantly ashamed and inadequate.

At termination, Gina and Paul were a committed couple who owned
a home and had a child. Gina had maintained sobriety for 4 years and
was certain of her heterosexual orientation. She and Paul were loving
and devoted parents. They had achieved harmony, if not marital bliss.
They knew they were capable of having coitus, even though they usually chose not to. Sexual contact was infrequent but was not a primary
source of anguish or marital conflict. Gina and Paul were more than
pleased with the outcome of therapy. I was less so.

This case is a poignant reminder of how an early history of abuse
and neglect can disrupt sexual functioning. Gina was not sexually abused
but she was physically abused, repeatedly and traumatically. She could
never quite relax at the prospect of physical intimacy and could never
totally trust a male, despite significant progress in both realms.

For Gina, sexuality was intrinsically dangerous and "penetration"
was to be avoided at all costs. It is a credit to her emotional resiliency
that eventually she was able to accomplish successful intercourse and to
have a child. Nevertheless, she never quite resolved her feelings of dis-
taste for and suspicion about sex. While she could see the importance of
sex for procreation, its ability to provide pleasure, comfort, or soothing
was slight.

Paul was also sexually insecure. Although his sexual drive was greater
than Gina's, he, too, was fearful about the destructive, as opposed to
the pleasurable, aspects of sex, and so he hesitated about resolving the
sexual impasse that had characterized their marriage for more than a
decade. His fear of eliciting anger and/or rejection from Gina prevented
him from taking an active stance in regard to her alcoholism until it
became absolutely necessary. In a similar fashion, he avoided taking an
active position with respect to their sexual difficulties, preferring to "make
do." At termination, it appeared that I was more upset about the lack of
sexual frequency than were either Gina or Paul.

Vaginismic couples are often a challenge but satisfying to work with. Typically, treatment is *ultimately* successful, even if it appears to be slow going at times. Although most cases are not as chronic and complex as the case presented, this one is illustrative of the kinds of issues and interventions that characterize treatment. While the goal of therapy is the resolution of the phobic response to penetration via a program of graduated dilation and relaxation exercises, treatment typically includes considerable emphasis on marital issues. The partner ought to be included in therapy as his fears and anxieties usually contribute directly to the ultimate success or failure of treatment.

When treatment is successful, as it often is, it is extremely gratifying for both the couple and the clinician. Months or years later, the therapist often learns that what once had been a dyad has become a triad.

REFERENCES

Hawton, K. (1982). The behavioral treatment of sexual dysfunction. *British Journal of Psychiatry, 140,* 94–101.

Lazarus, A. (1989). Dyspareunia: A multimodal psychotherapeutic perspective. In S. R. Leiblum & R. C. Rosen (Eds.), *Principles and practice of sex therapy* (2nd ed.): *Update for the 1990s* (pp. 89–112). New York: Guilford Press.

Leiblum, S. R., Pervin, L. A., & Campbell, E. (1989). The treatment of vaginismus: success and failure. In S. R. Leiblum & R. C. Rosen (Eds.), *Principles and practice of sex therapy* (2nd ed.): *Update for the 1990s* (pp. 113–138). New York: Guilford Press.

Masters, W. H., & Johnson, V. E. (1970). *Human sexual inadequacy.* Boston: Little, Brown.

Spector, L., & Carey, M. (1990). Incidence and prevalence of the sexual dysfunctions: A critical review of the empirical literature. *Archives of Sexual Behavior, 19,* 389–408.

15

Sex Therapy following Treatment by an Exploitive Therapist

S. MICHAEL PLAUT

INTRODUCTION

The ethical standards of medicine and of the mental health professions have long recognized the potential harm of sexual contact between provider and client (Gabbard, 1989; Gonsiorek, 1995; Peterson, 1992; Rutter, 1989). The power differential inherent in such relationships renders the patient vulnerable and thus unable to participate in such a relationship as a truly consenting person. In such a trust-based relationship, therefore, the responsibility for maintaining boundaries resides in the professional. Although boundary violations occur in all four gender combinations, reports involve male providers and female patients in about 90% of cases.

As Schover (1989) has indicated, it is unusual for qualified sex therapists to become sexually involved with their patients. However, reports of sexual exploitation by professionals in general have increased markedly over the last decade. Patients victimized by such professionals are thus increasingly likely to seek help from therapists, either for assistance in addressing the exploitive incident itself or for the problem for which they originally sought help from an exploitive therapist.

Joyce and Glen came to me for treatment with no knowledge that I had a professional interest in this field, not only in an academic sense (Plaut & Foster, 1986) but also as one who was frequently involved in disciplinary cases, both as an expert witness and as a member of a state licensing board. However, if that experience played a role in their therapy at all, it was probably an attitude of restraint rather than intervention with regard to their former therapist's exploitive behavior.

Professionals learning of an alleged sexual exploitation fall along a spectrum of possible responses, ranging from disbelief and mistrust of the complainant to anger at the alleged offender. Expression of neither serves the patient's best interests. For example, it is not helpful for the therapist to encourage a patient to bring charges if she is not so inclined. Doing so can only revictimize the patient, and there are many good reasons why a victim may not wish to bring formal charges—at least immediately, and sometimes not at all (Ameringer & Plaut, 1993). She may be reluctant to face the offender in a hearing or courtroom or may be convinced that no one would take her seriously. She may feel that he helped her despite his exploitive behavior. She may blame herself for her participation in the sexual relationship. Or, she may just want to put it all behind her. The new therapist can provide information about ethical standards or legal options and can refer the patient to support groups or experts in the field. Perhaps the most important roles of the therapist are to help the patient understand that she is not at fault and to help her enhance her sense of empowerment, so that whatever decisions she makes are clearly hers. As was true in the present case, the victim's partner may need support as well.

It may also be important to help the patient understand that her well-being must be based on how effectively she addresses her own issues, and not on the outcome of a legal case. The wishes of the patient can range from not wanting to destroy the career of someone who was otherwise helpful to an expectation that the therapist will be removed from the profession, or even imprisoned. However, there are often alternatives between these extremes, and there are many factors that determine the outcome of a legal case, most of which are out of the hands of both the patient and the therapist.

The exploitation case of Joyce and Glen was not among the more serious from an objective point of view (Gabbard, 1989). It did not involve a long therapist–patient relationship, nor did it result in hospitalization, divorce, or suicide, as many unfortunately do. The couple made a firm and timely decision to report Dr. S to appropriate authorities. However, the relatively "mild" nature of this case makes its example all the more poignant and the coercive power that we all have over our patients all the more weighty a consideration in how we do our work

(Levine, 1992; Peterson, 1992; Rutter, 1989). The influence of Dr. S clearly wove itself throughout the entire therapeutic process with me and has had a lasting impact on both members of the couple.

CASE HIGHLIGHTS

Glen was a 35-year-old white male referred by an internist. He had experienced difficulty either achieving or maintaining erections with all previous partners, although masturbatory erections had never been problematic. His poor self-esteem and passive style led him to accept the apparent inevitability of his problem. However, Joyce, his 35-year-old wife of 7 years, was becoming increasingly impatient about her failure to become pregnant and insisted that they seek professional help.

They had originally been referred by a physician to Dr. S, a psychologist who was not known in the professional community as a sex therapist. Unfortunately, Dr. S made a number of inappropriate interventions, including sexual overtures toward Joyce during one of a number of individual sessions. By the time of their first session with me, Joyce and Glen had reported Dr. S to the state licensing board. However, the incident with Dr. S had clearly compromised the couple's "trust in professionals in this field," prolonged their therapy, and is still an issue for them as of this writing, 5 years later.

Although Joyce and Glen were highly motivated and cooperative for the most part, the therapy was complicated further by Glen's difficulties in relating to women, Joyce's impatience with Glen's passivity, a number of family crises, and stresses related to Glen's work and Joyce's return to graduate school. As with many couples seeking help with sexual problems, Glen and Joyce also had to address and overcome certain sexual stereotypes. For them, a significant obstacle (reinforced by their previous therapist) was the notion that a man was not a man unless he could have successful intercourse in the male superior position. I saw Glen and Joyce a total of 39 times over a 24-month period, with a 7-month hiatus after the first 25 sessions, by which time they were having consistently successful intercourse in the female superior position. They returned to therapy after a relationship crisis and terminated the week after they learned that Dr. S's license had been revoked.

EVALUATION AND TREATMENT OF ERECTILE DYSFUNCTION

Initial evaluation of an erectile problem should determine the circumstances under which erections may or may not occur (e.g., upon wakening, during masturbation, during contact with all or with specific partners, or at times of stress), the extent of erection as observed by both the male and his partner, and situations surrounding the onset of the problem (e.g., high alcohol consumption, termination of a previous relationship, or moving in with the partner).

The evaluation should account for the possibility of a medical basis, and any doubt that the symptoms are not purely psychogenic should lead to referral to a urologist who is knowledgeable of and skilled in the appropriate methods of medical evaluation. Any patient whose erectile dysfunction was gradual in onset, whose erection is partial or nonexistent under all conditions, or who discloses a history of illness or medication known to cause erectile failure should be referred to an appropriate physician.

A complete description of an appropriate medical workup is beyond the scope of this chapter. Frequently used techniques for the evaluation of erectile dysfunction in addition to a genital and prostate exam may include determination of nocturnal penile tumescence and buckling pressure in a sleep laboratory or with the aid of a home monitor; measurement of penile blood flow using Doppler techniques and imaging; glucose tolerance tests; levels of testosterone, follicle-stimulating hormone, luteinizing hormone, prolactin, and thyroid hormone; and perhaps electromyography, a corpora cavernosagram, and an arteriogram. Using the right combination of tests, the physician can determine the extent to which the disorder may have a neurological, hormonal, or circulatory basis (Spark, 1991).

It is always possible that there is a psychogenic component to a medically based erectile dysfunction or vice versa, and it is important for physician and sex therapist to maintain close contact so that the patient is treated most appropriately. Even a primarily medical intervention, such as a penile implant, may require counseling, which involves the partner as well as the symptomatic patient.

Medical interventions are becoming increasingly sophisticated. There are a few types of penile implants, ranging from inflexible to inflatable, varying in cost and risk of malfunction. Self-injection of papaverine or prostaglandin E has been recently introduced as a therapeutic technique appropriate for some men, as has the use of a vacuum pump. The latter has a chamber placed over the flaccid penis from which the user pumps air. The penis becomes erect in the rarified environment of the chamber, and the erection is maintained by a constricting band once the chamber is removed. Choice of these methods depends on a number of factors, including etiology of the dysfunction, cost, and the tendency of the patient to comply with one method or another.

In many cases, as in the one reported here, there is no evidence of a medical basis for the problem, and Glen had, in fact, been referred by a physician for psychotherapy. Specific aspects of the psychosexual evaluation and treatment techniques are presented in the context of the case description.

CLINICAL CASE DESCRIPTION

Sexuality is still a difficult issue for many people, "sexual revolution" notwithstanding. As a society, we do not learn about sexuality well, we do not communicate about it easily, even with those with whom we are close, and we therefore tend to go through life with relatively narrow, stereotypical, and tentative ways of defining and expressing our sexuality.

Therefore, a therapist's first obligation to his/her patients is to help them feel comfortable discussing these difficult issues and looking at their sexuality in a way they may never have done before. This can best be done if the therapist appears to be both comfortable and nonjudgmental in how the subtle but often important details of history are gathered, and in how behavioral assignments are handled. A tasteful level of light-heartedness and encouragement helps to relieve anxiety and create a comfortable, accepting environment. All this was especially important in the present case, as the couple had every reason to be initially suspicious because of their experience with Dr. S.

Therapy is conducted as much as possible with the couple, allowing opportunities for individual evaluation and therapy sessions as appropriate. As Masters and Johnson (1970) first demonstrated so well, the solution to a sexual problem can be greatly facilitated by the shared commitment of the relationship itself. In the present case, for example, Joyce's motivation, resistance, observations, preoccupations, and support all contributed prominently to the therapeutic process, even though it was Glen who had presented with the sexual symptom of erectile dysfunction.

The primary goal of therapy is to alleviate the presenting symptoms following a cognitive-behavioral approach, focusing on what Kaplan (1974) has called the "immediate causes" of the sexual problem (e.g., performance anxiety or difficulties with fantasy). Patients may be invited to reassess their therapeutic goals as they redefine important issues for themselves. When "deeper" issues need to be addressed, they are, either with the couple or through concurrent or subsequent referral for individual therapy. In the present case, for example, issues in the relationship clearly contributed to the sexual symptoms and these were addressed in therapy. However, as Althof (1989) has written, there is a danger in doing "too much too soon." It is most effective to focus primarily on issues relevant to the presenting problem—issues with which the couple can easily identify—modifying the focus as necessary.

Evaluation

General Procedures

Before the first appointment, two copies of a Background Information Questionnaire, modeled after one used by the Masters and Johnson Institute, are mailed to the couple. This questionnaire is used to provide basic demographic data, referral source, living status, religious preferences and practices, names and addresses of relevant physicians, current medications, previous therapy for the presenting problem, and a brief statement of why they are coming for therapy and what they hope to accomplish by this process. Most of this information is covered again in the diagnostic interview. However, the form provides some documentation, encourages the couple to give some thought to what they are about to do and why, and gives me an idea of how each member of the couple sees the issues at hand.

I begin the first session by establishing rapport with the couple, finding out a bit about who they are and some basic information about their relationship (are they married, living together, how long, who lives with them, etc.). My interview style follows the basic outline proposed by Kaplan (1983), that is, description and history of the chief complaint, sexual status examination (to be described below), brief medical and psychiatric histories, family and sexual history, and relationship history and status. Glen was not referred for further medical evaluation because it was clear that he was able to achieve firm erections consistently in masturbation.

The sexual status examination involves a detailed description of recent sexual and/or relationship experiences, including specifics of planning, setting, thought, conversation, behavior, and perceptions. In this way, the subtle things that so often get in the way of successful sexual activity can be more readily identified and addressed. The sexual status examination is generally performed near the beginning of each therapy session in order to provide a detailed assessment of responses to the previous week's behavioral assignments and any other sexual or relationship issues that have come up. In addition to providing important clinical data, the expectation of providing this information each time helps the couple to focus on aspects of their sexuality and their relationship of which they may have been relatively unaware.

I see each member of the couple individually for at least part of one session in order to determine anything that might be of importance to an assessment of the problem but which each person may not feel comfortable sharing with his/her partner. This may include aspects of history, concerns about the relationship, affairs, or fantasy material. With the knowledge of both partners, I may schedule additional individual sessions as needed.

The Couple

Glen and Joyce were both observant Roman Catholics who had grown up in the Midwest. They met each other in college, were then geographically separated for a couple of years, but maintained a correspondence friendship over that time. Their marriage was generally a close, caring, and even playful friendship, and Joyce had remained dutifully accepting of their only rare occurrences of sexual intercourse until she began to feel the advances of the "ticking clock." Her increasing frustration at their inability to conceive and at Glen's reluctance to seek help expressed itself in temper outbursts and what he privately termed "belligerent, smart remarks" that further threatened his already poor self-esteem.

As is often the case in sex therapy, the sexual problem was symptomatic of other issues in the relationship that tend to play out in a sexual context. Joyce complained privately that Glen had difficulty expressing affection in general, and that he also was reluctant to express anger—a concern that she would express more powerfully a few weeks into the therapy.

Both Glen and Joyce had experienced dysfunctional family backgrounds. He was the youngest of four brothers, all sons of a physically abusive father. Glen had come to realize that intimate times shared by his parents typically followed quarrels involving physical abuse, which led Glen to associate sex with violence and to become convinced that he could never function as a man should. At one time he thought that he would never marry. He was a sensitive, gentle, somewhat passive person who had an almost naive, poetic way of looking at his life experience—a part of him that endeared him to Joyce despite his passivity. Yet, in describing a sexual encounter with Joyce, he would often refer to her in the third person (e.g., "It feels so good to touch a woman").

Joyce was an only child raised by an alcoholic, physically abusive, frequently absent father and a mother with whom she had always been close. She was a considerate, generous person in many ways but tended to press appropriate therapeutic boundaries, even in conjoint sessions, by her almost excessive warmth and attention toward me, even to the point of asking mildly personal questions. She once said, "I think of you as a friend as well as a counselor." She was clearly frustrated sexually and had said privately that she had even considered going outside the relationship. In addition, the tension resulting from their sexual problems led the couple to cancel many of their social engagements, leaving them in a somewhat isolated state.

At the time they came for therapy, Joyce and Glen were also experiencing concerns about their respective careers. He worked as a data analyst for a consulting firm, where he felt stiff competition for advancement. She was a math major who was doing secretarial work and had just decided to seek her master's degree in secondary education. She was not happy with her program, however, and was still uncertain about her career direction.

The Previous Therapist

Joyce and Glen terminated their work with Dr. S about 6 months before being referred to me. Following a pattern often seen in sexual exploitation cases, Dr. S began to see Joyce and Glen in separate sessions soon after an evaluation of their sexual concerns. Although this might have been appropriate under some circumstances, exploitive therapists often use such a device to sabotage the couple's relationship while gaining access to their intended victims. During one session, after telling Joyce that his wife would not have sex with him, he opened his fly and invited her to perform fellatio on him. She declined, paid her fee, and left, never to return. It was a number of weeks before she could tell Glen what had happened and why she had terminated therapy.

Dr. S also made a point of setting certain sexual standards for the couple, including the expectation that "real men" have intercourse in the male superior position, perpetuating a myth that was to haunt both members of the couple throughout much of their therapy with me.

Treatment

Kaplan (1974) has suggested that a useful initial assignment is to "prescribe the symptom." That is, the couple is encouraged to accept—at least for the present—that the problem is there and to stop trying to do something that just does not work. This assignment tends to result in a sense of relief and reduces anxiety enough that the couple can begin to focus more on alternatives to intercourse. (On occasion, this practice even results in erections.)

Behavioral assignments may involve reading, videos, exercises, and/or fantasy, depending on the needs of the couple and the moment. There is an effort to be flexible and innovative in developing productive homework assignments, designing each assignment in accord with the comfort level of the couple and their immediate therapeutic goals. Behavioral prescriptions can be diagnostic as well as therapeutic, and they can even be somewhat provocative at times. For example, couples often have difficulty "finding time" for their assignments, and one member of the couple may, initially at least, be reluctant to take the initiative in proposing a sexual session. In such cases, I may suggest that the more resistant member of the couple take the initiative during a given period. It is also sometimes necessary to give one member of the couple greater control over specific activities, such as initiating intercourse.

Sex therapy typically involves some teaching and reframing of the patient's concept of sexuality, and the use of mnemonic devices and metaphor facilitates this process. For example, the possible functions of sex may be outlined using the "four R's"—reproduction, recreation, relationship, and release. A patient experiencing loss of erection may be reminded that "there's always another bus around the corner." Such devices tend to be both permission giving and anxiety reducing. Patients tend to remember them, often repeating them back to the therapist and to their partners later in the course of therapy.

Four areas of focus were ultimately important in the present case. A behavioral and cognitive reframing of Joyce and Glen's concept of sexuality helped them to look at their sexual expectations with a more realistic perspective. Forming an alliance with Joyce and encouraging her to be more patient and supportive of Glen helped facilitate the therapeutic process and their sexual interactions. Discussion of the family issues helped both of them understand their role in Glen's conceptualization of himself as a man and in his image of Joyce as a woman. Finally, their experience with the previous therapist produced an undercurrent that prolonged the therapy for a number of reasons, making this one of the longest sex therapy cases I have encountered.

Phase I: Deceptive "Progress"

I recommended two books to this couple. Zilbergeld's *The New Male Sexuality* (1992) is often quite useful in normalizing a common human activity that is so often subject to distorted perceptions. In asking Glen one day what he was learning from the book, he referred to what he termed "the myth of the hard-driving f**k." It was clear that he was beginning to get the message.

The second book, which I often find useful for sex therapy patients, is *Touching for Pleasure* (Kennedy & Dean, 1986). This well-illustrated and tastefully written book discusses sensuality, touch, body image, genital anatomy, and related issues. It also provides a number of exercises, many of which can serve as a useful adjunct to therapy, more often because they provide the couple with ideas and with "permission" than because any one particular exercise is recommended. The use of bibliotherapy can also be diagnostic. Whereas one person might say, for example, "Oh, I knew all that stuff," another might say, "I never thought you could get so involved in just caressing your partner's face." Joyce and Glen were much closer to the latter.

As Althof (1989) has said, rapid "progress" in sex therapy can often be deceiving. In a way, this should not be at all surprising. Part of the diagnostic feature of the behavioral exercises often used in sex therapy is that the level of anxiety is titrated in such a way that the specific thresholds that are difficult to cross become quite apparent as they are reached under relatively controlled conditions. In this case, that threshold occurred at the point of genital–genital contact.

The first three levels of behavioral treatment went surprisingly well. Joyce and Glen were not only compliant with suggestions but comfortable and playful with each other in an intimate setting. Assignments began with nondemand sensate focus exercises in which each partner touches the other in turn, with the emphasis being on the sensations experienced by the *active* partner, thereby minimizing performance anxiety (Kaplan, 1974; Masters & Johnson, 1970). At this first level, genitals and breasts were off limits to touch.

At the second level, prescribed the following week, genital touch was permitted but in context with the rest of the body and not with the intent of inducing sexual excitement. That is, breasts and genitals are "normalized" by encouraging them to touch these areas essentially as they would any other area of the body, and certainly not as an area that one only "leads up to." They were comfortable at this level as well, and Glen was sometimes having erections during the exercises. He did raise some concern about how Joyce provided feedback to him when she was not comfortable with the way he touched her, saying that he felt "reproached."

The third level added the opportunity to stimulate the partner to orgasm either manually or orally, but with intercourse still prohibited. Both partners had orgasms through manual stimulation, the only problem being Glen's concern with rapid ejaculation. For the fourth week, therefore, Glen was taught how to do the Semans (1956) stop–start exercises in masturbation, so that he could gain greater control over his level of excitement as he approached the point of "ejaculatory inevitability." This brief experience was useful in helping him feel more confident about his body awareness. For the couple, I recommended genital–genital contact with Joyce in the superior position, stimulating Glen to orgasm, but with no attempt at penetration. Although this went well the first week, it was a different couple that returned after a 2-week holiday break.

Phase 2: Setback and Reorientation

"We fell into bad habits," reported Glen, saying that he was finding himself distracted in sexual situations and was unable to have either erections or orgasms consistently with manual stimulation. He was anxious about the prospect of genital contact and had been losing sleep over it. In tears, he said, "I feel stalled. I feel like a prisoner of my problem."

Joyce was furious, and her anger generalized to other situations that she had been previously unable to discuss in his presence. "He's too agreeable," she said. "I wish he'd be more assertive and stand up to me more!" For the first and only time in therapy, she talked of divorce. To their credit, they returned to the first level of sensate focus exercises on their own, and that began to restore their confidence. As they climbed back through the behavioral sequence over the next few weeks, Joyce became more supportive, and Glen was increasingly able to see her as his lover rather than as the generalized "woman" to whom he did not know how to relate.

Guided imagery was used to help Glen with his discomfort and guilt regarding sexual fantasy and his tendency to become distracted. These exercises, performed with both members of the couple in session, invited them to focus on sensual settings of their choice and to enhance, in turn, whatever sensory modalities increased the effectiveness of the imagery. Such exercises can help increase comfort with fantasy and help the patient realize the level of control he/she has over the nature, intensity, and variety of fantasy experiences. I often suggest an analogy of a library of fantasy "tapes" that we each carry in our heads, that we can make and edit for ourselves and select from at will. I also encourage the couple to identify and respond to characteristics or behaviors in each other that were "turn-ons," whether these were physical attributes, a style of walking, or a specific article of clothing. Thus, it became easier for each of them to "become" their partner's fantasy.

About 6 weeks into this phase of therapy, there was a perfectly timed happy accident, as the couple took a weekend trip over a holiday weekend. They picked a hotel room with a Jacuzzi, and the escape from work, school, and home was just enough to take them past a critical point in their therapy. They sat through their next session holding hands. Two weeks later, Glen experienced his first lasting vaginal intromission.

Phase 3: Improvement and Consolidation

I suggested a review of the couple's therapeutic goals. Although their goals were quite realistic and perceptive, they occasionally recalled the stated expectation of Dr. S that intercourse in the male superior position was to be expected of any man. The legal case against Dr. S was also developing at that point as those involved were being interviewed by the state's investigators, and Glen and Joyce were beginning to work with their very supportive prosecutor from the Office of the Attorney General. Unfortunately, they were only able to come in every other week over the next few months, so that what they accomplished in those 14 sessions might have taken less time with more concentrated work.

Glen continued to experience successful intromission and was able to cope comfortably with any loss of erection, having learned that another one would come along in due time—just like the bus. This attitude was aided by his increasing focus on Joyce's sexual needs, now that his confidence was improving. He continued to work on fantasy and was now able to have erections with kissing, no longer requiring direct penile stimulation. He also took an increasingly supportive role as Joyce was struggling with problems in her course work.

A remaining problem was Glen's difficulty ejaculating intravaginally. It was suggested that he masturbate in Joyce's presence as a way of bridging his ability to ejaculate alone and during intercourse. It was then suggested that he masturbate in Joyce's presence and place some of his semen in her vagina. He did and was able to have successful intercourse in the female superior position that same week. A month later, Joyce commented, "You never miss now." They decided to terminate after the next session, having experienced another romantic weekend away. They talked about having moved "from the era of Dr. S to an era of good feeling." Their accomplishments and remaining goals were then reviewed, including the advisability of referral for individual therapy. However, their immediate concern remained their desire for children, and it was on that objective that they wanted to place their energy.

Phase 4: Return to Treatment

A few months later, Glen called from a phone booth. Things were in crisis, he wanted to return to therapy, but Joyce had refused, saying that therapy was just "a crock." Glen was invited to come in alone, which he did. He said that sex was going well, at least mechanically, but that Joyce had still not gotten pregnant and was insisting that they have sex in the male superior position, which was still not possible for Glen. I suggested that fertility testing might be appropriate at this point, and I invited the couple to return to therapy in order to discuss the issue further.

Three weeks later, they came together for the first of 14 sessions spread over an 8-month period. Joyce was so focused on having intercourse every day with the single objective of pregnancy that she had lost the patience for romantic sex and for Glen's continuing inability to have intercourse in the one position she had become convinced was necessary for fertilization to occur. I suggested that they go through a brief sensate focus refresher. The following week, Joyce said, "I had forgotten how relaxing it really was." Improvement continued over the next week, when the couple also reported that the hearing on the case of Dr. S had been scheduled for the following month—an impending event that caused some anxiety for both members of the couple, each of whom would be expected to testify in some detail. Even though Joyce had always been certain of who was at fault, she knew she would be challenged, as such victims typically are, about her possible role in instigating the actions of Dr. S.

Much of the time during these months was spent discussing a number of challenges that Joyce and Glen were facing during that period, including the hearing, a major math exam for Joyce, and a confrontation between Glen and his older brother that gave him a sense of autonomy within his family that he had never before experienced.

A second area of focus was on the romantic aspects of their relationship. They improved in their ability to identify and respond to the things about each of them that each had experienced as seductive and became more playful with each other (e.g., "clowning around naked in the kitchen"), and Glen reported enhanced orgasms as he became more immersed. They experimented with different intercourse positions and discovered the rear entry position. When attempts at male superior intercourse failed, they were able to recover and do what worked. "We wonder why we ever had problems," said Glen one day. "It's just so good." One day they asked for a referral to a fertility program—something I had recommended to them at least 8 months earlier. The following week they learned that Dr. S's license had been revoked and said they were ready to terminate therapy. Sex was not yet "perfect," but they felt they had the tools to continue on their own. Whatever they had gained in their work with me, their first priority remained the one that had brought them in 2 years earlier—having a baby.

Follow-Up

About 2 years after termination, I made a follow-up call, simply asking how things were going. Glen answered and immediately called Joyce to an extension phone. They volunteered information in a number of areas, and no detailed questions were posed. Their fertility problem was still unresolved and they were now working with a different clinic. However, they had become comfortable with the possibility of adoption if things did not work out. More important, they spoke of a "marital renaissance," describing their sex as "vibrant," and saying that "we do it when we feel like doing it." Joyce volunteered that she was just now getting to the point where she could discuss her experience with Dr. S with close friends. I was tempted to do a complete sexual status exam—to find out whether they could have intercourse in the male superior position. But it really did not matter. About a year after that call, I received a birth announcement in the mail.

EPILOGUE

This case illustrates many of the important considerations in sex therapy, and psychogenic erectile dysfunction in particular—the need to understand and respect the patient's therapeutic goals and, in particular, the frequently consuming nature of concerns about infertility; the importance of attending to the needs and responses of both members of the couple; the frequent merit of assessing and reframing the patient's sense of sex and self; the timing and use of behavioral assignments for both diagnostic and therapeutic purposes; and the value to the couple of occasionally escaping from daily stresses but, at the same time, the need to integrate sexual growth with their busy and demanding lifestyle.

What was unique about this case, however, was the profound impact of a boundary violation that was perceived by both patients (and by the profession) as a serious betrayal of trust. It can never be known whether treatment would have been of shorter duration or more "successful" if that incident had not happened. What is known is the extent to which the incident made its presence felt throughout the therapeutic process—in its description by both members of the couple in the original background information form; in the frequent references to the former therapist's inappropriate sexual performance expectations for Glen and the tendency for both members of the couple to retain these expectations as a "standard" of success; in Joyce's difficulty discussing the incident, first with her husband and then with friends, for so long a time; and in the apparent coincidence of their return to therapy a month before the hearing and termination within 1 week of the license revocation. All of this underscores both the gravity of such a violation and the role that the mental health professional can play in supporting those who are victimized and helping them to reestablish their trust in those from whom they would seek professional help.

ACKNOWLEDGMENTS

My style of doing sex therapy has been greatly influenced by the people whose personal teaching, supervision, example, inspiration, and encouragement have affected me along the way. Primarily these people have included Ellen Hollander, Helen Singer Kaplan, Stephen Levine, Anne C. Lewis, William Masters, Judith M. Plaut, Richard Sarles, Mark Schwartz, and Linda Weiner. I attribute to them a good part of my skill, perspective, and confidence as a therapist. Responsibility for clinical judgment is mine alone.

I am deeply indebted to Peter Fagan, Susan E. Hetherington, Stuart L. Keill, Anne C. Lewis, Sharon Nathan, Catherine D. Nugent, Judith M. Plaut, and James W. Thompson for their helpful comments on the manuscript.

REFERENCES

Althof, S. E. (1989). Psychogenic impotence: Treatment of men and couples. In S. R. Leiblum, & R. C. Rosen (Eds.), *Principles and practice of sex therapy* (2nd ed., pp. 237–265). New York: Guilford Press.

Ameringer, C. F., & Plaut, S. M. (1993). Advising patient–victims of sexual misconduct by mental health professionals. *Maryland Bar Journal, 26,* 42–44.

Gabbard, G. O. (Ed.). (1989). *Sexual exploitation in professional relationships.* Washington, DC: American Psychiatric Press.

Gonsiorek, J. C. (Ed.). (1995). *Breach of trust: Sexual exploitation by health care professionals and clergy.* Thousand Oaks, CA: Sage.

Kaplan, H. S. (1974). *The new sex therapy.* New York: Brunner/Mazel.

Kaplan, H. S. (1983). *The evaluation of sexual disorders.* New York: Brunner/Mazel.

Kennedy, A. P., & Dean, S. (1986). *Touching for pleasure.* Chatsworth, CA: Chatsworth Press.

Levine, S. B. (1992). *Sexual life: A clinician's guide.* New York: Plenum Press.

Masters, W. H., & Johnson, V. E. (1970). *Human sexual inadequacy.* Boston: Little, Brown.

Peterson, M. R. (1992). *At personal risk: Boundary violations in professional relationships.* New York: W. W. Norton.

Plaut, S. M., & Foster, B. H. (1986). Roles of the health professional in cases involving sexual exploitation of patients. In A. W. Burgess & C. Hartman (Eds.), *Sexual exploitation of clients by health professionals* (pp. 5–25). Philadelphia: Praeger.

Rutter, P. (1989). *Sex in the forbidden zone.* New York: Fawcett Crest.

Schover, L. R. (1989). Sexual exploitation by sex therapists. In G. O. Gabbard (Ed.), *Sexual exploitation in professional relationships* (pp. 139–149). Washington, DC: American Psychiatric Press.

Semans, J. (1956). Premature ejaculation: A new approach. *Southern Medical Journal, 49,* 353–358.

Spark, R. F. (1991). *Male sexual health: A couples guide.* Yonkers, NY: Consumers Union.

Zilbergeld, B. (1992). *The new male sexuality.* New York: Bantam.

16

A Case of Premature Ejaculation: Too Little, Too Late?

RAYMOND C. ROSEN

INTRODUCTION

Premature ejaculation is a highly prevalent, frequently misunderstood, and sometimes debilitating male sexual dysfunction. Prevalence estimates of this common disorder have ranged from 20–50% of American males. For example, in their classic survey of 100 "happily married couples," Frank, Anderson, and Rubenstein (1978) found that 36% of males reported difficulty in controlling ejaculation or ejaculating too rapidly on most occasions. In our own recent study of 263 male medical students (Leiblum, Rosen, Platt, Cross, & Black, 1993), 26% of the sample reported ejaculating too rapidly on at least half of all intercourse experiences. Other surveys have reported that as many as 60% of males have intermittent concerns about rapid ejaculation (Reading & Wiest, 1984). Although there is some evidence of a decline in the number of cases of premature ejaculation presenting to sex therapy clinics in recent years, (Spector & Carey, 1990), it continues to be an important and challenging clinical problem.

A major limitation has been the lack of a clear-cut definition or diagnostic criteria for the disorder. Masters and Johnson (1970) initially defined premature ejaculation in terms of the male's ability to delay ejaculation until his partner had been sexually satisfied on at least 50% of intercourse attempts. Noting the lack of objectivity in this definition, other authors have emphasized the average duration of intercourse (Cooper & Magnus, 1984; Kilmann & Auerbach, 1979; Strassberg, Kelly, Carroll, & Kircher, 1987) or number of thrusts following penetration (Colpi, Faniullacci, Beretta, Negri, & Zanollo, 1986; Segraves, Saran, Segraves, & Maguire, 1992). A third approach has been to emphasize the degree of voluntary control that the male has over ejaculation (Kaplan, 1974; McCarthy, 1989). This approach assumes that voluntary control of ejaculation is a necessary prerequisite for sexual satisfaction of both partners. None of these definitions is entirely satisfactory, as is illustrated by the imprecise and relatively ambiguous diagnostic criteria of the fourth edition of the *Diagnostic and Statistical Manual of Mental Disorders* (DSM-IV):

A. Persistent or recurrent ejaculation with minimal sexual stimulation or before, on, or shortly after penetration and before the person wishes it. The clinician must take into account factors that affect duration of the excitement phase, such as age, novelty of the sexual partner or situation, and frequency of sexual activity.
B. The disturbance causes marked distress or interpersonal difficulty. (American Psychiatric Association, 1994, p. 511)

Several typologies of premature ejaculation have been proposed. For example, Cooper, Cernovsky, and Colussi (1993) have distinguished between primary or lifelong premature ejaculators, and those with secondary or situational premature ejaculation. In support of this dichotomy, these authors found that men with primary premature ejaculation were generally younger and had higher levels of sexual anxiety and increased libido. In contrast, patients with secondary premature ejaculation had a higher incidence of erectile dysfunction and other performance difficulties.

Learning factors have been strongly implicated in the development of premature ejaculation. Early experiences with masturbation, in particular, have been linked with a sexual style that is "penis-focused, goal-oriented, rapid and intense" (McCarthy, 1989). Early experiences with partner sex can also foster early ejaculation, as many adolescent males function autonomously and without much need for sexual stimulation from their partners. High levels of sexual excitement in combination with high anxiety, in many instances, lead naturally to rapid ejaculation. According to McCarthy (1989), the majority of males begin their sexual lives as premature ejaculators. Whereas some men develop skill and ejaculatory control in later years, others fail to progress.

Treatment approaches for premature ejaculation have ranged from the early stop–start and squeeze techniques (Semans, 1956; Masters &

Johnson, 1970) to the more recent use of pharmacological agents, such as alpha-adrenergic antagonists (e.g., phenoxybenzamine) or serotonin uptake inhibitors (e.g., fluoxetine and clomipramine). Whereas initial reports suggested that conditioning techniques (i.e., stop–start, squeeze) are successful in more than 90% of cases (Kaplan, 1974; Masters & Johnson, 1970), more recent studies indicate a much lower overall success rate (Hawton, Catalan, Martin, & Fagg, 1986; Kilmann, Boland, Noton, Davidson, & Caid, 1986). According to one study, almost all the posttherapy gains had been lost by the time of a 3-year follow-up (DeAmicis, Goldberg, LoPiccolo, Friedman, & Davies, 1985). Several explanations have been offered for the apparent decrease in effectiveness of sex therapy treatments for premature ejaculation, including the greater availability of self-help materials and resulting decrease in "straightforward" cases presenting for sex therapy, as well as methodological limitations of earlier studies (Zilbergeld & Evans, 1980).

In recent years, strong interest has developed in the use of pharmacological agents for the treatment of premature ejaculation. Serotonergic antidepressants, such as Prozac (fluoxetine) and Anafranil (clomipramine) have been especially recommended. Assalian (1988), for example, reported a series of five case studies in which chronic premature ejaculation was successfully treated with clomipramine (25 mg), taken on a once-daily basis. Several of these patients had been previously unresponsive to conventional sex therapy. Similarly, Segraves et al. (1992), in a double-blind study of clomipramine and placebo, found increased ejaculatory control with clomipramine in seven out of eight men with premature ejaculation. In this study, clomipramine (25 mg) was taken 6 hours before intercourse. According to the authors, the mean ejaculatory latency increased from 30 seconds on placebo to 9.9 minutes on clomipramine.

More recently, Althof, Levine, Corty, Risen, and Stern (1994) conducted a double-blind, crossover evaluation of placebo and two doses of clomipramine (25 and 50 mg) in 15 men with a chronic history of premature ejaculation. Ejaculatory latencies were increased from 77 to 202 seconds in the 25-mg condition, and to 458 seconds in the 50-mg condition. Withdrawal of the drug resulted in an immediate return to baseline values. Significant improvements in sexual satisfaction were reported by both male patients and their partners, whereas only the men reported improvements in relationship satisfaction. The authors recommend combining clomipramine with conventional sex therapy approaches. It can also be concluded that the drug is effective when taken both in single doses (i.e., about 3–6 hours before intercourse) or on a daily basis.

Despite the promise for efficient and cost-effective treatment of premature ejaculation with these drugs, several limitations and possible drawbacks should be considered. First, serotonergic drugs may be associated with diminished arousal or desire in some patients (Hollander & McCarley, 1992; Monteiro, Noshirvani, Marks, & Lelliott, 1987). For patients with premature ejaculation and erectile difficulties, in particular, these drugs are strongly contraindicated. Additionally, patients may encounter other adverse effects, such as sedation, dry mouth, and constipation. Finally, little attention has been given to the psychological implications of drug therapy for this disorder and the possible effects of long-term medication use on psychological dependency or lack of self-esteem (McCarthy, 1994).

In the following case, both conventional sex therapy and drug treatment (clomipramine) were used in the management of primary premature ejaculation. The long-term impact of the sexual disorder on the couple's marital and sexual relationship was a major concern, and the wife's response to therapy was a critical factor in determining treatment outcome. Overall, the case illustrates the complex interaction of sexual and relationship issues in an apparently straightforward case of premature ejaculation. The case also demonstrates the potential value of drug treatment (Anafranil) as an adjunct to traditional sex therapy for this disorder. The way in which the couple responded to this intervention and the need for ongoing couple therapy are key points in the case. Finally, the case illustrates the potential impact of factors outside the relationship (i.e., affairs and job changes) on the course of therapy.

CASE STUDY

Max and Rita J are an attractive Jewish couple in their early 40s, who were referred by a local urologist for treatment of Max's long-standing problem of premature ejaculation. Although the problem dated back to his first sexual experience at age 19, Max's lack of control had worsened notably in the past 5 years. "I don't know why this is happening to me," he stated, "but I seem to have lost complete control of the problem." During the past 6 months, the couple attempted intercourse only three times, and Max ejaculated prior to penetration on two of the three occasions. He felt frustrated and ashamed of his total lack of ejaculatory control and had virtually ceased initiating sexual contact with his wife. In turn, Rita felt angry and resentful that Max had delayed seeking help for their problem for so many years. She had virtually lost all interest in further sexual contact.

At the time they entered therapy, the couple had been married for 18 years and had two teenage sons, ages 14 and 11. They began dating in high school, and neither had had any prior sexual experiences. Rita was initially attracted to her husband's "good looks and easy personality" and recalled their early dating experiences as positive. Although Max ejaculated rapidly during their first intercourse experience (both were still virgins), neither perceived this to be a particular problem at the time. They attended the same college together and were engaged to be married during Max's senior year. The marriage was strongly encouraged by Rita's parents, who perceived Max to be "ideal husband material" for their daughter. By this time, Rita was aware of feeling less physically and emotionally attracted to Max but felt strong pressures to get married from both her parents and her fiance.

During the early years of their marriage, sexual relations were sporadic and relatively unsatisfying for both. Max would typically initiate sexual encounters, and intercourse occurred after a brief (i.e., 5–10 minutes) period of foreplay. At times, Max was able to delay his orgasm for several minutes, but more frequently he would ejaculate after 5 or 10 thrusts. Rita experienced little arousal and no orgasm during intercourse but waited almost 2 years before expressing her frustration to Max. When the issue finally surfaced, he responded defensively and blamed Rita for being "frigid" and unresponsive in bed. Several heated arguments ensued, although no resolution was achieved. Rita states that she simply "gave up" on trying to change or improve their sexual relationship. In turn, Max blamed their sexual difficulties on his wife's lack of interest or experience, and believed that "things would naturally improve" over time.

In other respects, the early years of their marriage were relatively satisfactory. Max completed his graduate degree in business administration and began working for an investment banking firm. During this period, Rita worked part-time as a substitute teacher and became active in community affairs. She remained close with her parents, who lived in the next town, and spent many afternoons visiting with her mother and sister. At times, Max complained that his wife was too closely tied to her parents and family and that the couple had little or no time for themselves. She responded that he "cared more about his job than his marriage," and resented his attempts to come between her and her parents.

With the birth of their first child, the couple enjoyed a period of renewed closeness. Max was an attentive and involved father who had no difficulty in adapting to his new role. Similarly, Rita was delighted with her newborn infant. Although the couple was sexually inactive for several months prior to and following the birth, neither felt much discomfort at the lack of sexual contact. When Max finally began to initiate sex again, the twin difficulties of his premature ejaculation and Rita's lack of arousal returned in full force. Both had secretly hoped that the problem might have been resolved in the interim, resulting in a strong sense of mutual disappointment and frustration. In particular, Rita recalls feeling "trapped and helpless" in the face of her husband's unwavering denial and refusal to confront the problem. "I kept wondering what was wrong with me," she states, "and if this was all there was to sex in marriage."

In reviewing the couple's history to this point, two basic issues need to be addressed: First, what factors might account for Max's lifelong pattern of premature ejaculation and complete failure to develop control over time? Second, why was this couple so unable or unwilling to confront their sexual and relationship difficulties more directly? In some respects, Max and Rita seemed to be colluding actively in maintaining the sexual status quo. What factors in each of their respective backgrounds might account for this pattern of mutual avoidance and emotional distance?

Backgound Information

Max's Story

Max was the youngest of two sons in an upper-middle-class, suburban Jewish family. Always a good student at school, Max saw himself as his mother's favorite. He felt distant and alienated from his father, however, who traveled frequently on "business trips" and showed little interest in the family. In his early teens, Max discovered that his father had been involved in a series of extramarital affairs over the years. His mother had suffered from a wide range of medical conditions during this time, including stomach ulcers, hypertension, and migraine headaches, all of which she blamed on her husband's infidelity. The lack of communication and emotional distance between his parents placed a significant strain on Max. He dealt with the family conflict by immersing himself in his schoolwork and withdrawing emotionally.

Not surprisingly, sex education was virtually nonexistent in this family environment. Aside from a few biologically oriented lectures at school, Max received little or no information on the topic. He began to masturbate at age 12 and usually felt anxious and guilty about this activity. Although he was unaware of difficulty in delaying or controlling orgasm, he recalls ejaculating rapidly on most occasions: "I felt it was wrong, and wanted to get it over with as soon as possible." In his early dating experiences, Max was shy and unassertive. He felt relieved when Rita took the lead in their relationship during his senior year in high school. He became highly aroused during their petting experiences and ejaculated in his pants on several occasions. He recalls feeling embarrassed and uncomfortable when this occurred. The couple's first intercourse took place after several months of dating, and Max ejaculated rapidly as described earlier.

Rita's Story

Rita describes herself as a "typical Jewish princess," growing up in the affluent suburbs of a large metropolitan area. Her father was a highly successful businessman, and the family enjoyed a comfortable lifestyle throughout her childhood and adolescence. Rita was the middle of three children (older brother, younger sister) in a closely knit, traditional family. She describes her father as a strong-willed and domineering man who was nevertheless physically affectionate with both his wife and his children. In contrast, Rita perceived her mother as self-effacing and submissive in the relationship and a "real pushover" for the family. At times, Rita felt intimidated by her father's judgmental attitudes, and she often felt pressured to seek his approval. This was especially true when Rita began dating in high school, as she was warned repeatedly against getting involved with the "wrong types." She dated sporadically prior to meeting Max and had no experience of intercourse or orgasm. She was attracted to Max's good looks and quiet personality and was especially pleased with the ready acceptance he received from her parents. In fact, Max began working in her father's office during his second year in graduate school.

In part, she blames the pressure she felt from her parents to marry Max, as well as the absence of prior dating experience, for her failure to address the intense sexual frustration in their relationship. "If only I had known better at the time!" Rita stated wistfully in our first individual interview, "I would never have married him if I knew what lay ahead." Like many women in this situation, she naively assumed that their sexual relationship would naturally improve over time. And, like her mother, she felt uncomfortable when confronting her husband on this or any other topic.

After joining a woman's group in her mid-30s, Rita became orgasmic during masturbation. When she attempted to guide Max in stimulating her toward orgasm, however, he became defensive and angry. As their sexual script became increasingly restrictive and goal directed, Rita felt herself becoming less and less aroused. Sexual contact diminished to once a month or less, and Max's premature ejaculation became even more severe.

The Affair

A major turning point occurred when Rita became involved in a sexual relationship with Joe, the husband of a neighborhood friend. Rita's relationship with Joe developed gradually during the course of a summer in which both were involved in managing their sons' soccer team. Several times Joe and Rita went out for coffee following an afternoon game, and Rita found herself becoming increasingly attracted to Joe. Unlike her husband, Joe seemed genuinely interested in Rita's feelings and opinions and talked openly about his difficulties in his own marriage. Their meetings became more frequent during the fall, and Rita offered little resistance when Joe suggested they visit a motel one afternoon after lunch.

The ensuing affair lasted for 14 months and represented a "sexual awakening" for Rita. She found Joe to be a confident and passionate lover. In marked contrast to Max, he had no difficulty in controlling ejaculation and Rita was able to experience, for the first time, protracted and mutually satisfying intercourse. Although limited by the need for secrecy, the couple continued to meet at least once weekly throughout this period. Despite increasing guilt and anxiety about their involvement, Rita felt herself to be "magnetically drawn" to Joe, and could not imagine ending their affair.

How did Max react to these changes in his wife? Surprisingly, he seemed oblivious to the detachment and moodiness that characterized Rita's behavior during the first few months of her affair. His suspicions were aroused, however, when Joe's wife made comments on several occasions about "how good Joe and Rita looked together." During this period, Rita also showed increasing disdain and disinterest in Max's sexual advances, and eventually she refused any sexual contact whatsoever. After discovering that she had lied one afternoon about having lunch with her mother, Max hired a private detective to have his wife followed.

Events moved rapidly from this point. Within 3 weeks, the detective agency reported to Max that it had photographic proof of his wife's sexual infidelity. Max immediately confronted Rita, who then confessed completely to her involvement with Joe over the past year. After several stormy exchanges, Rita finally agreed to end her relationship with Joe if Max would stop having her followed. As his initial anger subsided, Max decided not to leave the marriage and to give his wife "a second chance." He acknowledged that their sexual relationship had been disappointing and frustrating to both of them, and he agreed to enter therapy for his premature ejaculation.

For her part, Rita wonders whether she made the right decision in staying with Max. "Even though sex was great with Joe, I couldn't bring myself to break up my family." She was also apprehensive about the potential effects on Joe's family and pleaded with Max not to tell Joe's wife about their involvement. Again, Max agreed to this request if Rita would promise to end their affair permanently. At this point, the couple made a decision to enter therapy. It should be emphasized that all these events occurred *before* the couple actually began treatment. Much of the early phase of therapy consisted of processing these events with the couple and with each of them individually.

Sex Therapy: The Initial Evaluation

Max asked to be seen alone for the first several sessions. He appeared tense and withdrawn, at first, and sought frequent reassurances that he had "done the right thing" in confronting his wife on the subject of her affair. He blamed himself for the sexual and emotional distance in their marriage and regretted not coming for therapy earlier for his premature ejaculation. "If only I hadn't put it off so long," he exclaimed, "none of this would have happened!" The goal for therapy, according to Max, was simply to gain better control of his ejaculation. If this could be accomplished, he was certain that Rita would be sexually satisfied, and that other problems in the marriage would be resolved. He acknowledged feeling intimidated by his wife, both sexually and emotionally, although he seemed reluctant to explore this aspect of their relationship further.

Following three individual sessions with Max, I requested to see Rita alone. While acknowledging that Max's premature ejaculation was indeed a major source of frustration for her, Rita raised two additional problems:

1. Her continuing anger and mistrust of Max because of his "spying" on her during the affair. Rita stated she was not sure that Max had stopped having her followed, and had twice recently felt she was being "watched."
2. Her sexual interest and attraction to Max had been steadily declining since the early years of their marriage. She complained of increasing difficulty in becoming lubricated or aroused, and she was experiencing a degree of sexual aversion in their recent sexual contacts.

With my encouragement, Rita agreed to confront these issues more directly in the next conjoint session.

Over the next several months, I gradually introduced couple communication and sensate focus exercises. Although the couple made limited progress in alleviating Max's performance anxiety and in increasing Rita's level of trust, she continued to find his approach awkward and a sexual "turn-off." In an individual session after 3 months of couple therapy, Rita confessed that her level of sexual interest in Max had declined still further and that she was having great difficulty in participating in their sensate focus exercises. Moreover, she was unable to express physical affection for her husband and felt repulsed by his occasional efforts to hold or embrace her. Rita stated that she felt "trapped" and "suffocated" in the marriage. I recommended that she address these issues in the next couple session.

Phase 2: The Separation

Shortly after this session, the couple made a decision to separate temporarily. In fact, the final impetus for separation came from Max, who had become increasingly frustrated and angry with his wife's continuing rejection. Despite his repeated attempts to bridge the sexual and emotional gap between them, Rita was acting colder and more distant than ever. In desperation, Max suggested that they separate for a period of several months, or at least until a more permanent solution could be reached. After lengthy discussion, and despite some reservations on Rita's part, they developed a plan for Max to move out at the beginning of the summer, immediately after their two sons left for camp.

Surprisingly, Max made a rapid adjustment to living alone. He rented a furnished apartment, joined a health club, and started dating Anne, a 33-year-old, single woman whom he had recently met at work. Max felt relatively comfortable with his new sexual partner and began practicing the various techniques he had learned about during the course of couple therapy. After several dates, the relationship progressed rapidly to sexual intercourse. Although Max ejaculated after only 2 or 3 minutes, he experienced a greater sense of ejaculatory control than he had previously with Rita. Moreover, he was especially gratified at his ability to arouse his new partner, even bringing her to orgasm on two separate occasions. The resulting change in his mood and self-esteem was striking.

For her part, Rita spent much of the time during the separation visiting with her mother and sister and doing routine chores around the house. She went out occasionally with friends but did not date at all during this period. At one point, she briefly considered taking a part-time job but could find nothing that suited her interests or qualifications. As the summer wore on, Rita found herself increasingly bored and lonely. She looked forward to seeing Max, even if their conversations were perfunctory and limited to discussions about the children and household matters.

One evening toward the end of the summer, Max stopped by the house on his way home from work. They began talking and Rita suggested that he stay for dinner. Later on that evening, the couple had intercourse for the first time in several months. Although Max ejaculated rapidly, both partners described the experience in more positive terms. Rita felt that Max was more attentive to her needs than usual, and he was pleasantly surprised by her level of sexual arousal and apparent enjoyment of the experience. The following day, Rita suggested that Max return home at the end of the month. He gladly accepted her offer.

In a follow-up individual session, Max discussed his reasons for making this decision. "I believe we can work out our sexual problem, together," he stated, "and I am not prepared to be the one to break up the family." Max had always been committed to maintaining the marriage, and this commitment had not changed with his relationship with Anne. Despite his positive feelings toward Anne, and his enjoyment of their sexual encounters, he did not view it as grounds for refusing Rita's offer to return home. He again requested my assistance in overcoming their sexual difficulty.

Phase 3: Reconciliation and Anafranil Treatment

Soon after Max returned home, the couple began sex therapy treatment again. They resumed sensate focus and guided touching exercises, in addition to the initial stages of the stop–start procedure (McCarthy, 1989). As before, they also used cognitive therapy techniques. A strong emphasis was placed on couple communication issues, and I encouraged Rita to express directly any negative or hostile feelings she was experiencing. This was to diminish the likelihood of her "acting out" these feelings in their sexual relationship. She responded positively and agreed to participate as fully as possible. After 2 weeks of couple therapy, however, during which the ground rules and a therapy contract were negotiated, Max urgently requested an individual session.

In the course of this session, Max expressed his growing frustration and sense of desperation over the sexual problem. He had ejaculated almost immediately during the first stop–start exercise and felt ashamed and demoralized as a result. As in the past, Rita responded critically to his failure, stating that she found the therapy exercises to be "cold and clinical," and had begun to lose her sexual desire again.

At this point, Max inquired whether treatment by any other means, including acupuncture, hypnosis, or drugs, might be available. Although he acknowledged the impact of Rita's responses on his increasing anxiety and difficulty in ejaculatory control, he felt powerless to break the cycle. When informed about the possible use of drug therapy (i.e., clomipramine), he expressed strong interest in this treatment option. With some cautionary statements regarding possible side effects and limitations, I referred Max to our consulting psychiatrist for a medication evaluation.

After a brief medical and psychiatric evaluation, Max was provided with a prescription for Anafranil (25 mg), to be taken approximately

4 to 6 hours before intercourse. This dosage is similar to that used by other authors (Althof et al., 1994; Segraves et al., 1992) and has been recommended for use on a single-dose basis (R. T. Segraves, personal communication, 1994). The physician gave Max a prescription for 12 tablets, with instructions to recontact him after completion of the tablets or in the event that he encountered side effects. Couple therapy was also to be continued.

On the first occasion that he used the drug, Max opted not to inform Rita ahead of time. His rationale for not telling her, he explained, was to avoid disappointment if the medication was ineffective. In fact, the couple had not planned to have intercourse that night and were supposed to engage in sensual massage and stop–start exercises. However, shortly after the massage began, Max initiated intercourse. Although she was only moderately aroused, Rita permitted Max to enter her. She stated subsequently that she was unprepared and surprised by his insistence on initiating intercourse.

Although Max lasted longer than usual (about 3 to 4 minutes), Rita was angry and disappointed when she learned that Max had taken the drug earlier that day. She felt "tricked" and manipulated by him and enjoyed the resulting intercourse *less* than usual. Moreover, she complained that Max's deception had violated the ground rules of maximum openness in their relationship. Max responded defensively to these charges, and meekly countered that he had misread her response to the situation.

We reviewed the issue in detail during two additional couple therapy sessions, and we made plans for mutual decision making in regard to future use of the medication. Despite her apparent acceptance of this agreement, Rita stated that she had lost sexual interest during three of the next four intercourse attempts. For his part, Max complained on several occasions about adverse side effects of the drug, particularly drowsiness and sedation. Max and Rita made a mutual decision to temporarily discontinue his use of Anafranil.

Given that Rita's resistance was the central issue at this point in treatment, we scheduled two individual sessions with her. During these sessions Rita expressed her continuing lack of sexual attraction to Max, as well as occasional "flashbacks" to her relationship with Joe. We discussed her need to place or maintain Max in a submissive role in the relationship. She wondered whether she would be able to remain in the marriage but did not wish to take responsibility for its dissolution.

Treatment Follow-Up: An Uneasy Equilibrium

In the following months, the couple made modest gains in the nonsexual aspects of the relationship. Rita reported that Max had learned to be a

"better listener," and he found her to be more affectionate and supportive. Max received a promotion at work and felt buoyed and confident
at his new business prospects. The couple also planned a major addition
to their home, and they spent much time in meetings with architects and
builders. Based on these improvements in the relationship, the couple
requested a "vacation" from therapy. Accordingly, a follow-up appointment was scheduled for 3 months.

At this time, it appeared that an uneasy equilibrium had been reached
in the couple relationship. Whereas Rita continued to be generally unresponsive to Max's sexual overtures, and still found him to be awkward
and mechanical, she appreciated his greater sensitivity and attentiveness
both in and out of bed. They used the medication twice during this period,
with positive effects of the drug on ejaculatory latency. Sex was still "far
from great" in her opinion, but Rita was noticeably less angry than in
the final phase of therapy. Her attitude toward the medication seemed
also to be more accepting. For his part, Max felt more confident and
assertive in the relationship, although his lack of ejaculatory control was
still troubling. He appreciated the positive change in Rita's attitude and
felt confident that they would continue to make progress in their relationship during the months to come.

In a brief telephone follow-up at 1 year, Rita reported additional
improvements in the intervening months. The couple had continued
to use the medication on an intermittent basis, with moderate success
in ejaculatory control. She also reported a gradual increase in her level
of sexual desire and arousal, which still appeared to be less than her
husband's. Max and Rita were having intercourse about once every 2 to
3 weeks, almost always at Max's initiative. Finally, they had continued
to make modest progress in the nonsexual aspects of the relationship.

COMMENTARY AND DISCUSSION

This case illustrates several points, including the ever-present role of
individual and couple issues in sex therapy, the potential difficulty in
treating lifelong or primary premature ejaculation, and the complications
associated with the use of drug therapy for this condition. Motivational
and couple communication issues were a major consideration throughout, as the couple was seldom in agreement on the major goals for change.
From the outset, Max viewed his premature ejaculation as the major
stumbling block in their sexual relationship. In turn, Rita felt little desire
or physical attraction for her husband and complained frequently about
his awkward and clumsy approach to lovemaking. Clearly, Rita's critical and rejecting attitude played a major role in the maintenance of the
problem, although Max showed little interest or desire for change prior

to her affair. It could be argued that both partners were engaged in a mutual avoidance of sexual and emotional intimacy through their unwillingness to seek help for the problem.

Extramarital affairs and events outside the relationship played a significant role in determining the outcome. It was Rita's affair with Joe and the aftermath thereof that brought the couple to therapy, and it was Max's affair during the summer of their separation that led him to attempt intercourse with Rita again. Max also obtained a significant promotion at work during the follow-up phase of treatment, which may have contributed to his positive outlook at this time. It also underlined for Rita the financial stability and related benefits of the marriage. Finally, both partners were strongly committed to their roles as parents, and the desire not to disrupt the family was a major determinant of their decision to stay together.

The case illustrates the potential value of pharmacotherapy (Anafranil) in the treatment of primary premature ejaculation. In fact, the drug increased the latency of Max's ejaculation by approximately 10 to 15 minutes. Equally significantly, however, the conflicts and tensions surrounding their use of the drug also exemplified the underlying dynamics of the couple's relationship. In his typically unassertive way, Max failed to inform Rita of his initial use of the drug. Her critical and hostile reaction typified her responses to his sexual problem in the past, and her basic message, "Look what I have to put up with," had not changed. Max's use of the medication also reinforced his role as the identified patient and deflected attention from Rita's ongoing contribution to the problem.

On a more positive note, the combination of traditional sex therapy and medication use did result in moderate improvements in the sexual relationship over time. Although Rita's lack of sexual desire and attraction was a central issue throughout, positive changes were noted at the 1-year follow-up. This is particularly encouraging considering Rita's complete absence of sexual attraction to her husband in the past. As we recently noted (Rosen & Leiblum, 1995), lack of sexual attraction to the partner is among the most difficult problems to treat. According to Rita, her increased interest in sex was related to Max's greater assertiveness and confidence in lovemaking rather than a direct effect of his ejaculatory control.

Finally, this case illustrates clearly the need for couple therapy in conjunction with medication use in cases of primary premature ejaculation. As noted recently by Althof et al. (1994), female partners are less likely than males to be sexually satisfied following drug therapy alone for premature ejaculation. These authors also noted that the benefits of drug therapy were rapidly reversed (i.e., ejaculation latency shortened) following withdrawal of the drug. Accordingly, Althof et al. (1994) have recommended a combination of traditional sex therapy and pharmacological intervention for premature ejaculation. I used couple communication training, sensate focus exercises, and stop–start techniques extensively in the present case, and they remain valuable treatment approaches in the management of this highly prevalent disorder.

ACKNOWLEDGMENT

The assistance of Myron Gessner, M.D., in providing adjunctive pharmacotherapy for this case is gratefully acknowledged.

REFERENCES

Althof, S. E., Levine, S. B., Corty, E., Risen, C., & Stern, E. (1994, March). *The role of clomipramine in the treatment of premature ejaculation.* Paper presented at the 19th annual meeting of the Society for Sex Therapy and Research, Atlanta.

American Psychiatric Association. (1994). *Diagnostic and statistical manual of mental disorders* (4th ed.). Washington, DC: Authors.

Assalian, P. (1988). Clomipramine in the treatment of premature ejaculation. *Journal of Sex Research, 24,* 213–215.

Colpi, G. M., Faniullacci, F., Beretta, G., Negri, L., & Zanollo, A. (1986). Evoked sacral potentials in subjects with true premature ejaculation. *Andrologia, 18,* 583–586.

Cooper, A., & Magnus, R. (1984). A clinical trial of the beta blocker propranolol in premature ejaculation. *Journal of Psychosomatic Research, 28,* 331–336.

Cooper, A. J., Cernovsky, Z. Z., & Colussi, K. (1993). Some clinical and psychometric characteristics of primary and secondary premature ejaculators. *Journal of Sex and Marital Therapy, 19,* 276–288.

DeAmicis, L., Goldberg, D., LoPiccolo, J., Friedman, J., & Davies, L. (1985). Clinical follow-up of couples treated for sexual dysfunction. *Archives of Sexual Behavior, 14,* 467–489.

Frank, E., Anderson, A., & Rubenstein, D. (1978). Frequency of sexual dysfunction in "normal" couples. *New England Journal of Medicine, 299,* 111–115.

Hawton, K., Catalan, J., Martin, P., & Fagg, J. (1986). Prognostic factors in sex therapy. *Behaviour Research and Therapy, 24,* 377–385.

Hollander, E., & McCarley, A. (1992). Yohimbine treatment of sexual side effects induced by serotonin reuptake blockers. *Journal of Clinical Psychiatry, 53,* 207–209.

Kaplan, H. S. (1974). *The new sex therapy.* New York: Brunner/Mazel.

Kilmann, P. R., & Auerbach, R. (1979). Treatments of premature ejaculation and psychogenic impotence: A critical review of the literature. *Archives of Sexual Behavior, 8,* 81–100.

Kilmann, P. R., Boland, J. P., Noton, S. P., Davidson, E., & Caid, C. (1986). Perspectives of sex therapy outcome: A survey of AASECT providers. *Journal of Sex and Marital Therapy, 12,* 116–138.

Leiblum, S. R., Rosen, R. C., Platt, M., Cross, R. J., & Black, C. (1993). Sexual attitudes and behavior of a cross-sectional sample of United States medical students: Effects of gender, age, and year of study. *Journal of Sex Education and Therapy, 19,* 235–245.

Masters, W. H., & Johnson, V. E. (1970). *Human sexual inadequacy.* Boston: Little, Brown.

McCarthy, B. W. (1989). Cognitive-behavioral strategies and techniques in the treatment of early ejaculation. In S. R. Leiblum & R. C. Rosen (Eds), *Principles and practice of sex therapy* (2nd ed., pp. 141–167). New York: Guilford Press.

McCarthy, B. W. (1994). Etiology and treatment of early ejaculation. *Journal of Sex Education and Therapy, 20,* 5–6.

Monteiro, W. O., Noshirvani, H. F., Marks, I. M., & Lelliott, P. T. (1987). Anorgasmia from clomipramine in obsessive–compulsive disorder: A controlled trial. *British Journal of Psychiatry, 151,* 107–112.

Reading, A., & Wiest, W. (1984). An analysis of self-reported sexual behavior in a sample of normal males. *Archives of Sexual Behavior, 13,* 69–83.

Rosen, R. C., & Leiblum, S. R. (1995). Hypoactive sexual desire. *Psychiatric Clinics of North America, 18,* 107–121.

Segraves, R. T., Saran, A., Segraves, K., & Maguire, E. (1992). *Clomipramine versus placebo in the treatment of premature ejaculation.* Paper presented at the annual meeting of the International Academy of Sex Research, Prague, Czechoslovakia.

Semans, J. (1956). Premature ejaculation. *Southern Medical Journal, 49,* 352–358.

Spector, I. P., & Carey, M. P. (1990). Incidence and prevalence of the sexual dysfunctions: A critical review of the empirical literature. *Archives of Sexual Behavior, 19,* 389–408.

Strassberg, D. S., Kelly, M. P., Carroll, C., & Kircher, J. C. (1987). The psychophysiological nature of premature ejaculation. *Archives of Sexual Behavior, 16,* 327–336.

Zilbergeld, B., & Evans, M. (1980, June). The inadequacy of Masters and Johnson. *Psychology Today,* pp. 29–43.

17

It's Not All in Your Head: Integrating Sex Therapy and Surgery in Treating a Case of Chronic Vulvar Pain

LESLIE R. SCHOVER

INTRODUCTION

One of the more stubborn sexual dysfunctions to treat is dyspareunia, or pain with sexual activity. Dyspareunia is a common problem for women. Although reliable data are lacking, surveys of unselected women in the community suggest that 8 to 23% have coital pain (Osborn, Horton, & Gath, 1988; Spector & Carey, 1990). A large recent study of women coming for routine care to either a university-based women's clinic or a family medical center at the same institution found that 16% had experienced dyspareunia in their lifetimes (Walker et al., 1991). We do not know how often these problems have an organic basis. It is important to remember, however, that women's reproductive lives involve a number of routine events that can contribute to dyspareunia, such as the initial dilation of the hymen with first sexual activity, healing from childbirth, the temporary hormonal changes during breastfeeding, and the atrophy of the vagina that can occur at menopause.

Most typically, sex therapists receive referrals of women with dyspareunia after a gynecologist has performed an examination to rule out organic causes for the pain (Lazarus, 1989). Evaluation of the contribution of medical versus psychological factors to dyspareunia is difficult, however. Many medical causes of dyspareunia are subtle and not easily recognized by the average gynecologist, for example, Bartholin's gland infections (Sarrel, Steege, Maltzer, & Bolinsky, 1983), pathology in the uterine ligaments (Fordney, 1978), or an unusual remnant of hymenal tissue (Schover, Montague, & Youngs, 1993). Patients have often consulted several gynecological specialists about the pain, receiving varied diagnoses and treatment plans. This experience produces confusion and distrust.

The referral for sex therapy is typically made with the implicit or explicit message that the pain is "all psychological." Not only are most patients who have sought medical help for a sexual problem skeptical of such a pronouncement, but women with pelvic or genital pain are particularly likely to reject a psychological explanation. These patients often meet criteria for full-scale somatization disorder (Peters et al., 1991; Reiter, Shakerin, Gambone, & Milburn, 1991). With histories that include a higher than expected rate of depression, chemical dependency, and traumatic sexual experiences (Walker et al., 1988), women with pelvic pain usually expect to find a medical cause and treatment for their dyspareunia. Engaging them in sex therapy presents a special challenge.

One approach is to recommend a comprehensive treatment program designed to address both medical and psychological factors. A research study in the Netherlands recently demonstrated that women with pelvic pain improved significantly more often when randomized into a treatment program including psychological therapy, nutrition, and physical therapy than when assigned to a traditional gynecological format with pelvic examinations and laparoscopy to rule out or treat medical factors (Peters et al., 1991). Sex therapy thus might be better accepted when prescribed as a component of a complex therapeutic regimen.

This chapter focuses on a particular genital pain syndrome that involves detectable tissue damage. In the past few years, gynecologists have focused increasingly on a specific subtype of genital pain, chronic vulvar pain (McKay et al., 1991). Many woman with vulvar pain are now diagnosed as having the syndrome of vulvar vestibulitis, a chronic inflammation of the delicate tissues of the vaginal vestibule (Friedrich, 1987; Marinoff & Turner, 1991). The vulvar soreness and burning are often quite severe, especially on attempts at vaginal penetration during sexual activity. After intercourse, pain may persist for hours or even several days. The pain is most typically localized to the area immediately surrounding the vaginal entrance.

Gynecologists who are not familiar with the syndrome of vulvar vestibulitis may miss the characteristic physical findings on routine pelvic examination. Sometimes the tender areas appear reddened to the naked eye, but often the tissue does not seem abnormal with a cursory inspection. If the gynecologist takes a cotton swab and touches gently in a circular pattern around the vaginal entrance, however, typically several areas will be exquisitely painful. Gynecologists also use a mild solution of acetic acid (similar to vinegar) to paint the area, highlighting areas of inflamed tissue while scanning the vulva with a special magnifying instrument called a colposcope. If these areas of tissue are removed surgically and examined by a pathologist, the usual findings are of chronic inflammation. No clear cause for the irritation, such as a bacteria, virus, or environmental irritant, has been identified.

Women with vulvar vestibulitis are usually in their reproductive years (ages 20 to 40) and have been sexually active until the pain interfered (Schover, Youngs, & Cannata, 1992). It is rare to find the syndrome in African American or Asian women, though some cases have been reported. A fair complexion or sensitive skin may be a risk factor (Friedrich, 1987). When a careful examination does not reveal skin changes associated with vulvar vestibulitis, vulvar pain may represent a type of neuralgia. In such cases, low-dose antidepressant therapy has been tried with some success (McKay et al., 1991).

Not only are the causes of vulvar vestibulitis uncertain, but the type of treatment most effective is a matter of debate (Marinoff & Turner, 1991). The most radical approach is a surgery called perineoplasty, removing a fairly wide area of tissue around the vaginal entrance. To cover this area, the bottom end of the vaginal lining is freed from its underlying tissue and pulled forward (Friedrich, 1987). The success rate for this surgery in completely alleviating pain is about 60% (Friedrich, 1987).

At the opposite end of the spectrum, several European groups report curing vulvar vestibulitis with sex therapy alone (W. C. M. Weijmar-Schultz, personal communication, January 1994). Sex therapy in such cases usually includes exercises to relieve pelvic floor muscle tension; the use of lubricants, anesthetic gels, and graduated sizes of vaginal dilators; and treatment of attitudinal or communication problems.

In my collaboration with a gynecologist, Dr. David Youngs, we searched for the most conservative treatment that would be effective for vulvar vestibulitis. Evaluation of women's psychological status suggested that most had experienced specific emotional stressors at the onset of the problem that could contribute to a chronic pain syndrome (Schover et al., 1992). Therefore we were enthusiastic about attempting sex therapy. The case I describe in this chapter was one of several that tempered our optimism about the success of purely psychological treatment, however.

Over several years we developed a multidisciplinary treatment program. If women did not have lesions typical of vulvar vestibulitis, we did not offer surgery but instead recommended sex therapy as the treatment of choice. For women who did have lesions on colposcopy, we recommended a combined approach involving psychological evaluation to identify contributing emotional factors followed by a conservative surgery that only removed small areas of tissue surrounding the vaginal entrance (Schover et al., 1992). The tissue removed included skin and the underlying glands that are involved in the chronic inflammation. It was not necessary to undermine the entrance of the vagina. The surgery was performed on an outpatient basis. After healing was complete, we initiated brief sex therapy, including instruction on pubococcygeal muscle exercises and the use of vaginal dilators. For women whose pain did not resolve within several months, antidepressant therapy was usually prescribed.

Initial success rates for pain relief were 56% of women reporting their pain as much better and 44% as somewhat better (Schover et al., 1992). At the time of our first follow-up study, only 16 women had completed the full treatment program, however. A longer-term follow-up is currently in progress. Initial data confirm that over half the women have almost complete pain relief, and another quarter of the sample have had some improvement. About a quarter of the women continue to have chronic, severe vulvar pain.

The case that follows illustrates the syndrome of vulvar vestibulitis and the use of sex therapy and surgery in a complex treatment program. This particular patient hoped to avoid surgical treatment, and so we began with the hope that sex therapy alone would be effective in relieving her pain. Demographic information has been changed to avoid identifying details.

CASE HISTORY

Background Information

Teresa was an attractive, 25-year-old graduate student in music. The daughter of a Cuban American couple who both worked in professional jobs, Teresa was living in the Midwest while completing her education. Her family lived in Florida. She was engaged to be married to Steve, a chemist, also age 25, who worked for an industrial company. Teresa and Steve both felt their relationship was ideal. Despite different ethnic and religious backgrounds, both shared a dream of creating a warm family life as a two-career couple. The only flaw in this picture was Teresa's severe pain with intercourse. When her vulvar pain began, Teresa immediately sought medical help, but repeated treatments for "yeast infections" did nothing but increase her symptoms. Steve reassured Teresa that he still wanted to marry her. "I would never leave you because of this," he repeated, but she feared that a marriage would fail if she were unable to enjoy intercourse. Both partners remained frustrated and mystified by the pain. After 7 months of severe vulvar burning, Teresa was referred to our gynecologist for an evaluation.

A careful examination, including colposcopy revealed that she had typical lesions of vulvar vestibulitis. As was routine, Teresa was asked to fill out questionnaires, including the Sex History Form (Schover & Jensen, 1988), Dyadic Adjustment Scale (DAS; Spanier, 1976), and Brief Symptom Inventory (BSI; Derogatis & Melisaratos, 1983). A psychological evaluation interview was also scheduled.

Teresa's DAS score of 124 showed high satisfaction with her relationship in general. No areas of major couple conflict were evident. The BSI was completely within normal limits, with no indication of psychological distress. On the Sex History Form, Teresa indicated that she felt sexual desire about twice weekly and engaged in sexual activity about that often. Foreplay lasted for 16 to 30 minutes, but she felt dissatisfied with the variety of stimulation in the couple's lovemaking routine. Sexual communication between the partners was typically nonverbal. Teresa reported good subjective and physiological sexual arousal and denied having negative emotions, such as guilt or anxiety, during sex. Although she could still reach orgasm easily, genital pain during sex was severe, always interfering with her pleasure.

Initial Assessment Interview

Teresa and Steve were interviewed jointly for their first session. They met in college and had been dating steadily for the past 3 years. They appeared very happy together, making eye contact with each other consistently and collaborating in telling their story without interruptions or contradictions. At one point they held hands. They reported that they rarely argued. If a minor disagreement came up, Teresa was more likely to verbalize her anger while Steve tended to withdraw from conflict. This had not interfered with their ability to compromise, however. Expression of affection in nonsexual situations was satisfactory to both partners. They continued to hold each other, kiss, and caress even when intercourse became impossible.

After Steve finished college, he moved to the Midwest for his job. Teresa saw him long distance for the next year, until her own graduation. She then chose a graduate program close to where he was living. The partners still lived an hour's drive apart, so they spent weekends together only during the school year. Although they missed each other, both had the capacity to get quite absorbed in their work, which helped them to bear their separation. When treatment began, Teresa was on summer break and was spending most of her time at Steve's apartment. They shared common leisure interests in hiking, computers, and photography. They had not yet set a date for their wedding but were planning to marry when Teresa finished her master's degree. As a pianist, she anticipated a career in music education.

During Teresa's childhood and adolescence, her mother attempted to provide her with specific facts about sexuality, for example, preparing her for the onset of menstruation. Teresa described her mother as giving her a book about "the facts of life." "You can ask me questions after you read it," the mother said sternly. Teresa never asked. The family was strongly religious, and Teresa's Catholic education included a clear message that sex was wrong outside marriage.

Teresa dated in high school and college but never yearned to try intercourse until she fell in love with Steve. She had no history of traumatic experiences with sex as a child or teen. After her first experience of genital caressing from a partner at around age 19, she decided to try masturbation. She was easily able to reach orgasm through her own self-touch or through clitoral caressing from a man. One date in college attempted to coerce her into sexual activity, but she was assertive and ended the interaction without any violence or lasting emotional impact. "I just didn't go out with him again," she recalled.

Steve was raised in a white, Protestant, Southern family without a strong religious education. When he was age 10, his parents divorced and he lived with his father. He learned about sex mainly from reading or friends. He never liked the idea of casual sex and had only one previous sexual relationship before beginning to date Teresa. He reported no problems with erections or premature ejaculation.

After Steve and Teresa had been dating for a year, she told him that she was ready to progress beyond mutual manual or oral genital caressing. She had obtained oral contraceptives and wanted to try intercourse. Steve was surprised, knowing Teresa's beliefs against premarital sex. He was pleased, however, and agreed to explore penetration. "I was also a little scared about making it a special experience," Steve recalled. "I knew we would remember it all our lives."

Unfortunately, the couple's first attempts at intercourse were awkward and painful. Teresa consulted a gynecologist at the university health service, who informed her she had vaginismus. The doctor advised Teresa to have Steve use first one, and then two fingers to penetrate her vagina. With the help of a water-based lubricant and several weeks of practice, the couple was finally able to achieve penile penetration without pain.

"I felt on top of the world," Steve said. "Our sex life was just as I hoped it would be." Teresa agreed with his recollection. "Every now and then I felt a little guilty, but mainly when my parents would call." They continued to enjoy an active sex life for over a year before the sensation of vulvar burning began.

Pain began rather suddenly at a time of some stress in Teresa's life. After college graduation, she had been working at a music store and living near her parents and older sister. She was seeing Steve once every couple of months, as she was in Florida and he was in Ohio. She decided to enter graduate school and move up to Ohio herself. It was in the month or two before her move that she first experienced pain at penetration. Misdiagnosed with a vaginal infection, Teresa tried a series of antifungal medications. If anything, these creams exacerbated the pain.

Although Teresa's parents liked Steve, they had some reservations about the relationship. They were not upset about the ethnic difference but were regretful that Steve was not Catholic. They feared he would lead Teresa away from the church. Steve was supportive of Teresa's attending Catholic services but did not want to convert to Catholicism himself. Teresa's older sister had recently let the parents know that she was sexually active with her boyfriend. This had sparked overt conflict with Teresa's mother. Teresa was apprehensive about her parents' reaction to her decision to move to the same area as Steve.

Although the couple was not officially living together, Teresa spent weekends at Steve's apartment. She made some effort to conceal the situation from her parents; that is, Teresa would call them during the day and avoided answering Steve's phone at night in case they were looking for her. Both partners felt that Teresa's parents had become less cordial to Steve since Teresa moved to Ohio.

Teresa did not have vulvar discomfort in nonsexual situations except for a loss of her ability to use tampons comfortably. The couple was continuing to attempt intercourse twice weekly. Teresa had no pain with clitoral caressing. If the couple used a female superior position for intercourse and Steve did not thrust deeply or strongly, Teresa could still enjoy sex and achieve coital orgasm. Afterwards, she would have a day of vulvar burning, however.

Teresa was told about our combined treatment program of surgery and brief sex therapy. The rationale for sex therapy was described, including reports of its success for vulvar vestibulitis. Teresa wanted to see whether she could avoid having vulvar surgery. She and Steve were enthusiastic about beginning sex therapy, despite living 2 hours away from the clinic. We decided that they would schedule visits on a weekly basis to take advantage of their extra time together during the summer.

Sex Therapy Phase of Treatment

At the end of the evaluation session, the couple was provided with written instructions for the sexual rehabilitation program, including the use of water-based lubricants, vaginal dilators, and Kegel exercises to reduce pubococcygeal muscle tension. Teresa's homework assignment for the first week was to squeeze her pubococcygeal muscles for a count of three and then release the tension. She would perform 10 Kegel squeezes, twice daily. She already felt she knew how to identify the muscles and contract them voluntarily. I also asked the partners to perform two sensate focus exercises, exchanging body caresses without including the breasts or genitals. Each partner would have half an hour to receive touch as well as a turn at being the giver of touch. I asked them not to try to have orgasms together or to attempt penetration for sexual intercourse.

When Steve and Teresa returned for their second sex therapy session, they reported that the sensate focus exercises had been very enjoyable. They listened to music in their candlelit bedroom. "I really appreciated the chance to just relax without worrying about trying for intercourse and having all that pain afterwards," said Teresa. She had found herself quite concerned the first time, however, about pleasing Steve by doing a "good job." She was more able to focus on her sensations on the second try. In her individual assignment to practice Kegel squeezes, Teresa was surprised that she had trouble holding the muscle tension for a count of three. She noticed some improvement in her capacity over the week of practice.

In the therapy session, I used a three-dimensional model of the vulva and internal pelvic organs to illustrate female sexual anatomy and response. We again reviewed the syndrome of vulvar vestibulitis, including possible causes and treatments.

I also interviewed Teresa individually. She had little new information to add to the history that was taken conjointly. She verified that she felt quite attracted to Steve, and that he had been a supportive and skillful lover. She also acknowledged that her mother's negative view of sex outside of marriage was a source of guilt. "I've always been the good daughter who lived up to Mom's standards," Teresa said. "My sister is more the rebellious type. Sometimes I envy her, but I can't seem to confront my parents the way she does."

The next homework assignment was to continue with sensate focus exercises, allowing brief stimulation of the breast and genital areas as one small part of the experience. On the second occasion, Teresa was to give Steve a "guided tour" of her genital area, including feedback on where and how she preferred to be caressed. Before this second couple exercise, I asked Teresa to examine her own genitals in the mirror, identifying the areas we had discussed in reviewing the genital model and touching each part lightly to see where sensation was pleasurable versus painful. Orgasms together or attempts at intercourse were still off limits for the couple.

At session 3, the couple had again completed all their homework successfully. In her individual exercise, Teresa was able to find the remnants of her hymen and to locate the tender areas around her vaginal entrance. She was even able to put a finger into her own vagina without pain. When she showed her genital area to Steve she felt quite relaxed. "I really feel I'm making progress," she commented. "I don't think I could have imagined doing some of these things a year ago." Again both partners enjoyed the sensate focus touching without experiencing any negative emotional reactions.

Because debriefing the homework did not reveal any problems, we spent time focusing on psychodynamic issues, particularly Teresa's memories of her family history and her perceptions of her parents' view of her relationship with Steve. The story that was elicited shed additional light on the onset of the sexual problems. On the night of Teresa's graduation from college, her mother discovered a package of condoms in Teresa's purse. Both parents confronted Teresa with their disappointment that she and Steve were sexually active. Not only did Teresa cry for a week afterwards, but her parents did not invite Steve to their house for a full year. Since that time, Teresa's mother would speak to Steve but never was really warm to him. Teresa went on a trip to California after graduation. It was on her return that she moved to the Midwest and the pain began. The fact that this story was not revealed until after several attempts to take a history seemed significant. Teresa's shame about disappointing her parents was a source of deep ambivalence to her. I discussed this with both partners. Steve expressed to Teresa his fear that her family would ultimately interfere with their marriage, but she reassured him about her commitment.

In this session, I educated the couple about vaginal lubricants. I provided a sample of Astroglide (BioFilm, Inc., Vista, CA) for use in their next homework assignment, a sensate focus exercise including more prolonged genital caressing. Steve was to try gently slipping one lubricated finger into Teresa's vagina once she was aroused but before she had an orgasm, so that vaginal expansion and lubrication would be maximized. Teresa was advised to take some private time and practice putting one lubricated finger into her own vagina. If this was comfortable, she could try using two fingers. She was to continue practicing Kegels twice daily, as well as using a squeeze and relaxation before any attempt to put a finger into her vagina.

Session 4 was encouraging. Teresa felt that her vestibular irritation was decreasing. The tender areas seemed smaller to her and less reddened when she examined them in the mirror. During the sensate focus, she had used Kegels to enhance her arousal while Steve was caressing her genitals, finding that the muscle contractions made her orgasm more intense. Steve could feel a definite increase in the strength of her voluntary vaginal contractions. He was able to insert a finger into her vagina without causing pain or even triggering soreness after the sexual activity. Astroglide was helpful in minimizing friction and irritation.

Teresa linked the progress to a talk she had with Steve about her loss of self-esteem since the sexual problem had begun. She realized that her family's perfectionistic standards affected her judgment of herself. She saw her pain as a personal failure rather than as a medical problem. Steve's emotional support and reassurance that he loved her helped Teresa to feel more confident.

Teresa then obtained a set of four latex vaginal dilators of graduated size (Milex, Chicago, IL) from her gynecologist. During this session, Teresa was given homework with the dilators. She was to lubricate the smallest dilator and try to slip it into her vagina, using a Kegel squeeze and release while holding the dilator at her vaginal entrance. Thus she could ensure that her muscles felt relaxed before she touched the dilator to the vaginal entrance. If it felt tight or uncomfortable to insert the dilator, I instructed her to hold the dilator at that point, without removing it, and squeeze and release her muscles again. After relaxing the muscle, she could advance the dilator further.

A second step, once she could insert and remove the smallest dilator without discomfort, was to insert the dilator and hold it still in her vagina for about 5 minutes. When she could accomplish the second step, the third task was to wiggle the dilator gently up and down or in and out of her vagina, to experience movement without pain. When she could achieve all three steps with the smallest dilator, she could begin again with step one using the next size of dilator. She was to spend 15 minutes or less on these exercises every other day. This schedule was designed to reduce genital irritation or emotional frustration from prolonged attempts to insert dilators and to allow a day for any local irritation to clear before the next try. Dilation should be frequent enough, however, so that the exercise did not loom as a dreaded event to be done once a week just before the next therapy session.

When the couple returned for their next visit, Teresa said she found working with the smallest dilator easy until she got to the step of moving the dilator in her vagina. Then she experienced pain at the vaginal entrance. In contrast, she had no discomfort when Steve used one finger to caress her vagina internally for several minutes during the sensate focus exercise. We discussed the possibility that sexual arousal acted to reduce

Teresa's threshold for pain (Whipple & Komisaruk, 1988). When she was working with the dilators in an unaroused state, the pain would be more noticeable.

After dilator use or after Steve's caressing, Teresa noted some mild vulvar burning for several hours. Teresa felt discouraged by her continuing vulvar irritation. Steve was supportive, however. "Remember that you're always being hard on yourself. Give it a chance," he told her. I asked Teresa to think about the sensate focus exercises as a time to feel relaxed and close to Steve, without expecting immediate pain relief. During the next week, she and Steve would continue practicing vaginal caressing with two of his fingers. Teresa would also continue working at a comfortable pace with her dilator exercises.

We discussed Teresa's fears that she would need surgery to cure her pain. I pointed out that we were doing our best to use a psychological approach. At least she knew there was another treatment option if our attempt was not successful. I suggested that Teresa use positive self-statements to prepare for the stress of using a dilator; that is, "I will spend a few minutes working on this, and can always stop if the pain becomes too uncomfortable." We also discussed using reinforcing cognitions to reward herself for each attempt; for example, "Today I was able to use the second dilator with less discomfort than last time. I am really working hard to solve my problem."

We planned to leave a gap of 2 to 3 weeks between sessions. In fact it was 5 weeks before Steve and Teresa returned for session 6. Teresa had begun her fall classes, taking away from her time with Steve. She felt somewhat uncomfortable using dilators in her dormitory room, as walls were thin and she could overhear other women. Intellectually, she knew she had privacy, but emotionally she felt ill at ease. She was having trouble relaxing the pubococcygeal muscles with the second of the four dilators. It felt more tight than painful to insert the dilator. Vulvar tenderness was increasing, however, especially during the week before the onset of her menses. "I feel like I'm back to square one!" she complained.

On weekends with Steve, she continued to enjoy the sensate focus exercises and to feel relaxed. The partners were not following the formal "giver and receiver" format anymore but continued to feel that they spent far more time on touch and communicated more openly about their preferences. Unfortunately, however, Steve was unable to use two fingers to caress Teresa's vagina without causing a good deal of discomfort. "I can tell that her muscles are much more relaxed than in the past when I just use one finger," he observed, "but I really feel bad because I know she'll be hurting the whole next day. She tries to hide it, but when she sits in the tub for forty minutes after sex, I know what's going on."

My impression was that Teresa and Steve enjoyed an excellent relationship in general. Although she had some guilt about disappointing her family by being sexually active before marriage, she had been able to enjoy sex for over a year before the pain began. Her parents were now expressing happiness with the couple's plans to marry the next summer. The sex therapy had enhanced the couple's knowledge about anatomy and each other. They felt their sexual communication was more open, but the pain had not improved. Therefore, Teresa decided to see the gynecologist for a reevaluation of her physical status. When he examined her, he noted lesions of vulvar vestibulitis that were unchanged despite our 3 months of sex therapy. He scheduled Teresa to have surgery to excise the inflamed area.

Postsurgical Sexual Rehabilitation

The next time Teresa and Steve were seen for therapy it was 2 months after her surgery and 6 months since their last visit. She had begun using the vaginal dilators again but was being quite cautious with them. The smallest dilator or one of Steve's fingers did not produce pain on vaginal insertion. The partners were continuing to engage regularly in noncoital caressing to bring each other to orgasm.

Teresa had not told her parents about her vulvar pain or her surgery. She and Steve were actively planning their wedding, however, and Teresa's mother was enthusiastic about the process. The couple were going to be married in a Catholic ceremony. Teresa felt less stressed by her graduate school and was happy about her success in eating a healthy diet and exercising regularly. She felt her life was more under her control. She was encouraged to speed up her progress with the dilators. We agreed to talk on the phone in 6 weeks to check on how things were going.

At the follow-up time, Teresa said she had recently been able to use the largest of the four dilators without pain. She and Steve were not yet ready to try penile penetration but were talking about it. They had been given a set of transitional exercises, including having Steve insert the dilators, staying at least a size below the one Teresa was using individually. At first Steve was simply to place his hand over Teresa's while she inserted the dilator. Then she was to guide Steve's hand while he put the dilator in. Finally, he would insert the dilator without her help but with her telling him when she was ready.

After Steve could insert all four dilators, as well as being able to caress Teresa's vagina with two fingers without causing pain, the couple could try penile penetration of the vagina. Teresa was instructed to straddle

Steve's body, sitting down slowly onto his penis. She could use Kegel squeezes and releases to make sure her muscles were relaxed during penetration. The first goal was penetration without any movement or thrusting. On a subsequent attempt, Teresa could move gently and slowly while Steve stayed still. Finally, the couple could experiment with more thrusting or different coital positions. Again we agreed to talk on the phone in 1 month to review the couple's progress.

By the next phone call, Steve and Teresa had been able to have intercourse on two occasions with both partners thrusting. Teresa still felt some tightness but had no pain during intercourse or afterwards. Both partners agreed that they still would like sex to be more spontaneous, as it had been before the pain interfered. The couple was scheduled to marry in 5 months. "I hated the idea of surgery," Teresa said, "but I think it really has helped. I'm so relieved to feel normal again. I still find myself worrying after each time we have sex, though, that the pain will come back."

One year later, Teresa filled out follow-up questionnaires. A BSI revealed even less psychological distress than on initial assessment. On both occasions, her scores were a standard deviation below the mean level of distress for women in a community normative sample. She reported that she had no vulvar pain in sexual activity or daily life. The couple was engaging in intercourse twice a week. Teresa was almost always orgasmic, either through clitoral caressing or from penile thrusting. Steve included a note in the questionnaire packet. "I just wanted to say thanks for all your help. It was so frustrating to feel like something was physically wrong, but be told there was nothing there. I feel like we also learned a lot about communication. I would still like sex to be a little more spontaneous, but it's slowly getting there."

COMMENTS

Although the outcome in this case was quite successful, it may be asked whether sex therapy alone for a longer duration might have alleviated Teresa's pain. Perhaps the availability of surgery provided a temptation to abandon psychotherapy prematurely. I doubt that more sex therapy would have made a difference, however. This young couple was highly motivated and quite diligent in fulfilling their homework assignments. They felt their sexual relationship improved in general from the exercises. Despite several months without attempting intercourse, the vulvar lesions remained unchanged on physical examination. As soon as Teresa attempted to place an object larger than a finger in her vagina, her vulvar irritation grew worse.

In terms of psychodynamic issues, the guilt induction from Teresa's family of origin was significant. She was able to overcome her initial vaginismus and to enjoy sex as long as she did not discuss her sexual relationship overtly with her mother. The revelation that she was no longer a virgin also coincided with her decision to separate geographically and emotionally from her close-knit, Hispanic family. Perhaps her guilt about leaving the family interfered with her sexual arousal once she and Steve were together. Vaginal dryness and muscle tension could then have contributed to the onset of vulvar inflammation. The discomfort she felt at using dilators in her dormitory room suggests that Teresa's guilt about sexual issues was not completely resolved by the sex therapy. Perhaps getting married was necessary for Teresa to feel totally comfortable with sex. These are hardly unusual issues, however, and the vast majority of young women negotiate them without developing vulvar vestibulitis. Despite her strong religious background, she had been able to enjoy masturbation and noncoital caressing with dating partners. Teresa's general psychological coping skills and relationship skills were excellent. She also had the advantage of a very loving and supportive partner. Thus I believe that some organic vulnerability or pathogen also is involved in the etiology of vulvar vestibulitis. Once the inflammation is chronic, it rarely heals by itself.

Teresa was not typical of most women with dyspareunia in that she wanted to avoid surgery. Thus, she was highly motivated to try sex therapy. In most cases, the preoperative psychological assessment also has the agenda of reframing the problem for the woman as an interaction of emotional and physical factors. For women with vulvar vestibulitis in particular, it is important that women go into the surgery with realistic expectations that complete pain relief will probably involve several months of working with muscle relaxation and dilators after surgery. It has been very helpful to have a structured treatment program to offer to women with vulvar vestibulitis, with some empirical information available on outcome.

For women whose dyspareunia does not have a readily treatable physical cause, the largest barrier to effective sex therapy is usually the woman's perception that she has an undiagnosed medical condition and is being denied the proper surgical or medical treatment. Sex therapy is then viewed as a poor alternative, unlikely to be effective. Difficulty in obtaining insurance coverage for mental health services and the fact that treatment takes a number of sessions and a commitment to do "homework" are other factors that decrease women's enthusiasm. Many women evaluated in our clinic do not return for the recommended course of sex therapy. As clinicians we mitigate our frequent disappointment by remembering the success stories like Teresa's and Steve's.

In summary, while the causes of vulvar vestibulitis remain unclear, removing the affected tissue is a helpful therapy for many women with this form of chronic pain. The sessions before surgery prepared Steve and Teresa for surgery and allowed them to continue sexual rehabilitation afterwards with minimal therapist contact, employing a written, self-help program. My clinical experience suggests that the highly successful outcome of this case not only reflects our treatments but the absence of a history of sexual trauma or significant psychopathology for either partner. Teresa did not have other psychosomatic illnesses or chemical dependency. Because this couple relationship was emotionally supportive, with open communication, Teresa and Steve did not need intensive professional intervention. More complex cases require far more psychological preparation and follow-up, even when medical or surgical treatments are part of the plan.

ACKNOWLEDGMENT

I would like to acknowledge the clinical assistance of David D. Youngs, M.D., who played a crucial role in the medical and surgical treatment of this case.

REFERENCES

Derogatis, L. R., & Melisaratos, N. (1983). The Brief Symptom Inventory: An introductory report. *Psychological Medicine, 13,* 595–605.

Fordney, D. S. (1978). Dyspareunia and vaginismus. *Clinical Obstetrics and Gynecology, 21,* 205–221.

Friedrich, E. G. (1987). Vulvar vestibulitis syndrome. *Journal of Reproductive Medicine, 32,* 110–114.

Lazarus, A. A. (1989). Dyspareunia: A multimodal psychotherapeutic perspective. In S. R. Leiblum & R. C. Rosen (Eds.), *Principles and practice of sex therapy* (2nd ed.): *Update for the 1990s* (pp. 89–112). New York: Guilford Press.

Marinoff, S. C., & Turner, M. L. (1991). Vulvar vestibulitis syndrome: An overview. *American Journal of Obstetrics and Gynecology, 165,* 1228–1233.

McKay, M., Frankman, O., Horowitz, B. J., Lecart, C., Micheletti, L., Ridley, C. M., Turner, M. L. C., & Woodruff, J. D. (1991). Vulvar vestibulitis and vestibular papillomatosis: Report of the ISSVD committee on vulvodynia. *Journal of Reproductive Medicine, 36,* 413–415.

Osborn, M., Hawton, K., & Gath, D. (1988). Sexual dysfunction among middle aged women in the community. *British Medical Journal, 296,* 959–962.

Peters, A. A., van Dorst, E., Jellis, B., van Zuuren, E., Hermans, J., & Tribos, J. B. (1991). A randomized clinical trial to compare two different approaches to women with chronic pelvic pain. *Obstetrics and Gynecology,* 77, 740–744.

Reiter, R. C., Shakerin, L. R., Gambone, J. C., & Milburn, A. K. (1991). Correlation between sexual abuse and somatization in women with somatic and nonsomatic chronic pelvic pain. *American Journal of Obstetrics and Gynecology, 165,* 104–109.

Sarrel, P. M., Steege, J. F., Maltzer, M., & Bolinsky, D. (1983). Pain during sex response due to occlusion of the Bartholin gland duct. *Obstetrics and Gynecology, 62,* 261–264.

Schover, L. R., & Jensen, S. B. (1988). *Sexuality and chronic illness: A comprehensive approach.* New York: Guilford Press.

Schover, L. R., Montague, D. K., & Youngs, D. D. (1993). Multidisciplinary treatment of an unconsummated marriage with organic factors in both spouses. *Cleveland Clinic Journal of Medicine, 60,* 49–55.

Schover, L. R., Youngs, D. D., & Cannata, R. (1992). Psychosexual aspects of the evaluation and management of vulvar vestibulitis. *American Journal of Obstetrics and Gynecology, 167,* 630–636.

Spanier, G. B. (1976). Measuring dyadic adjustment: New scales for assessing the quality of marriage and similar dyads. *Journal of Marriage and the Family, 38,* 15–28.

Spector, I. P., & Carey, M. P. (1990). Incidence and prevalence of the sexual dysfunctions: A critical review of the empirical literature. *Archives of Sexual Behavior, 19,* 389–408.

Walker, E., Katon, W., Harrop-Griffiths, J., Holm, L., Russo, J., &Hickok, L. R. (1988). Relationship of chronic pelvic pain to psychiatric diagnoses and childhood sexual abuse. *American Journal of Psychiatry, 145,* 75–80.

Walker, E., Katon, W., Jemelka, R., Alfrey, H., Bowers, M., & Stenchever, M. A. (1991). The prevalence of chronic pelvic pain and irritable bowel syndrome in two university clinics. *Journal of Psychosomatic Obstetrics and Gynecology, 12,* 65–75.

Whipple, B., & Komisaruk, B. R. (1988). Analgesia produced in women by genital self-stimulation. *Journal of Sex Research, 24,* 130–140.

18

The Critical and Demanding
Partner in Sex Therapy

BERNIE ZILBERGELD

INTRODUCTION

Although the case discussed here includes both erection and desire problems, the main reason for presenting it is to address one of the most
important and neglected issues in sex therapy: the role of the critical and
demanding partner. I think the ideal case for sex therapists, the kind we
dream about, is one in which the partner without the problem is supportive, cooperative, and ready and able to do whatever is necessary to
help. Whether that partner is male or female, this means he/she does not
pressure the partner with the problem to do what he/she can't do, is
willing to make do with whatever frequency and activities are possible,
and does not attack, blame, or criticize the partner for having the problem. Because sexual intercourse is usually the most difficult act for the
partner with the problem, the ideal partner without the problem is also
willing to be satisfied with nonintercourse sex until the problem is
resolved.

While such ideal partners are rare, of course, many real partners
manifest to some extent the required characteristics. However, there are
also many cases in which the partners are very far from ideal. They are
scornful, sarcastic, and demanding. These are the cases we have nightmares about. I see many such cases myself and many are also brought to
me for consultation. It is my impression that they are becoming the norm

in sex therapy. Yet I have found few extended discussions in the sex therapy literature of such couples. Masters and Johnson (1970) did not address the issue. Others, such as Kaplan (1974) and LoPiccolo (1992), have discussed the contribution of couple dynamics to causing and maintaining sex problems, but even they did not focus on critical partners.

That such discussion is needed is obvious. Aside from making relationships unpleasant and difficult, critical partners can cause a sex problem or make resolution of existing problems difficult or impossible. This happens in a number of ways. A critical attitude virtually always has the effect of increasing the already high level of anxiety in the partner with the problem and with anxiety at such high levels resolution may be impossible to attain.

The most dramatic example I have in this regard involved an extremely demanding woman who became so upset when her 64-year-old partner lost his erection in their hotel room one night that she had a screaming fit lasting for over 15 minutes during which she threw ashtrays, baggage, and the telephone against the wall. People in adjoining rooms assumed that she was being abused and called hotel security. Within minutes, the naked man, feeling humiliated and trying to get his partner to calm down while she screamed what a rotten lover he was and continued to throw things, was faced with security people knocking at the door demanding he open it immediately and threatening to use their own key if he did not. In discussing his erection problem with him months later, I asked what thoughts he had when anticipating sex with her. His answer: "As soon as I think of sex or we start playing around, I remember that night and get scared. I know it could happen again. My arousal goes right out the door."

A critical partner not only evokes anxiety but other feelings as well— sexual inhibition and lack of interest, anger, and resentment. In a case involving a woman who had difficulty having orgasms with her husband, he frequently called her frigid and, when stimulating her, made comments such as, "How long is this going to take? I'm getting tired," and, "This sure isn't my idea of fun." She expressed the effects of his attitude during a session: "Your comments are ruining any chance of therapy working. I don't look forward to having you touch me. The stimulation itself feels good, but my fear of what you're going to say gets in the way. And I'm angry. I'm doing my best and I need support and encouragement. Instead I get nothing but shit. So I feel, 'OK, I know me not having orgasms hurts you, makes you feel less of a man. Since you demean me and make me feel less of a woman, I'll get back at you by not having orgasms.' I know it's childish and self-defeating, but that's where I am."

The causes of the criticalness and anger of the partner may be seen as stemming mainly from relational determinants or from personality and personal history dynamics. Relational causes are illustrated by a case in which the woman refused to have sex with her husband and was harshly critical of him. Yet this was a woman who was timid and deferential with other people. Her behavior with her husband, it turned out, was due to his numerous affairs and the demeaning ways he treated her. There are other cases, however, in which the partner is not the main cause of the anger. A man I saw, for example, was able to admit after a few sessions that although he usually found convenient rationalizations for his blaming and critical treatment of his girlfriend, the truth was that he treated most people the same way and had been doing so as far back as he could recall.

However we conceptualize the causes of the criticalness and demandingness, they need to be dealt with if therapy is to succeed. Although there are many methods available—anger management, reviewing family-of-origin issues, empathy and forgiveness exercises, antianxiety and antidepressant medications—the question remains, how and when to most effectively use them.

Because I believe discussion of the critical partner is important and long overdue, I present a case where such a partner was a major feature of the clinical picture. It's not that I have all the answers. In fact, I have more questions than I do answers and the case to be presented was not an unqualified success. I feel in need of help in this area myself and I hope presenting a case that raises the issue and is open to the scrutiny and critique of others will be of value.

There are also other interesting aspects to the case: penile injections that didn't help, an antidepressant that did, and the timing of the sessions. For reasons over which neither the clients nor I had control, the frequency and length of our meetings were somewhat unusual and I believe the outcome may have been affected as a result.

For clarity in the presentation, I put both my thinking during the sessions and my reflections afterward in italics.

BACKGROUND INFORMATION ON COUPLE

The background information given here was obtained in four 2-hour sessions held on 4 successive days. In the first and last of these meetings, I saw the couple together. In the second, I met with the wife alone; in the third with the husband.

Norm and Linda are both 44 and have been married 15 years, the first marriage for him, the second for her. For many years they have worked and spent most of their time abroad in a third-world country, returning to the United States for a 2½-month vacation each year. Linda called to ask if I would be available immediately to work with her and her husband, who had low sexual desire and erection problems. They would be available for therapy for only 9 weeks. This was also going to be their last extended visit for a long time. They had decided to sell their house here and make their permanent home in the country in which they worked. I arranged to see them the following day.

Individually, they are very different. Linda is attractive, vivacious, impulsive, and very critical. She throws out words seemingly without thinking about them and without understanding the effect they might have on others. I know I felt criticized by her from the first phone call. Even though I gave them an appointment less than 18 hours after her call and at a time when I don't usually see clients, she said several things on the phone and during the first session that indicated I could have done better. And there was also a sense of urgency and demandingness, a kind of why-is-this-taking-so-long-and-why-can't-you-do-it-quicker-and-better attitude.

Linda grew up in a lower-middle-class family where, according to her, nothing anyone ever did was good enough. Her mother constantly criticized her father for not making more money; her father constantly criticized her mother for not doing a better job of managing the house and the children. And both criticized their three children for their looks, their grades, their behavior, and just about everything else. The father was physically abusive—slaps with an open hand and hits with a hairbrush—to his wife and the children. Looking back, Linda believes her father was "just a crude, angry man" and her mother was both anxious and depressed. Because her bedroom was next to her parents' and she could hear most of what went on in there, she knew from an early age that her parents had an active sex life. She often heard her father say to her mother that he was "going to fuck her hard" or "tear into her" and her mother extolling the virtues of his "big, hard cock." From what she heard, Linda believed that both of them enjoyed their sexual play. But because of the frequent complaints by both parents and the physical abuse, when Linda was 8 or 9 she asked her mother why she didn't leave. Her mother responded tearfully, "Because despite all the bad things, he loves me and he makes me feel good." Linda says the main attitude she got from her parents was that nothing she or anyone else did was enough. And in prior therapy, she realized that in her childhood she had learned to equate good sex with love, even though the insight had availed her nothing.

Although Linda did well in school and college and has a successful career, she has long been aware that people feel pressured and negatively judged by her. Despite her attractiveness, many men she was interested in stopped calling after a few dates. And women whose friendship she desired and both men and women colleagues have tended to keep their distance. Over the years she tried various therapies to deal with these issues, but she reports that the results were "marginal."

When I asked what attracted her to Norm, she said it was his intelligence ("I'd never been close to anyone who was so smart.") and his gentleness ("I've been with lots of guys who were good fucks but they were mean, irresponsible, liars and cheaters, and I knew he could never be like that. Unfortunately, I was right all the way. He's never been mean, but he's never been a great fuck either.").

Norm appeared to be the "nerd" he later called himself. He seemed generally timid and reluctant to express his feelings in front of his wife, spoke slowly and usually only after some time, and then said only nice things in a nice way, and he struck me as being depressed.

Both of Norm's parents were quiet and bookish people, his father a professor and his mother a teacher. He was the only child and while he felt loved as a youngster and treated with respect, there wasn't much physical contact with his parents. He couldn't recall his father ever hugging or kissing him and couldn't recall his parents ever hugging or kissing each other. Sex was never mentioned in their house. Norm says he's "pretty much like they were, living more in my head than in my body, not very comfortable with new people, somewhat fearful of personal confrontations, very different from my wife." These differences were obvious even in what seemed like similarities. Both, for instance, were interested in watching sports, but from very different perspectives: "I'm all in my head, analyzing the strategy, trying to see what each team or player is trying to do and how well they're succeeding. With Linda, on the other hand, it's only the combat and conflict that are appealing. She yells when her team wins, cries when they lose, and takes issue with everything the coaches, the players, and the referees do."

During the first session, it was apparent that Norm and Linda had a serviceable relationship in many ways. Neither had close friends and tended to rely on each other for support and companionship. They shared a number of common interests and held similar values about most things.

The only problem, as far as they were concerned, was sex. When they first met, Linda was far more sexually experienced than Norm. She was surprised that a man could have had so little knowledge and experience. He, on the other hand, was somewhat intimidated by her experience and knowledge. But he tried to be a good student and they enjoyed frequent lovemaking at the beginning, although not as frequent or as passionate as she would have liked.

Over the years, however, Norm gradually lost interest in sex and developed erection problems. Either he wouldn't get an erection or he would lose it before or during insertion. Norm sought help from a urologist who, although he found nothing physically wrong, gave him an

injection of papaverine in his penis, which produced an erection that
lasted for 3 hours.

But neither Norm nor Linda was overjoyed by the idea of him taking injections. Norm had always been fearful of needles and almost
fainted when the urologist gave him the first injection. Linda didn't like
the needles either. In her mind, they weren't "natural or normal." For
Norm to have to take shots to get erections meant that he didn't love
her or wasn't aroused by her.

They both went to see the urologist, who opined that injections were
the only reasonable option. There were no sex therapists in that country
and besides, he insisted, sex therapy was a time-consuming and expensive process that often failed. Whatever their feelings, the fact was that
the injections did give Norm good erections. They had no choice but to
use the injections unless Norm wanted to get a penile prosthesis.

The results of the injection therapy were mixed. At times Norm got
a good erection and they had intercourse. But more than half the time
the injections did not produce an erection. This led to more visits to the
urologist to determine whether Norm was injecting himself properly and
whether the papaverine was still potent. Each time he got an injection at
the urologist's office, he had a good, long-lasting erection, although the
same was not true at home. The injections did nothing for Norm's desire.
Linda was still the initiator virtually 100% of the time and many times
when she did initiate, Norm seemed uninterested.

The introduction of penile injections into Norm and Linda's life
actually made the situation worse. As Linda put it, "Before I had gotten
to the point where I wasn't expecting anything. I think I actually shut
down sexually. But with the shots, even though I still think the whole
idea is ridiculous, I had the hope that sex would get back to normal. So
I opened myself up again and then there's all this failure and frustration.
I hate it! Now it's hard to have any hope at all." Norm also felt frustrated and discouraged. "If these injections don't work, what will?"

Linda appeared to be hurt and angry in my individual session with
her. "I read your book and I know you're so sympathetic toward men
with erection problems. But what about me! I feel totally defeminized.
How can I feel loved or desirable when he can't get it up for me? You
don't have any idea what that's like. Even with the help of modern chemistry, he can't do it for me. It's obvious he doesn't want me, doesn't desire
me. Even at my age, other men look at me and want me. But not my
husband. I feel like shit."

For Linda, a man wanting her sexually, proved by him coming after
her for sex and having an erection, was the evidence she needed that she
was attractive, desirable, and loved. This deeply ingrained notion had
caused her to endure 4 years of an emotionally and physically abusive

marriage. As she related the story: "I knew it was a horrible relationship and I had to get out. He criticized me constantly and often hit me. But as soon as I said I was leaving, he would say he needed me and would pull out his hard cock; as soon as I saw it I would melt, we'd screw like crazy and I'd be hooked in again." Although she had a few sessions of counseling to try to get out of the marriage, she was unable to do it. The marriage ended only after her husband left her.

In my session with Norm, he repeated several times that he loved Linda and wanted to stay with her. When I asked if he found her sexually attractive, he hesitated and then said yes. When I asked about the hesitation, he was silent for a few moments and then said, "No, it's nothing. I am turned on to her." Further prodding on my part yielded nothing, but I thought his arousal was not as unambivalent as he said. As we continued our discussion, I asked how he felt when he was first dating her. He began by saying how beautiful he found her and how surprised he was that a woman like her would take an interest "in a nerd like me." When I asked what else he felt at that time, he answered, "To tell the truth, I was frightened by her experience and sexual openness. It was like I was in kindergarten and she was a professor. I'm not sure I've ever gotten over that. I've always felt at least a little inadequate. And things really got bad after I started having trouble with erections." I wanted to know more about how their sex had been before the erection problem. He said that it had been good and added in a voice so low I could barely hear his words, "She was always teaching and correcting me. Somehow I wasn't able to do exactly what she wanted. I didn't touch her right, my erections were never as hard as she liked, and when we had intercourse, I wasn't passionate enough."

When I inquired about the first time he hadn't gotten an erection with her, he started crying. "I felt so humiliated, just like I felt as a child when my mother caught me stealing a quarter from her purse. I felt like I had done the most horrible thing in the world and been found out. I was tired that night—I was working 10 to 15 hours a day—but I always thought I had to have sex when she wanted it. Anyway, after she stimulated me a few minutes and nothing happened, she blew up and screamed, 'I want a hard-on, not some little squishy thing.'" When I asked how those words affected him, he said, "Just terrible. They have haunted me ever since. When I think of them, or other choice ones she's used over the years, I get totally turned off."

Here was the reason for Norm's ambivalent arousal toward Linda. He was attracted to her sexually but memories of the "choice" words she'd hurled at him in the past interfered. Although he had in effect said this, he didn't quite understand it yet.

I then asked Norm whether he felt Linda was generally supportive or critical. To my surprise, he said she was a supportive partner. When I asked whether he considered the phrase about hard-ons and squishy things supportive, he quickly answered that that was an aberration and she was usually supportive.

I realized I had made a mistake and pushed him too far. Norm was very fearful of being critical of his wife. He was more open and critical when with me than he had been when she was in the room, but there were limits I would have to respect. He was not yet ready to acknowledge how critical she was or, I suspected, how angry he was at her because of it.

I retreated to another subject. Norm sometimes woke up with an erection and he almost always had one when he stimulated himself. He rarely masturbated to orgasm, but often stroked himself a minute or two "just to see if the thing still works." And work it did, whether he was standing up in the shower or lying or sitting on the bed. These self-induced erections lasted as long as he continued stimulation and often for a few minutes after he stopped. This information confirmed the urologist's impression. There was nothing seriously physically wrong with him.

When I asked Norm what he made of the fact that he almost always had erections with himself and often did not with his wife, even with the injections, he thought for a while and said, somewhat sadly it seemed to me, "I just don't know."

By this time, the answer was obvious. But here again Norm showed that he was not yet willing to acknowledge his wife's role in his problem.

When I asked about his desire for sex, Norm said that Linda had always wanted more than he did. When they were first together, he felt he had to have sex when she desired it no matter how he felt. And he always tried no matter how tired or uninterested he was. He started to say something that sounded like, "She would be furious if I wasn't interested," but took it back and I couldn't get more out of him on the subject.

I told Norm that he seemed depressed. He immediately agreed, saying he had had problems sleeping for months yet wanted to sleep all the time, didn't have much appetite for food or sex, and was quite discouraged about the possibility of resolving the erection problem and keeping the marriage. I had him take the Beck Depression Inventory (Burns, 1980) during our session. His score of 28 confirmed my impression of moderate to severe depression. He agreed to see a psychiatrist I recommended and made an appointment for the following day. The psychiatrist gave him a prescription for Prozac (fluoxetine).

In our fourth session, the second conjoint session, the problem became clearer. Norm winced and seemed to shrink to half his size as Linda said she couldn't live like this and wanted a divorce if the therapy wasn't successful. His response to her, given in a very controlled voice, was typical for him: "Honey, I'm sorry you're so upset. I know you've been through a lot but I hope you can be patient. I'm sure the doctor can help us." At which point she exploded, "Us doesn't need help. You do! I'm ready, willing and able. There are plenty of men who'd give anything to have me. You're the one who doesn't want me, who can't fuck me." Then, turning to me, "I'm sorry, doctor. I didn't mean to be so loud, but I'm just saying how I feel."

I asked what happened on the occasions when he couldn't get or lost his erection. Both agreed that that ended the sexual activity. Norm said he would like to satisfy Linda orally or manually but she had become less and less interested in these activities although she was easily orgasmic with them. She added, "It's high school stuff. I want the real thing. If I can't have it, I'd just as soon pack it in."

My formulation after the first four sessions (8 hours) was as follows. Linda had a deep need to be sexually desired and ravished by a man. This was her way of knowing she was loved and desirable. The more often he wanted her, the harder his erection, and more lusty he was, the more secure she felt. Norm was good for her in many ways. She had been attracted by his intelligence, his gentleness and thoughtfulness, and the common interests they shared. But sexually he could not give her the assurance she needed. Because of the anxiety this evoked in her, she became increasingly critical of him. I suspected that her criticism is what caused him to lose interest in sex in the first place. As for his erection problem, anxiety about her reaction was probably paramount, but I also suspected that his unacknowledged anger at her and his fear of losing her played major roles.

How to proceed with this information was the problem. The situation was complex and time was limited. It turned out that although they didn't have to return to work for 8 more weeks, 2 of those weeks had already been committed to visiting relatives and friends in other parts of the United States. So we had only 6 more weeks. I hoped for some help from the Prozac but realized it often took up to 2 weeks to have an effect. In any case, I knew it wouldn't be a complete answer. Norm had lost interest in sex and had developed erection problems long before he became depressed. I discounted the usefulness of the penile injections. His anxiety and anger were usually sufficient to undermine their effect. And the fact that he could get erections on his own, even while depressed, strongly suggested that the main problem was Linda's words and their effect on him.

TREATMENT

In order to give the Prozac a chance to take effect, I told them it would be of great help if they could take one of the trips to visit relatives now instead of later. They agreed and left 2 days later for a 6-day visit. I gave a few body rub exercises (Zilbergeld, 1992) as homework to be done in their motel while on the trip, in addition to bans on intercourse and genital stimulation, and made arrangements to keep in touch by phone.

The body rubs went better than I anticipated. There was a tenderness involved that had been lacking in our joint sessions and in their interactions in the past years. Both said that doing them, whether giving or receiving, made them realize how much they loved each other and how much they had to lose. By the end of the week away, Norm reported feeling somewhat better.

We had our next session, the fifth, the day after they returned from their trip. Norm and Linda were more affectionate than I had seen them before and reiterated what they had told me on the phone about realizing how much they loved one another and how much they wanted resolution of the sex problems. The Prozac had clearly been working for Norm and he was looking and feeling much better.

Their closeness and positive mood encouraged me to carry out the plan I had devised while they were gone. I spent a long time thinking about them before this session. I have always had difficulty in cases in which I believe that the attitude of one partner is causing or maintaining the problem of the other because I know such things are hard to hear. Despite the many different ways I've tried to bring up this issue, the partner frequently feels blamed and gets defensive and the mate will often come to the partner's defense or say nothing at all, leaving me alone to deal with the angry partner. The result is that some of these couples terminate therapy. Even when they don't, the one whose behavior was discussed is often wary, suspicious that I am not on his/her side. It is especially difficult for me when the partner whose behavior I feel is problematic is a woman. I don't want to blame women for men's problems or even to seem to be blaming them. Despite these misgivings, I didn't see an alternative to putting out this information to them. Exactly how to do it was the big question. I knew from past experience that the process went better and created fewer bad feelings if the couple rather than me came up with the explanation. Could I lead them to this point?

I told Linda and Norm that the most perplexing question was this: How was it that Norm almost always had good erections on his own and with the injections in the doctor's office but not when the two of them wanted to have sex? I said I needed their help to understand this issue because if we could understand it, we could probably resolve the difficulties.

Norm looked perplexed, but Linda reacted quickly and angrily. "I see where this is going. You're going to make me out to be a demanding, castrating bitch, that I'm the reason he can't get it up. Just get me out of the picture and he'll be hard all the time." Norm looked alarmed but didn't say anything.

This is exactly what I feared, that Linda would get angry and defensive and that Norm wouldn't say anything, leaving me to deal with her. But this is what often happens in these cases, so deal with her I would.

After we took a short break so we could all regain our composure, Linda apologized. She said that although Norm never mentioned it, she had heard it all before since childhood. Friends, colleagues, relatives, and former lovers had accused her of being "critical, nasty, sarcastic, and intimidating." She allowed there was truth to these allegations, but she didn't know what to do. "I'm just saying how I feel, isn't that what I'm supposed to do? Do you want me to just keep everything bottled up inside like some chickenshit wimp? Do you want me to be like my husband who never comes out with anything except for this polite facade like he's above it all. Well, I'm not above it all. I have feelings! And I think I've been very supportive and patient. God, do you know when we first met, he didn't know the first thing about fucking a woman. I taught him everything. He made progress, but he's still not the world's greatest lover. All I want is some good lovemaking. Is that asking too much!"

After acknowledging Linda's upset feelings, I asked her to look at Norm, who once again seemed to have sunk into the chair and shrunk to half his size. When I asked what she made of that, she surprised me by saying, "Yeah, I got it. I really shrunk him down."

Although Linda was angry and defensive, she was also more receptive than I expected. Clearly she already knew that her behavior was affecting Norm. After all, she was the one who brought it up. (Her ability to quickly recover after being angry and defensive and to see the effect she was having was a major strength of her personality and was to be demonstrated many times during the course of our work. Without it, treatment would have been even more difficult. Most of the critical partners I have worked with are not blessed with this characteristic.) Given what I took as a window of opportunity, I was encouraged to proceed with my plan.

Linda said yes when I asked whether we could continue, although I warned she'd be hearing some things that were hard to hear. After getting Norm's agreement to point out any places where my explanation wasn't true for him, I gave my thoughts. I started off by saying that I wasn't blaming Linda but was just trying to understand what was causing the problem and what needed to be done about it. I agreed that Linda had a right to have and express feelings. The problem, I noted, was that there is a cost to expressing oneself. One's expressions may have effects one doesn't want on those who hear them. I then gave them the formulation I had after our fourth meeting, frequently stopping to ask Norm whether I was correct. He said yes each time.

The reason for giving the formulation myself instead of trying to get it out of Norm is my experience that people as fearful of criticizing their partners as he is simply can't do it. In fact, if pushed, they end up denying reality and defending their partner. But if I correctly express what they feel, this often gives them the courage to elaborate on or repeat in their own words what I have said. And this is what Norm was able to do.

When I finished I asked for their reactions. Norm spoke first: "Honey, I think he's right. I've always been afraid of you in sex, always afraid that what I do won't be right or won't be enough for you. I think I started losing interest when I realized that no matter how hard I tried, I couldn't satisfy you. I'd never be enough. It was easier not to even bother than to try and fail. And he's right about the `squishy thing' comment. That's been on my mind ever since. I'd like to get over it and move on, but haven't been able to."

Linda took Norm's hand and softly said she was sorry. I asked them to go home and think about what had been said and decide if they wanted to continue. They called a few hours later and said yes, so we met again the following morning.

During that session I said I agreed with what Linda said about wanting to be able to express her feelings. I thought both of them should express themselves. The manner in which this was done, however, was crucial. I thought it was fine if Linda told Norm that something he did or didn't do disappointed her or made her feel frustrated, provided it was done in a civil manner. I added that this would be difficult for her because I was asking her to talk about her feelings rather than acting them out. I also thought it would be helpful and appropriate for Norm to tell her how what she said and did affected him. I added that this would be difficult for him because he probably hadn't even acknowledged to himself some of the feelings he had toward her and, in any case, wasn't used to expressing feelings to her.

Although this is standard sex therapy fare for me (Zilbergeld, 1992), I did it at the start of the session for several reasons. The most important is that I knew Linda would like having permission to express her-

self and I felt I needed to give her something after what she went through the night before. I also wanted to plant the distinction as early as possible between talking about feelings and acting them out. And I wanted to give Norm the idea as quickly as I could that he needed to start being more expressive.

I suggested to Linda that she might want to get therapy for herself to deal with her criticalness and with her need for erections and sex to feel good about herself. Given the time constraints, I didn't think there would be enough time in our sessions to do that. Although she agreed she had a clearer understanding than before of her effect on Norm, she resisted the advice. She also resisted my suggestion to have a consultation with a psychiatrist to determine whether an antianxiety or antidepressant drug might help her be calmer. She said she was committed to doing what was necessary but only in the context of our work. I could not get her to budge on this.

During the rest of our sessions I gave fairly standard assignments for men with erection problems (Zilbergeld, 1992) and worked with Norm and Linda individually and together. With Norm, I worked toward his being more assertive and expressive with Linda (e.g., telling her the effect her words had on him as soon as possible). Because this was difficult for him, I role-played scripts for him, things he might want to say in various situations, and then had him try them using more of his own words. I also tried various ways of decreasing the effect of those words. Because I knew he read science fiction, I suggested an image of a force field he could have around him whenever he felt the need so that her critical words would bounce off it. He would hear the words and know what she was saying, but they wouldn't affect him the way they had in the past. This appealed to him so I guided him into a relaxed state and described the force field and how he could use it. I gave him a recording of this relaxation and imagery exercise and recommended he listen to it as often as possible.

Because Linda's "squishy thing" comment still haunted him, I did a combination desensitization and neurolinguistic programming (NLP) exercise with him. When he was relaxed, we went through a list of the critical comments she had made to him in the traditional behavioral manner, with squishy thing being the last one dealt with. We also played games with the items following NLP conventions (Bandler, 1985), such as changing their speed, playing silly music as he heard them, and seeing Linda in diapers as she said them. He had fun with the exercise—he laughed for the first time in my presence when I asked him to visualize Linda in dirty diapers as she made her critical comments—and it definitely reduced the impact of those memories.

I attempted to explore with him what I assumed was unacknowledged anger toward Linda but got nowhere. Frustrated and a little annoyed was as much as he would concede, but anger, never! Because time was short and because dealing with this issue seemed so difficult, I dropped it.

I suspected that Norm suffered from a coping style common in some men, a flattening of intense affect of any kind. He simply could not acknowledge, let alone express, the presence of a strong feeling such as anger or lust. He always spoke about sex in gentle ways using only the terms "making love," "sex," or "intercourse" and when discussing what he enjoyed about sex he mentioned closeness, sharing, and expressing love. When in several individual sessions I tried to talk with him about the joys of fucking, taking her, or even just going after what he wanted without worrying about what she wanted, his eyes glazed over as if I were speaking an alien tongue. This style would need to be overcome for him to be a better lover for Linda and to get more for himself out of sex, but I didn't pursue it because of the lack of time.

With Linda I employed various ways of helping her to calm down, including relaxation tapes and exercises, of helping her to feel good and loved no matter what happened in sex, and of trying to get her to accept and enjoy stimulation other than intercourse. I hammered away at the idea that she was attractive, lovable, and loved whether or not her husband was interested in sex that day, whether or not he had an erection. I also suggested to her many times that a really sexual woman could enjoy sex in many ways and was not totally dependent for her gratification on a man's penis. Additionally, I tried to get her to accept the lemonade idea (if God gives you lemons, don't be upset; make lemonade), pointing out that any fool can have good sex if everything goes perfectly but the sign of a mature woman is making the best with what you have at the moment. She liked the idea, so I asked her to review each day before going to sleep, picking one event or experience, which didn't have to be sexual, that didn't go as she wanted, and to think of a way she could have improved the experience by "making lemonade." This exercise proved to be especially beneficial to her.

All these suggestions and methods seemed to help to some extent. As the couple did the genital stimulation exercises, Norm's interest increased and he started having better and longer-lasting erections. A clear pattern emerged. He almost always had more interest, better erections, and more pleasure in the hours or days after Linda was not critical and had allowed him to stimulate her to orgasm by hand or mouth. He was initiating sex more than he had since the very early days of their relationship (though still not as much as she would have preferred). And within 3 weeks they were having enjoyable intercourse (though still not as lustful as she wanted). But on those days when Linda "lost it" (her words), he wouldn't do as well. At times he would employ his force-field image and also tell her how he felt about her words. When he did, everything went better. But at other times, he forgot to use the image or didn't express himself. Usually things did not go as well at these times. But at least now they were able to get together within a few hours and talk about what happened, a technique I had suggested to them several times. Linda was invariably apologetic, Norm invariably tender and loving, and things tended to get back on track within a day.

Three weeks before their departure, they agreed that the sexual situation was improved although far from perfect. Linda said, "I really got it. It's so clear now that how I act has an immediate negative influence on him and his penis. I don't like exploding, I really don't, and I feel like hell afterward. Really guilty and terrible. I do it less often than before, but sometimes I can't stop myself." I again suggested the possibility of medication, but she again refused, saying, "I hate the thought of taking drugs."

Things got hectic during the last 3 weeks—unexpected difficulties had arisen regarding the sale of their house, which meant they had to spend a lot of time dealing with real estate agents and lawyers—and we weren't able to meet as often as I would have liked. During the last week they were so busy with meetings and packing up all their belongings that we met for only 1 hour. But the pattern established in the prior weeks continued.

In our last meeting, Linda and Norm were both thankful and guarded. They felt they had come a long way but still had a long way to go. We spent most of the session going over ideas and methods they could employ to maintain and expand their gains. Two large impasses remained. Norm said he was initiating sex as often as he desired to and he could do no more unless Linda wanted him to fake it as he had in earlier times. And the joys of more lustful sex still seemed beyond him. Linda, of course, was not happy about these matters but at least she was not as angry and upset about them as before.

In all, treatment consisted of 35 hours, including 4 hours over the telephone during the 2 weeks they were out of town, spread over 9 weeks.

FOLLOW-UP

I received two long letters from the couple over the next 2 years, one from each of them. The improvement made in therapy has been maintained but not significantly expanded. Linda wrote: "I guess I've made peace with my lot. I'm trying to make lemonade. Norm is a good, loving, responsible man who treats me better than I've been treated by anyone. I'm finally getting it that he really loves me and I sometimes even get it that I deserve that love. I know I could find a better fuck, but I also know I couldn't find a better husband. Because of your help, we are having better sex than ever. His erections are usually good—except after I lose it, of course—and I enjoy making love with him. I sometimes fantasize about a hard fuck or a man who's crazed with desire for me, but I know I can't have that with him. It's just not his nature. So I try to look more on what I have and less on what I'm missing. It usually works, but then there are those awful times when I forget myself and yell at him. I feel so deprived at those times. I don't think I'm asking for a lot, but I guess no one gets everything they want. I'm still working on that and hope to get better."

Norm wrote: "The situation is better than before. I'm happy with the sex we have but it saddens me that Linda isn't. I wish I could be more interested in sex and I wish I could be more passionate to give her what she wants. It's not clear when, if ever, we will be back in California. If we do return, I'd like to see you again to work on these issues. Perhaps I could make some changes. I love Linda very much and even though I know she's happier with our sex life than previously, I would like to make her even more content. Anyway, for now I can say that the force field works a good percentage of the time, helped of course by the fact that she doesn't criticize as much as before. The diaper image also helps when I remember to use it.

"We had a big problem some months back. She got crazier than ever one night—I had been working 12-hour days again, was extremely tired and not interested in sex, but I forgot what you said and tried to do it for her and of course didn't get hard—and I didn't have an erection for three weeks afterwards. I got so worried that I went back to the urologist and got a batch of a new medicine, prostaglandin, but it didn't help. I tried to think what you might recommend. Relaxation seemed like a good idea so I listened to your tapes and suggested we go back and do the genital massage exercises. We did and in a few weeks things were back to normal again. The last few months have been good and I hope we never again have another episode like that. But with the two of us, it's hard to be sure."

DISCUSSION

I'm ambivalent about the outcome of this case. Some days I think that although it was only a qualified success, it probably went as well as it could have given what I had to work with and the time limitations. Other days I feel differently, thinking that had I only done some things differently, the outcome would have been more positive. The problem is that although I have a great many ideas as to what I could have done differently, I'm not sure any of it would have made any difference.

I certainly wish I could have had more time. Not necessarily more sessions, because we packed a lot of therapy hours into 9 weeks, but more weeks over which to spread those sessions. Both Norm and Linda were barraged with new ideas, and I asked for radical changes in both. I believe that more time to get accustomed to the ideas and more time for them to practice the relaxation, assertiveness, imagery, and other exercises under my guidance would have helped.

I do not regret laying it all out on the line during our fifth session. It was almost brutal but given the time constraints, I think it was the right thing to do. It worked for this couple—after all, they did continue in therapy and did make some progress—but I also know it doesn't work for every couple. Unfortunately, I'm not sure I know when to do it this way and when to take more time and be less direct and more gentle. Although I don't regret what I did in this regard, I'm not sure I did it the best way possible. There must be better ways of communicating this kind of information so that the client wouldn't feel as criticized and wouldn't get as defensive.

Getting Norm on Prozac was a crucial step. Without it, I'm certain we would not have made the progress we did. He would not have had the strength to be more assertive and expressive and his lack of interest would probably not have had a chance to improve. The value I give to Norm taking Prozac and my attempt to get Linda to a psychiatric evaluation may give the impression that I own stock in a pharmaceutical firm. I don't, but one lesson I have learned over the years is that I, like many other nonmedical therapists, did not pay enough attention to medical assessments and treatments. When I started paying more attention, I found that penile injections, vacuum pump devices, estrogen replacement therapy, and medications of various sorts (especially antianxiety and antidepressant agents) were helpful in many cases. Speaking of penile injections, Norm was one of the first men I treated who did not benefit from them and I learned that even powerful drugs like papaverine and prostaglandin could be neutralized by emotions such as anxiety and anger.

I tried a potpourri of methods, including some not mentioned here, and my sense is that a number helped to some extent, each adding a bit to the total effect. The lemonade idea and exercise, as well as the relaxation tapes, seemed especially helpful to Linda, while the force-field and Linda-in-diaper images and assertiveness exercises seemed to work well

for Norm. Our work on communication—especially on Linda's expressing her feelings of disappointment and frustration instead of acting them
out and the two of them getting together to talk about a recent conflict—
was also clearly helpful.

Sometimes I have wondered whether Norm and Linda should be
together. Although there is a lot of good in their marriage, sexually they
are on different wavelengths and will almost certainly remain so for the
rest of their lives. It's not just a matter of desired frequency of activity
but also of attitude and action. Whatever her motives, Linda is a far more
sexually expressive and open person than Norm. I do not consider her
desire for more lusty sex pathological. But Norm can't even grasp what
more lustful sex is. I have had cases where I was able to help men like
him become more lustful, but it takes a relatively long time and time was
the one thing we didn't have. Whether or not, even given the time, I could
have taken him to Linda's level is something I'll never know. But I do
believe some progress in this area was possible even though it would have
required him to overcome his long-standing and powerful fear of intense
feeling. I realize that sex is only a small part of a total relationship—
that's what Linda seemed to be realizing and accepting—but I sometimes
regret that this issue will never be fully resolved for this couple and will
probably remain a source of concern for all their days.

My main regret regarding this case is not having found a way to do
better work with Linda's need for Norm to desire her more and have
erections, and also with her critical and demanding attitude. I wish I could
have gotten her to go for a drug consultation. Although I had no reason
to believe she was depressed, I have had a number of cases in which an
antidepressant agent greatly reduced a client's anger and criticalness,
regardless of whether the client was depressed.

I wonder if it would have helped to explore in greater depth the roots
of her sexual needs and criticalness. Clearly these issues stemmed from
the dynamics in her family. She had explored them in previous therapy
without much benefit, but perhaps another go-around, or a different way
of dealing with the same issues, could have helped.

And this, of course, brings us back to where we began: how to best
work with critical and demanding partners. I now view such partners,
whether they be male or female, as typical in sex therapy. Over the years,
I have seen fewer and fewer couples in which the partner without the
problem is supportive and cooperative and increasing numbers of those
in which the partner is unsupportive and even downright hostile.
Although some progress was made with Norm and Linda, I believe it is
incumbent upon us to present more cases like this and develop better
ways of dealing with them. This is especially important in light of the
fact that the results obtained in this case were greatly aided by Linda's

ability to quickly recover from her bouts of anger and criticalness and to understand the effect of her words on Norm. Most critical partners do not have this ability and that makes working with them and their partners much more difficult.

ADDENDUM

Long after seeing Norm and Linda, I learned about and received training in eye movement desensitization and reprocessing (EMDR), a method I have since used with good results in a number of cases of sexual dysfunction and dissatisfaction where anxiety was a significant factor. I will not describe it here because interested readers can turn to Shapiro's (1995) complete discussion. I wish I had known about EMDR when Norm and Linda were in treatment. From my experience with other cases, I believe it would have helped in a number of ways. I am reasonably certain EMDR would have more quickly and more completely reduced the emotional charge for Norm of Linda's past derogatory comments and more effectively reduced his anticipatory anxiety about future comments. Because I have used EMDR effectively with other clients who feared intense emotion, I think it could have helped Norm in this regard as well. After several long EMDR sessions, a male client whose fear of affect was at least as strong as Norm's said, "I don't know what the big deal was. Feelings are just feelings, sometimes good, sometimes bad, but usually not a problem." This kind of response is typical of clients who have used EMDR successfully.

Because I have had positive results with EMDR in several cases where the client behaved with anger when he/she felt anxious, I would have tried it to deal with Linda's insecurity (not feeling loved or desired unless she was regularly ravished). Obviously, any reduction in her inappropriate expression of anger would have had a dramatic positive effect on Norm's feelings and functioning, as well as on the couple system generally. Since Linda's demand (as contrasted to preference) for frequent, lusty, and absolutely functional sex seemed to be based to some extent on her insecurity, it is possible that EMDR might have influenced that as well. As a bonus, it has been my experience that when EMDR is successful, it has the overall outcome of calming people down, as if they had undergone months of relaxation training or meditation. And this is exactly what Linda needed.

In short, I believe that EMDR might well have made therapy more effective for this couple by helping to eliminate the obstacles to more frequent, more passionate, and more functional sex. Whether or not, with the obstacles eliminated, Norm would have turned into the lusty lover that Linda so much desired, and whether or not the couple would, therefore, have reached true sexual compatibility are, unfortunately, questions without answers.

REFERENCES

Bandler, R. (1985). *Using your brain—For a change: Neuro-linguistic programming*. Moab, UT: Real People Press.

Burns, D. D. (1980). *Feeling good: The new mood therapy*. New York: William Morrow.

Kaplan, H. S. (1974). *The new sex therapy: Active treatment of sexual dysfunctions*. New York: Brunner/Mazel.

LoPiccolo, J. (1992). Postmodern sex therapy for erectile failure. In R. C. Rosen & S. R. Leiblum (Eds.), *Erectile failure: Assessment and treatment* (pp. 171–197). New York: Guilford.

Masters, W. H., & Johnson, V. E. (1970). *Human sexual inadequacy*. Boston: Little, Brown.

Shapiro, F. (1995). *Eye movement desensitization and reprocessing: Basic principles, protocols, and procedures*. New York: Guilford Press.

Zilbergeld, B. (1992). *The new male sexuality*. New York: Bantam.

PART III

Sexual Addiction and Compulsion

Hypersexuality or complaints about sexual addiction and compulsion have increased markedly in recent years. Among the most common explanations offered for this increase are changing diagnostic practices, greater societal concern with sexual promiscuity, and a possible backlash againt the sexual freedom movement of the 1960s and 1970s (Levine & Troiden, 1988). The growth of "addictions medicine" as a new subspecialty field, along with the availability of safe and effective drugs (i.e., serotonin reuptake inhibitors) for treating compulsive behaviors generally, including sexual compulsions, has no doubt also contributed to this trend. As noted by Eli Coleman (Chapter 19), sexually compulsive behavior may be either paraphiliac or nonparaphiliac in orientiation; that is, the choice of sexual outlet involves either conventional or societally proscribed behaviors.

Little is known about the etiology or treatment of compulsive sexual behavior. Several authors have suggested that a history of early abuse or neglect may be important, while others have pointed to the difficulties with intimacy and emotional closeness that often underlie the disorder. Alcohol and drug use are frequent, although not inevitable concomitants, and some individuals show deficits in other areas of work or social functioning. Perhaps the only generalization to be made with certainty is that the vast majority of cases presenting for treatment are male. No satisfactory explanation has been offered, to date, for this striking gender imbalance.

From a treatment perspective, sexual compulsion or addiction is generally viewed as requiring long-term, intensive treatment. Pharmacological therapy, including either antiandrogens or serotonin uptake inhibitors, may be combined with individual or couple therapy interventions. Group therapy or referral to 12-step programs, such as Sexaholics

331

Anonymous or Sex and Love Addicts Anonymous, is also frequently recommended. A major treatment issue is the inability or unwillingness of many clients to make an adequate commitment to the therapy process. This problem is highlighted in the case studies by Sharon G. Nathan (Chapter 20) and John P. Wincze (Chapter 22) in this section.

Each of the chapters in this section presents a different perspective on assessment and treatment of sexually compulsive behavior. In Chapter 19, Coleman argues that anxiety-reduction mechanisms are pivotal in the etiology and maintenance of these behaviors, and that treatment should be aimed at interrupting the escalating cycle of psychological distress and sexual acting out. In the accompanying case, Coleman describes the use of psychotropic medication (fluoxetine), group therapy, and cognitive-behavioral techniques to achieve control of compulsive "cruising" behavior and extramarital sex. Successful outcome is similarly reported by Candace B. Risen and Stanley E. Althof (Chapter 21), following extended treatment of compulsive, fetishistic behavior in a 35-year-old physician. Risen and Althof view sexual paraphilias as disorders of masculine development, and treatment is directed at establishing a more secure masculine identity.

The final chapters by Nathan and Wincze powerfully illustrates some of the pitfalls and problems associated with treatment in this area. Nathan describes her attempted therapy with a 36-year-old, single actor, who presents for treatment with a long history of sexual addiction and substance abuse. In this fascinating case study, the author raises key questions about the nature of sexual addiction, in addition to the biases and prejudices that most therapists feel about these problems. In the final chapter of the book, Wincze describes a challenging and difficult case of sexual compulsion in a middle-aged, Protestant minister. This case illustrates the interpersonal dimensions of sexual addiction, as well as the fundamental intimacy deficits that frequently are at the root of the problem.

Among the authors in this section are several distinguished and experienced sex therapists. Coleman is the author of numerous articles and book chapters on the topic of compulsive sexual behavior. Nathan, Risen, and Althof are "master therapists," who have contributed widely to the theory and practice of sex therapy. Finally, Wincze is a nationally recognized sex researcher and clinician.

REFERENCE

Levine, M., & Troiden, R. (1988). The myth of sexual compulsivity. *Journal of Sex Research, 25*, 347–378.

19

Treatment of Compulsive Sexual Behavior

ELI COLEMAN

INTRODUCTION

Many terms have been used to describe the phenomenon of compulsive sexual behavior, including hyperphilia, erotomania, hypersexuality, nymphomania, satyriasis, promiscuity, Don Juanism and Don Juanitism, and more recently sexual compulsivity and sexual addiction. The terminology has often implied different values, attitudes, and theoretical formulations (Coleman, 1992).

Overpathologizing this disorder is an ever-present danger. Professionals with conservative or restrictive attitudes about sexuality are likely to impose a pathological label on normative sexual behavior. It is important for professionals to recognize and be comfortable with a wide range of normal sexual behavior. Many individuals may experience intense involvement with sexual behavior during their lifetimes, which should not automatically be viewed as disordered sexuality. In many cases, this intense involvement reflects normal developmental processes or may be short-lived, responding to some situational variable. Similarly, compulsive sexual behavior should not be confused with value conflicts within an individual or between a couple. Therefore, it is important to differentiate normative sexual behavior, behavior that is problematic, and that which is symptomatic of underlying psychological distress or a psychological disorder.

Compulsive sexual behavior (CSB) is defined here as behavior that is driven by anxiety-reduction mechanisms rather than by sexual desire.

333

The obsessive thoughts and compulsive behaviors reduce anxiety and distress, although they lead to a self-perpetuating cycle. The sexual activity provides temporary relief but is followed by further distress: guilt and remorse associated with engaging in unwanted obsessions and compulsions. Depending on the intensity of the disorder, this self-perpetuating cycle may be highly resistant to change.

Disagreement exists as to whether CSB constitutes an addiction (Carnes, 1983, 1989, 1991), "lovemap" pathology (Money, 1980, 1986), psychosexual developmental disorder (Levine, 1982; Stoller, 1975), impulse control disorder (Barth & Kinder, 1987), mood disorder (Kafka, 1991), or variant of obsessive–compulsive disorder (OCD; Coleman, 1990, 1991, 1992).

In my opinion, the obsessive–compulsive model leads to clearer understanding of CSB and the development of more effective treatment methods. Using recent advances in the understanding and treatment of OCD, effective treatment techniques have been developed that combine pharmacological and psychological therapies. Serotonergic medications have proven to be quite effective in treating a variety of CSBs (Cesnik & Coleman, 1989; Coleman & Cesnik, 1990; Coleman, Cesnik, Moore, & Dwyer, 1992; Federoff, 1988; Kafka, 1991; Kafka & Coleman, 1991). These medications interrupt the obsessive–compulsive cycle of CSB and assist patients to use therapy more effectively.

The most widely used medication in this regard is fluoxetine (Prozac). Fluoxetine is a potent serotonin reuptake inhibitor that was first approved for clinical use in 1987. Low doses (20 mg per day) have been found to be as effective as higher doses of Prozac. Prozac's most common uses at this time are for dysthymia (chronic, low-grade depression falling short of major depression), anxiety disorders, OCD, and impulse control disorders (Kramer, 1994). In our clinical experience, the newer serotonergic medications such as Zoloft (sertraline) or Paxil (paroxetine) are producing similar results in cases in which patients cannot tolerate the side effects of Prozac. For the most part, the advantages of the newer serotonergic drugs over the tricyclics, monoamine oxidase inhibitors, or antiandrogens are their broad efficacy and reduced side effects. Obviously, more controlled studies are needed to substantiate claims that serotonergic medications may be specifically effective in treating CSB.

TYPES OF COMPULSIVE SEXUAL BEHAVIOR

Nonparaphiliac Behavior

Any sexual behavior or its avoidance can become compulsive. The compulsive behavior may involve behaviors that are considered normal by sociocultural standards. Therefore, nonparaphiliac CSB involves conventional and normative sexual behavior taken to a compulsive extreme (Coleman, 1992). One example of nonparaphiliac CSB is given in the fourth edition of the *Diagnostic and Statistical Manual of Mental Disorders* (DSM-IV; American Psychiatric Association, 1994) under the category of Sexual Disorders Not Otherwise Specified. DSM-IV describes nonparaphiliac CSB as "distress about a pattern of repeated sexual relationships involving a succession of lovers who are experienced by the individual only as things to be used" (p. 538).

Other forms of nonparaphiliac CSB include compulsive cruising and multiple partners, compulsive fixation on an unattainable partner, compulsive autoeroticism, compulsive multiple love relationships, and compulsive sexuality in a relationship (Coleman, 1991, 1992).

Paraphiliac Behavior

Paraphilic behavior involves socially unacceptable behavior that society considers to be perverse or deviant. Money (1986) defines paraphilia as

> a condition occurring in men and women of being compulsively responsive to and obligatively dependent upon an unusual and personally or socially unacceptable stimulus, perceived or in the imagery of fantasy, for optimal initiation and maintenance of erotosexual arousal and the facilitation or attainment of orgasm (from Greek, para- + -philia). Paraphilic imagery may be replayed in fantasy during solo masturbation or intercourse with a partner. In legal terminology, a paraphilia is a perversion or deviancy; and in the vernacular it is kinky or bizarre sex. (p. 267)

In Greek, the term *para* means "beyond, alongside of, aside from, modified from, subsidiary to, and faulty," and *philos* means "loving, dear."

The most common examples of paraphiliac behavior are exhibitionism, fetishism, frotteurism, pedophilia, sexual masochism, sexual sadism, transvestic fetishism, and voyeurism. While only these eight paraphilias are listed in the DSM-IV, Money (1986) has identified more than 40 such paraphilias. In the DSM-IV, the essential features of paraphilias are defined as

> recurrent, intense sexually arousing fantasies, sexual urges, or behaviors generally involving 1) nonhuman objects, 2) the suffering or humiliation of oneself or one's partner, or 3) children or other nonconsenting persons, that occur over a period of at least 6 months (Criterion A). . . .
> The behavior, sexual urges, or fantasies cause clinically significant distress or impairment in social, occupational, or other important areas

of functioning (Criterion B). (American Psychiatric Association, 1994, pp. 522–523)

CASE ILLUSTRATION

Presenting Complaint

John, a 38-year-old married man, presented himself to the sexual disorders clinic with concerns that he might be "sexually compulsive." He had been referred by the local health department's sexually transmitted disease (STD) clinic. John had been married to Barbara for 11 years; they had two children, ages 6 and 8. John was highly educated and a successful businessman in the local community. Recently, he contracted gonorrhea and told his wife that she needed to be tested and treated. This revelation confirmed Barbara's suspicions that John had been sexually active outside the marriage. He had always denied her accusations. She was furious and immediately demanded that he leave the house; she also planned to file for divorce. In an attempt to save their marriage, John decided to be honest with Barbara and revealed that he had had numerous sexual encounters, usually during the course of his many business trips.

History and Onset of the Problem

In the early years of the marriage, John was not terribly concerned about his extramarital sexual activity. He felt that his encounters with other women were relatively innocent and did not adversely affect his relationship with his wife. His rationalization at this time was: "What she doesn't know won't hurt her." However, as years went by, he began to feel more driven to seek these encounters. Increasingly, he found himself constantly scanning his environment for available sexual partners. He skipped business meetings, lying to his wife and coworkers about his whereabouts. For the past 3 or 4 years, John had begun to recognize that he had little or no control over this behavior. He made pledges and promises to himself to avoid these encounters but found himself becoming obsessed and compelled to "score." He spent most of his time in singles bars, strip shows, and "adult" bookstores. During this time, he continued to be sexual with his wife on a regular basis. While he found this mildly pleasurable, his main intent was to persuade his wife that her suspicions of his infidelity were unfounded. His sexual encounters with his wife were perfunctory, and much of his time was spent obsessing about other women with whom he had been sexual.

Three years earlier, he became sufficiently concerned to contact a 12-step support group for "sex addicts." While he found consolation in this group, his compulsive behavior continued to escalate.

John avoided safer sex practices during his sexual encounters and worried incessantly about contracting an STD and passing it on to his wife. He received testing at an anonymous STD testing site on a monthly basis. Until his recent diagnosis, John had never contracted an STD and his numerous HIV tests had all been negative.

Assessment Process

Because John presented with concerns about his CSB, it was not difficult for him to identify behaviors that troubled him. In other clinical situations, the presenting complaint may conceal problematic or compulsive sexual behavior. Therefore, the clinician should routinely ask questions related to CSB. The following questions may be asked to identify patients who are experiencing symptoms of CSB:

1. Do you, or others who know you, find that you are overly preoccupied or obsessed with sexual activity?
2. Do you ever find yourself compelled to engage in sexual activity in response to stress, anxiety, or depression?
3. Have serious problems developed as a result of your sexual behavior (e.g., loss of a job or relationship, sexually transmitted diseases, injuries or illnesses, or sexual offenses)?
4. Do you feel guilty and shameful about some of your sexual behaviors?
5. Do you fantasize or engage in any unusual or what some would consider "deviant" sexual behavior?
6. Do you find yourself constantly searching or "scanning" the environment for a potential sexual partner?
7. Do you ever find yourself sexually obsessed with someone who is not interested in you or does not even know you?
8. Do you think your pattern of masturbation is excessive, driven, or dangerous?
9. Have you had numerous love relationships that are short-lived, intense, and unfulfilling?
10. Do you feel a constant need for sex or expressions of love in your sexual relationship?

If the answer is yes to any of the above questions, the clinician should explore further to make a differential diagnosis. These questions are not sufficient to make a diagnosis but are screening questions with which the clinician can explore further as needed.

In John's case, he answered yes to questions 1 through 6. The first five questions reflect general characteristics of CSB, the sixth question related more to his specific form of nonparaphiliac CSB—compulsive cruising and multiple partners.

As part of the assessment process, John was interviewed about his presenting complaint, history and onset, previous treatment, and current therapy goals. A complete sex history was taken including family background, family attitudes about sexuality, sex education, early sexual experiences, masturbation, fantasies, body image, history of intimate relationships, and sexual functioning. Questions were asked regarding traumatic experiences, current health status, use of alcohol or other drugs, and current psychosocial stressors. A psychological assessment was conducted to assess general mental, interpersonal, and occupational functioning and evidence of psychiatric disorders. To assist in the evaluation, a number of nonstandardized questionnaires (sexual behavior survey, sexual compulsivity inventory, compulsive sexual behavior inventory, history of other compulsive disorders, chemical use history, family of origin, current family functioning, sex history, current fantasies, previous treatment, and previous pharmacotherapies) and two standardized psychometric instruments, the Derogatis Sexual Functioning Inventory (Derogatis & Meyer, 1979) and the Minnesota Multiphasic Personality Inventory—II (Butcher, 1989), were administered.

It was important to consider potential neuropsychogenic causes for John's CSB. Compulsive sexual behavior can result from birth defects, trauma, surgery, illness, or prescribed or nonprescribed substances. Thus, CSB could result from a biological predisposition, illness, or injury or may develop as a result of environmental stressors. A variety of factors is likely involved in the development of CSB, as is the case with many other psychiatric disorders.

Assessment

John was in good health and had no history of birth defects or substance abuse. He had a suspected history of head trauma but no known neurological abnormalities. He had recently completed a full physical exam, and no health problems were noted.

It was evident that John was quite anxious and depressed and fit diagnostic criteria for dysthymia. A primary anxiety disorder stemming from childhood abandonment fears and physical abuse from his father was identified. His dysthymia was conceptualized as secondary to the underlying anxiety disorder. In turn, his CSB was nonparaphiliac and fit the category of compulsive cruising and multiple partners. As with most cases of CSB, John had low self-esteem and a history of abuse and had come from a background of restrictive attitudes about sexuality (Coleman, 1987).

Treatment Plan

Clinical experience indicates a wide continuum of severity for this disorder. Therefore, some patients who present with concerns regarding CSB respond to brief interventions and do not require pharmacological therapy. Understanding the severity of the CSB can lead to individualized treatment; some treatments might require psychological or psychoeducational interventions, while others require psychotherapy with or without psychotropic medications. In John's case, our clinic staff recommended a combination of pharmacotherapy and psychotherapy. The psychotherapy would involve weekly group psychotherapy and once monthly conjoint or family psychotherapy.

Pharmacotherapy

Based on an evaluation by the staff psychiatrist, John was given a prescription of 20 mg per day of Prozac. Within a week, John reported reduced anxiety and less frequent obsessional thinking. He continued to feel compelled to seek sexual encounters, however, and did so two to three times a week. He maintained the Prozac dosage throughout his treatment and reported reductions in anxiety, depression, obsessive thoughts, and compulsive behaviors.

Group Therapy

John participated in group therapy with six other men who had a variety of sexually compulsive behaviors. The group was led by a female cotherapist and me. While it is important for men to participate in a group with other sexually compulsive men, heterogeneity is preserved by having men with a variety of types of CSB, ages, socioeconomic backgrounds, and sexual orientations. The mixed-gender, cotherapy team provided an opportunity for John to explore transference issues with parental and opposite-gendered significant figures.

He reported having typical feelings of relief that "I am not the only one." At the same time, he felt that he could not identify with other members of the group because he saw them as more disturbed than himself.

Because he was in an ongoing therapy group, John was able to see individuals at different points in the therapeutic process and understand that people could and did change, which was hopeful to him.

Sex History

After brief introductions of group members, John was asked to begin the first therapeutic task: to trace his sexual biography in the context of his family upbringing and interactions with his environment. This was an important method to increase his cognitive understanding of the psychodynamics and etiology of his CSB.

Because most individuals with CSB come from highly dysfunctional family backgrounds, this is often a painful process. He was asked to talk about this history in the group setting. In many group sessions, John would relate other parts of his sexual history and would receive empathic, challenging, and insightful feedback from other group members. Through this process, John began to understand and to reconnect his feelings to memories of his childhood. This process was cathartic for him. He began to understand how he experienced this pain and how sexual activity was his primary coping mechanism. While he understood the disruptive effects of CSB on his life, he also realized that his obsessive and compulsive sexual behavior was not an effective means for solving his problems. John became increasingly motivated to understand the source of his fears and anxieties and to manage these in a healthier fashion. He began to understand the futility of his obsessive and compulsive behaviors and was ready to progress to the next phase of therapy.

Clarifying Boundaries of Healthy Sexual Expression

In the initial stage of therapy, efforts were made to bolster John's motivation to eliminate the most clearly self- or other-destructive sexual behaviors. This is not always possible given the nature of CSB and its resistant nature to change. However, trying to eliminate the most destructive elements, rather than trying to stop immediately all compulsive sexual behavior, is necessary. For example, in John's case, he knew that having sexual intercourse with another woman without a condom was risky for contracting an STD and potentially life threatening because of the current HIV epidemic. He was reluctant to use condoms because of reduced sensation and lack of spontaneity. However, he was obsessively fearful that he might lose even the slightest amount of pleasure during sexual activity. Even without a condom, John did not experience much feeling, and orgasms were quickly followed by a sense of guilt and remorse for yielding to his compulsion. Fears of contracting an STD dominated his thinking, and he spent the next few nights without sleep and urgently made an appointment with the STD clinic.

Therefore, it was clear that "unsafe sex" was an extremely unhealthy sexual behavior. We introduced the concept of setting a boundary around this unhealthy behavior, recognizing that there is always a gray zone of other behaviors that may have more or less unhealthy aspects to them.

Our success in helping John gain control of this behavior was assisted through pharmacotherapy. Having safer sex using a condom gave John some confidence in trying to look at other sexual behaviors over which he wished to gain control. Individuals with CSB tend to rationalize the unhealthy aspects of their sexual behavior or to stop abruptly all forms of sexual behavior other than sexual activity within the context of a relationship. In John's case, he immediately wanted to stop having sex with women outside his marriage and to stop going to strip shows and adult bookstores, viewing pornography, fantasizing about women he met, and having sex with his wife until he could prove to himself that he was "cured." The group encouraged him to set more realistic expectations for himself and to define more carefully what he considered to be CSBs. He received feedback that many of his sexual desires were normal and healthy, and he was encouraged to define healthy outlets for sexual activity. An analogy was used that you do not ask someone with an eating disorder to stop eating. Instead, you attempt to stop bingeing and purging at the same time that you learn healthy eating habits. Because John's relationship with his wife was strained and currently nonsexual, he was encouraged to consider masturbation as an alternative outlet for sexual expression. At this time in therapy, he had not masturbated in many years. John's attitudes about masturbation were very negative: He viewed it as selfish and sinful. Group members suggested that his attitudes toward masturbation might be rather restrictive and that most of his conflicts around masturbation involved a values conflict. The group encouraged him to begin masturbating in a self- nurturing way. He was instructed to read *The New Male Sexuality* (Zilbergeld, 1992) and to begin to reevaluate his attitudes and values around sexuality.

Risk Situations and Triggers

He was then asked to identify his obsessions and compulsions and to identify stressful situations, events, and environments that evoke unpleasant feelings. Through this exercise, John could better identify when and how he was at risk and begin using alternative coping strategies. The first step in breaking out of his pattern was to identify it.

In the process of therapy, we taught John a variety of relaxation exercises and ways to nurture himself and call upon sources of support to help short-circuit his obsessive and compulsive behaviors. Certain situations, environments, or events were unavoidable, and he needed to learn coping mechanisms to handle these situations with less stress. However, other situations were avoidable and unnecessary. For example, because of the dysfunctional relationship with his family of origin, his obsessions and compulsions were triggered whenever he visited his mother and father. He decided to stop seeing them for a time to avoid this stressor.

Managing Risk Situations

Seeing his family, being in a singles bar, being criticized, and having a fight with his wife were some of the risk situations he identified. He learned to recognize when he was "at risk" and to bypass avoidable risk situations (e.g., going to a strip show). John also began to employ some of his new coping techniques when faced with unavoidable risk situations. He noticed that since he had begun taking his medication, these risk situations did not trigger the intensity of negative emotions he had experienced in the past, and he could better handle these situations.

Gaining Control over Compulsive Sexual Behavior

Within about 8 weeks of beginning Prozac and group psychotherapy, John had identified his typical obsessions and compulsions and his arousal pattern and triggers; experienced improvement in his negative emotions in response to stressful situations, events, and environments; set boundaries around the most destructive elements of his obsessive and compulsive behavior and stayed within those boundaries; set boundaries around risk situations that he could avoid and avoided them; and developed some new coping mechanisms for unavoidable stressful situations.

Stabilizing the Marital Relationship

As I stated earlier, John's relationship with his wife was extremely strained. Along with the group psychotherapy, we began conjoint sessions. He told his wife what he had been learning in his therapy, his desire to resolve his problem, and his wish to work on their relationship and rebuild trust and intimacy. Since the disclosures of his extramarital sexual activities, his wife expressed intense hurt and anger. She felt that she could no longer trust him and doubted whether the relationship could be salvaged.

The goals of these sessions were to stabilize the marital relationship by engaging his wife in the process of therapy, suggesting individual therapy for her, and helping the couple to work on the issues in their relationship. It was essential for John to express his thoughts and feelings and to show genuine remorse and a sincere willingness to address his problems. This helped create some hope for Barbara that her husband might behave differently and that their relationship might eventually be restored. John had predictable feelings of impatience with Barbara's mistrust of him and pleaded with her to end the separation. Barbara felt resentful that he was more concerned about his feelings than hers. However, they were able to commit themselves to working on their relationship, and if it improved, she agreed to reevaluate her intentions to divorce him. Barbara was agreeable to seeing another therapist to understand her own issues, to deal with her grief and anger, and to clarify what she wanted in the relationship. I recommended a therapist who was experienced in working with partners of individuals with CSB.

In their joint sessions, I helped Barbara to understand CSB and how it is treated. I encouraged her to read articles and books on the subject, and John and I invited her to ask as many questions as she wanted. I told her that the process of resolving CSB was not remedied overnight and that rebuilding trust and intimacy—including sexual intimacy—would take some time. She was encouraged by John's progress in avoiding extramarital sex. We explained that John needed to address some of his family-of-origin conflicts before he could make further progress in rebuilding intimacy in their relationship.

Resolving Family-of-Origin Conflicts

John was now ready to address the next phase of the treatment process: resolving family-of-origin conflicts. Although he had gained control over his compulsions, he still struggled with occasional obsessive thoughts and had not addressed the underlying source of his anxiety, low self-esteem and difficulty in intimate relationships. In this phase of therapy, he began to recognize the origin of these difficulties by continuing to explore his sexual biography and to develop greater awareness of how spending time with his family triggered many of his negative feelings and activated his obsessions. When John had gained some control over his compulsive sexual behavior, he had more access to his feelings and was less guarded and defensive. In this way, he was better able to address therapeutic issues at a deeper level.

The group encouraged him to look into his relationship with his parents and siblings. He recalled how punitive his father had been. As a child, it seemed as if nothing he could do was right. His father held high standards for John's behavior and routinely punished him for his transgressions. He was severely disciplined with regular beatings. This discipline often occurred when his father came home drunk, but he also recalled that his father could explode easily and he never knew when this might occur. He remembers being hit in the face often, beaten, and kicked. One time, his mother took him to the emergency room for excessive bleeding caused by one of his father's beatings. His mother told the doctor that John had fallen accidentally, and the physician never suspected child abuse. John was too terrified of his father to tell the physician otherwise.

Although the physical beatings were painful, the verbal "beatings" were even more painful. His father constantly told John that he was a "bum" who would never amount to anything. His father was critical of everything John did. John desperately tried to meet his father's approval, but nothing seemed to satisfy him. John excelled in school, but his father ignored these positive achievements.

John's mother received similar treatment from his father. His parents fought constantly, and his father struck his mother and humiliated her in front of the children. His father suspected that she was having an affair and often called her a whore. John was always in doubt whether his parents would stay together. While he wanted them to remain together as a family, he often wished his mother would leave his father. In his therapy, John became aware of his intense anger toward his mother for her ineffectual attempts at protecting him from his father and her complacency about their dysfunctional relationship.

John was asked to bring other family members in for therapy. At first, he was reluctant and did not believe that his father and mother would be willing to come in. His mother agreed to come for a session, but his father told him that John should sort out his own problems. John feared his mother's rejection for his recent CSB. His mother always espoused a conservative and rigid morality around sexuality: Sex was permissible only in the context of marriage and should not be discussed. With great trepidation, John described his present difficulties to his mother and related some of his childhood memories. He was asked to describe aspects of his CSB. It was not necessary for him to go into great detail, but by talking about some of his shameful behavior, he had to confront his fears of his mother's abandonment. Because she had not known he was experiencing any difficulties, she was stunned and could hardly believe what she heard. However, she was able to corroborate the history of his childhood. She cried when he talked about going to the hospital and telling the doctor the lie about his injury. At the end of the first session, she told John that she was sorry for the hurt that she had caused but emphasized that she always loved him and, in spite of what she heard, she still loved him and expressed a willingness to do whatever she could to help him. He cried and the session ended with an embrace and many tears. She was able to encourage her husband to attend the next session. John's father was much more defensive than his mother had been but was able to listen and offered his support. Several more sessions were held with his parents separately. In these sessions, they were able to review their relationship, break down defenses, and talk about ways to improve their relationship. During one session, his father broke down in tears and told of his remorse about the beatings and emotional abuse. He talked about how his father had treated him in the same way. Since his treatment for alcoholism, he had come to understand the origin of his own problems and had improved his relationship with his wife, but he had been unable to bridge the gap in his relationship with his son or with John's siblings.

John was greatly relieved by these sessions. He now found that he could visit with his parents without strong negative feelings, and he experienced fewer sexual obsessions. His self-esteem was further enhanced.

Improving Healthy Sexual and Intimate Relationships

The next phase of therapy was to address current sexual and intimate relationships. When John's relationship with his wife had stabilized, the couple began to address their own individual issues. Within a month or so, Barbara decided to have John move back into their house. Therapy sessions continued monthly. At a behavioral and cognitive level, these sessions were designed to improve marital intimacy by teaching communication skills, negotiating roles and rules in their relationship, and improving conflict-resolution skills. At a deeper level, John and Barbara were able to understand the dynamics of their relationship and how these dynamics stemmed from their family-of-origin relationships. They expressed feelings about deep wounds created by the intimacy dysfunction in their relationship. These sessions were cathartic and resulted in greater trust and closeness.

Although they had resumed their sexual relationship when John moved back into the house, the couple was never fully satisfied with this aspect of their relationship. There were no performance difficulties but both perceived that their sexual relationship was rather perfunctory, uncreative, and "empty." Barbara felt it was important for her to act as "sexy" as she could to keep John satisfied. In this process, she neglected her own needs and felt as though she was "servicing" him. In turn, John felt guilty because he spent much of his time fantasizing and obsessing about other women while having sex with Barbara. I drew distinction between fantasizing about someone else and obsessional thinking. I encouraged the couple to talk about their fantasies and to move back and forth from fantasies to a focus on each other. John had developed a pattern of obsessional fantasies of other partners and had not learned to make an emotional connection with his wife while having sex with her. He had not learned to eroticize an intimate relationship.

At this point I used sex therapy exercises (e.g., sensate focus) that were standard in the treatment of sexual dysfunction. These exercises were helpful in improving the couple's sexual and intimate relationship.

During this phase of treatment, John and Barbara were encouraged to attend our Sexual Attitude Reassessment Seminar. This 2-day, psychoeducational and experiential seminar is designed to increase comfort with one's own and others' sexuality, to reevaluate one's attitudes and values, and to present some models of healthy sexual and intimacy functioning. This seminar was helpful to John and Barbara as a catalyst to enhancing their sexual and intimate relationship.

Maintenance Plan and Support System

At this point in his therapy, John had achieved control over his obsessions and compulsions and had improved his sexual and intimacy functioning. During periods of stress, however, he continued to obsess about partners. Sometimes these obsessional thoughts resulted in urges to act out sexually outside his boundaries. However, he was able to manage his obsessions, to use his newly learned coping strategies, and to avoid acting on his urges.

John was now ready for therapy termination. He was uncertain and fearful that if he stopped therapy, his obsessions and compulsions would return. However, he had gained enough confidence to leave the group and discontinue his marital and family therapy sessions. He had developed strong feelings of closeness within the group, and he expressed concerns over loss of their support and guidance.

The group encouraged John to map out his strategy for maintaining the gains that he had made and to articulate how he would handle difficult situations in the future. He was also asked to clarify his support system. He needed to identify people in his life who he could rely on for ongoing support. We recommended that this support group include a member of his family of origin, a few friends, and one or two group members. We also encouraged him to become a part of our aftercare group.

Aftercare

Recognizing the need for ongoing support, we have established an aftercare group that meets monthly and is open to all individuals who have completed our treatment process. John joined this group for ongoing support and consolidation of gains made through his therapeutic process. It also served as a place for him to discuss any difficulties he was experiencing and to help prevent them from becoming a source of relapse. Sometimes in the course of this process, individuals decide to reengage in therapy. John found the aftercare group sufficient for his needs and has remained a part of this group.

At this point John wondered whether he needed to continue his medication. Following consultation with our psychiatrist, he decided to taper off his medication and to reevaluate his functioning. He had no difficulty in reducing the medication, and he felt fine. However, within 4 to 6 weeks, he found himself becoming more irritable and had started obsessive thinking again. Upon consulting with our psychiatrist, he resumed his medication and his symptoms remitted. Continued medication was an important part of his maintenance plan.

DISCUSSION

New developments in the field of psychiatry are shedding light on the nature and treatment of compulsive sexual behavior. The advent of the serotonin reuptake inhibitors has made a significant impact on our ability to treat these disorders. This pharmacotherapy was clearly beneficial to John in his ability to gain control over his CSB and to engage in the process of psychotherapy. This, in turn, allowed him to resolve his underlying anxiety and intimacy disorder. It is impossible to determine retrospectively the relative contributions of the various components of this treatment process. Could John have improved with pharmacotherapy alone? Could he have improved with psychotherapy alone? Was family or group therapy necessary? Each case of CSB must have its own individualized treatment plan; however, the greatest success in treating CSB is achieved when the patient is motivated and has the resources to engage in the treatment components described here. John was fortunate to have a wife who loved him and was willing to work on her own therapeutic issues and the couple relationship. That his parents and siblings were willing to participate in the treatment process was also helpful. In many ways, this was an ideal case with a very positive outcome. Treating CSB is not easy and various twists, turns, and obstacles are usually encountered along the way. However, treatment can often be successful and results gratifying.

REFERENCES

American Psychiatric Association. (1994). *Diagnostic and statistical manual of mental disorders* (4th ed.). Washington, DC: Author.

Barth, R. J., & Kinder, B. N. (1987). The mislabeling of sexual impulsivity. *Journal of Sex and Marital Therapy, 13,* 15–23.

Butcher, J. N. (1989). *Minnesota multiphasic personality inventory (MMPI-II): User's guide.* Minneapolis: National Computer Systems.

Carnes, P. (1983). *Out of the shadows: Understanding sexual addiction.* Minneapolis: CompCare.

Carnes, P. (1989). *Contrary to love: Helping the sexual addict.* Minneapolis: CompCare.

Carnes, P. (1991). *Don't call it love: Recovering from sexual addiction.* New York: Bantam.

Cesnik, J. A., & Coleman, E. (1989). Use of lithium carbonate in the treatment of autoerotic asphyxia. *American Journal of Psychotherapy, 43*(2), 277–286.

Coleman, E. *(1987).* Sexual compulsivity: Definition, etiology, and treatment considerations. In E. Coleman (Ed.), *Chemical dependency and intimacy dysfunction.* New York: Haworth.

Coleman, E. (1990). The obsessive–compulsive model for describing compulsive sexual behavior. *American Journal of Preventive Psychiatry and Neurology, 2* (3), 9–14.

Coleman, E. (1991). Compulsive sexual behavior: New concepts and treatments. *Journal of Psychology and Human Sexuality, 4*(2), 37–52.

Coleman, E. (1992). Is your patient suffering from compulsive sexual behavior? *Psychiatric Annals, 22*(6), 320–325.

Coleman, E., & Cesnik, J. (1990). An unusual manifestation of obsessional gender dysphoria: Treatment with lithium carbonate and psychotherapy. *American Journal of Psychotherapy, 44*(2), 204–217.

Coleman, E., Cesnik, J., Moore, A. M., & Dwyer, S. M. (1992). Exploratory study of the role of psychotropic medications in the psychological treatment of sex offenders. *Journal of Offender Rehabilitation, 18* (3/4), 75–88.

Derogatis, L. R., & Meyer, J. K. (1979). A psychological profile of the sexual dysfunctions. *Archives of Sexual Behavior, 8,* 201–223.

Federoff, P. (1988). Buspirone hydrochloride in the treatment of transvestic fetishism. *Journal of Clinical Psychiatry, 49,* 408–409.

Kafka, M. (1991). Successful antidepressant treatment of nonparaphilic sexual addictions and paraphilias in males. *Journal of Clinical Psychiatry, 52*(5), 60–65.

Kafka, M., & Coleman, E. (1991). Serotonin and paraphilias: The convergence of mood, impulse and compulsive disorders. *Journal of Clinical Psychopharmacology, 11*(3), 223–224.

Kramer, P. D. (1994). *Listening to Prozac.* New York: Penguin.

Levine, S. B. (1982). A modern perspective on nymphomania. *Journal of Sex and Marital Therapy, 8,* 316–324.

Money, J. (1980). *Love and love sickness: The science of sex, gender difference, and pairbonding.* Baltimore: Johns Hopkins University Press.

Money, J. (1986). *Lovemaps: Clinical concepts of sexual/erotic health and pathology, paraphilia, and gender transposition in childhood, adolescence, and maturity.* New York: Irvington.

Stoller, R. J. (1975). *Perversion: The erotic form of hatred.* New York: Pantheon.

Zilbergeld, B. (1992). *The new male sexuality.* New York: Bantam.

20

Sexual Addiction: A Sex Therapist's Struggles with an Unfamiliar Clinical Entity

SHARON G. NATHAN

INTRODUCTION

Of all of the cases discussed in this volume, surely only those pertaining to sexual addiction/compulsion need to address the question whether the problem treated actually exists. That individuals could be addicted to sex, or repeatedly compulsively driven to engage in sexual activities they believe to be harmful to their well-being, evokes incredulity in some sex therapists and angry opposition in others. What are the sources of this waning, but still common, professional resistance?

Perhaps the strongest source of opposition comes from those who see concern with sexual addiction as the vanguard of the sexual counter-revolution. This case is fleshed out the most comprehensively by Levine and Troiden (1988), who argue from a sociological perspective that sexual addiction "constitute[s] an attempt to repathologize forms of erotic behavior that became acceptable in the 1960s and 1970s" (p. 349). They assert that labeling behavior "sexually compulsive" or "addicted" is simply applying a medical label to a behavior that is disapproved of for moral reasons. Because what is thought of as sexually appropriate varies from culture to culture and from one time to another, they see no warrant for making a disease out of a person's sexual choice. (Their argument applies with equal force to all, or almost all, the sexual dysfunctions, a point they readily acknowledge.) But from a clinical point of view, a behavior's relationship or adaptiveness to a patient's culture is not irrelevant. That cannibalism was normative in 19th-century Fiji does not bar defining such a practice as pathological (as well as illegal) in our culture, where the etiology and meaning of the behavior are bound to be completely different. Similarly, one can argue that recreational sex with multiple anonymous partners means something different today from what it meant in the pre-AIDS era. The behavior itself is no more immoral today than it was in the 1970s (unless the person is knowingly risking transmitting a venereal disease to another), but a person can no longer be considered to be simply following the crowd and doing the "done" thing when engaging in such activities today.

Even many sex therapists who would not go to the extreme of Levine and Troiden's "it's all relative" feel uneasy with some of the embedded notions of sexual addiction. Because the bulk of patients seen by sex therapists have problems stemming from overcontrol, guilt, and anxiety, we are used to reassuring people reflexively that sex is natural and good, nothing is wrong between consenting partners, most people disapprove of their own sexual fantasies, and so on. To consider instead that individuals may be doing themselves harm through their sexual behavior feels counterintuitive, and to work with a patient to curb his/her sexual activities (or, worse, to forsake all sexual activity—including fantasy—for a while) feels wrong. Yet pronouncing our liberal shibboleths is obviously inappropriate when we are confronted with patients whose sexual lives are as out of control as that of the patient discussed in this chapter. To tell someone that he must not condemn himself for his sexual desires (e.g., unprotected bathhouse sex with multiple partners each day) is one thing, but to actually promote such activity as harmless and good is entirely another.

Yet another source of resistance to the concept of sexual addiction/ compulsion (sexual addiction in particular) is that it derives not from sexology but from addictionology, a field with which many of us have virtually no familiarity. (The *locus classicus* of the sexual addiction concept is Carnes, 1983.) We do not know its proponents personally or professionally (the exception among the early explicators of the problem is Quadland, 1985); we question their credentials, assumptions, and knowledge of sexuality. (Would it surprise you to know that the suspicion is mutual? More than one colleague working in the addictions field has expressed to me the belief that sex therapists do not want to consider sexual addiction because many sex therapists are themselves sex addicts.) The 12-step model of recovery (in and of itself an alien term) is suspect because it seems more exhortatory and evangelical than medical or psychological; in such important ways we are not speaking the same language. And when practitioners coming from the addictions world try to frame their assumptions in our language (Carnes, 1990; Goodman, 1992), the result is often clumsy and imprecise (see Moser, 1993).

By and large, sex therapists seem more comfortable with the more medical term "sexual compulsion" than with "sexual addiction." Patients, however, seem intuitively drawn to "sexual addiction," and not, I think, just because it is a catchier phrase. Whether thinking of it literally or merely as a powerful metaphor, many patients see in the addiction concept ideas that speak to their own experience—the sense of being driven to do something even though they know they will regret it, the feeling of being "high" when engaged in acting out, the experience of painful withdrawal when trying to control sexual activity. The two locutions—sexual compulsion and sexual addiction—are not merely synonyms (Carnes, 1990; Coleman, 1990); they implicate different etiologies and treatments. However, it seems very early in the game to have to commit to one model or the other; each seems to suggest possibilities the other does not (e.g., sexual compulsion draws attention to the possible utility of psychotropic medications, sexual addiction to a consideration of abstinence), and far too little evidence has been gathered to know which is predictively more accurate (i.e., Can one recover, as a sexual compulsion model suggests, or is one always "recovering," as the addictions model would imply?).

What appears undeniable is that there are people who are troubled by a sense that they cannot curb, control, or modify their sexual behavior, even when they are aware of the negative social, medical, and/or financial consequences that attend their inability to do so. It is the fact that such patients have been presenting themselves to us for treatment—rather than any scholarly debates in our journals—that has led us to consider the phenomenon seriously. While a small subset of these patients may be merely guilt ridden about behavior that we deem perfectly normal, far too many seem truly out of control. Reassurances about their simply having a high sex drive ring hollow to therapist and patient alike.

As a practicing sex therapist I have struggled (and continue to struggle) with these issues. The case described here represents the state of that struggle at a point early in my work with sexual addiction patients. I chose this case because it demonstrates how someone trained as a sex therapist has to monitor and combat reflexes instilled by sex therapy training when treating a sex addict. Even though I was already a believer in the reality of sex addiction at the time I worked with David, I did not yet have an intuitive feel for the problem; when confronted with a manifestation for which I had not yet learned a specific sexual addiction intervention, I had a tendency to revert to my sex therapy roots—to the detriment of the treatment. Because I suspect that many sex therapists would operate in a similar fashion, I present my own errors and what I learned from them with the hope that this will prove useful to my colleagues.

CASE REPORT

While I was in session one winter morning, a man left a message on my answering machine, stating that his name was David K, that he had gotten my name from a hotline, and that he wanted to make an appointment to see me. I called him back immediately and arranged to see him that afternoon during what would have otherwise been a break in my schedule.

Many features of this presentation and of my responses to it are typical of initial encounters with patients who are sexually compulsive or addicted. They are almost always referred by sources that refer only sexually addicted patients: hotlines, colleagues working in the addictions field, and citations in books or articles about sexual addiction; they are almost never referred by the same sources that send sex therapy or psychotherapy patients: other psychotherapists, medical doctors, and former patients. This underscores the separation of sexual addiction from other sexual and psychological problems; although its label, "sexual addiction," contains references to both sex and addiction, in practice it is usually diagnosed as a kind of addiction rather than a kind of sexual problem. (This may account for the fact that many sex therapists deny that the entity exists because they have never seen a case of it; ironically, one seldom sees a case of sex addiction until one is trained and vetted to treat it, which, of course, implies that one already believes it exists.)

Also typical is my response to the phone message. I have learned that unless I return such a call immediately and set up an appointment within 24 hours (better yet, the very same day), I am unlikely ever to see the patient. There is a very small window of opportunity between the time the patient realizes that he must deal with this problem and the time he erases that knowledge by acting out again. I have also discovered that it is quite unimportant that the proposed appointment time be a "convenient" one; as with his acting out, the patient will keep the appointment if he is motivated even if it means disregarding a previous commitment, such as work.

The patient who arrived at my office was a 36-year-old actor and technical worker, short of stature and appealing in a kind of puckish way. David was divorced and also recently separated from a fiancee. He reported that he had had some success as a character actor in the past *but had not been employed in this line of work for some time although he hoped to get back into it. He now had a job in which he was competent but not interested. Despite earning a reasonable salary, he was $65,000 in debt, without credit, and so far behind in his rent that he was facing possible eviction from his apartment.*

Such chaotic life circumstances are quite common for patients with sexual addictions. Sexual preoccupations can become so compelling and time-consuming for the sex addict that he has little energy or attention left over for dealing with the activities of daily life. In addition, some forms of sexual addiction can be quite expensive in and of themselves—prostitutes, large pornography collections, phone sex, and so on.

When asked what led him to seek this consultation, David told me that he was a sex addict. He said he had previously been addicted to alcohol, marijuana, and cocaine, but that after a year and a half of inpatient rehabilitation, attendance at 12-step groups, and many lapses, he had finally achieved 10 consecutive months of abstinence from these substances.

While there is much controversy in the field about whether this problem is more properly labeled "sexual addiction" or "sexual compulsivity," I find that patients usually have a commitment to one term or the other, and I tend to use the term they prefer. In general, patients like David who have, or have had, other addictions prefer the term "sexual addiction," and their use of the term is significant because it condenses a lot of assumptions about the nature of the problem (a disease), its resolution (abstinence, sobriety, recovery), means of treatment (12-step groups, rehabs), and prognosis (difficult, but possible with everlasting vigilance) into one word. On the other hand, patients (although not necessarily therapists) who use the term "sexual compulsivity" tend to think of overcoming the problem in a more traditionally psychodynamic way—that is, they believe they need to understand the roots and meaning of their behavior for it to change, and they tend to be skeptical about treatment that focuses on the symptom.

David reported the manifestations of his sexual addiction as masturbation, peep shows, voyeurism, prostitutes, sex with female partners he did not pay, and preoccupations with sexual thoughts, fantasies, and plans. As David detailed this picture, it became clear that virtually his entire waking life was consumed by one form or another of sexual activity. David masturbated several times a day (including immediately after having sex with a partner); he appraised every woman he encountered (at work, at Alcoholics Anlnymous meetings, sitting across from him on the subway, etc.) in terms of her sexual availability and often picked up for sex those he considered amenable; he planned, or took advantage of, naturally occurring opportunities to peep at women in states of undress; he debated with himself endlessly whether to go to Times Square for a peep show or to Eighth Avenue to pick up a prosti-tute (a debate sometimes concluded by a decision to do so); and he thought about sex—what he would like to do, what he had done, why he should not do it, how he would do it—many hours a day.

To a sexually addicted/compulsive person, the world appears as if a template has been superimposed on reality, a template that highlights sexual opportunities and obscures almost everything else. For example, when most New Yorkers look out their apartment windows, they see buildings, traffic, an occasional tree, pedestrians, windows with various kinds of curtains and blinds, and so on. When a sex addict looks out his apartment window (and David is only one of several patients reporting the same thing), he frequently sees neighbors undressing, masturbating, and having sex in front of open windows—a private peep show that can recur with such regularity that a *TV Guide*-like schedule could be drawn up. Similarly, while most of the single patients I work with need dating services, personal ads, mixers, and introductions from friends in order to meet members of the opposite sex, sexually compulsive patients find partners wherever they are. In one 2-week period, David had sex with a woman from his Alcoholics Anonymous (AA) meeting, a woman he met on the subway on his way to work, a waitress who had served him lunch, and a woman in his workplace whose telephone he had been sent to fix. It does not seem to me as if sexually addicted people necessarily place themselves in situations in which sex is especially likely to happen; it is rather that they see the sexual possibilities wherever they are. Just as an ancient Native American hunter was said to be aware of the faintest signs that his prey has passed a certain way, so, too, does a sexual compulsive note manifestations of his quarry too subtle for the less experienced and less motivated to detect.

The range of sexual activities in which David was compulsively involved is somewhat broader than that of the average sexually addicted patient. Frequent masturbation is an activity common to most sexual compulsives, and to that most add one, two, or more other types of sexual expression. But no matter how many different types of sexual behavior the person employs, sexual thoughts and behavior (and efforts to control the sexual thoughts and behavior) come to fill a large part of the day.

David reported that he had made efforts to overcome his addiction. He repeatedly promised himself that he would stop these behaviors and had concretized this commitment by taking steps to make acting out less likely. He had thrown away his pornography collection and had not bought any replacements. And because he knew that when he got into a car, he felt almost compelled to drive to an area where he could pick up a prostitute, he forced himself never to borrow or rent a car. Despite all these quite sincere efforts, David had never been able to put together more than 16 consecutive days of sexual sobriety.

Most patients who seek treatment for sexual addiction have already made similar efforts to control their behavior. Although presenting for treatment takes place only when someone has come to label his behavior "addicted" and has learned that help for it is available—usually following seeing a television program or magazine article devoted to the topic—the afflicted person has usually been clear in his own mind for a long time that something is wrong with what he is doing. Attempts at control mostly involve what people in the addictions field call "white-knuckling it"—gritting one's teeth, hanging on tight, and vowing not to act out ever again. Such attempts do not succeed for very long because, unbeknownst to patients, the compulsive activities fulfill a function for which they currently have no suitable replacement available in their behavioral repertoire.

Does David's situation qualify as sexual addiction? Because the fourth edition of the *Diagnostic and Statistical Manual of Mental Disorders* (DSM-IV; American Psychiatric Association, 1994) does not recognize this entity and provide criteria for its diagnosis, sex therapists are on their own in making this determination. In practice, I think many of us employ an analogue of Justice Potter Stewart's comment about pornography: I may not be able to define it "but I know it when I see it." I myself try to formalize this somewhat by holding the patient's situation up to a variant of the 12-step movement's standards for addiction in general: powerlessness and unmanageability. Is the patient unable to make his/her behavior conform to his/her own standards of acceptability (provided that the standards are reasonable), and is this inability getting the patient into trouble? Utilizing these criteria helps extricate the sex therapist from a morass of quantitative considerations—that is, how many times a day or how many partners constitutes a problem? It also gives weight to the patient's subjective discomfort and to the issue of maladaptation. This is necessary to address the charges that the label "sexual addiction" is merely a way of stigmatizing or pathologizing a person with a high level of sexual desire, or that it is a way to make sound scientific what is nothing more than a disapproval of some lifestyles. (The only times that I have actually encountered this potential for misuse involved two cases in which husbands presented their wives for treatment of their purported sexual addictions; in each case the woman had had an extramarital affair, and the husband, unwilling to accept that his wife preferred another, sought to understand the wellspring of her behavior as illness rather than choice.)

Given these criteria, David's case easily qualifies as sexual addiction. David had been powerless in stopping or controlling his sexual behavior despite sincere efforts, and his sexual behavior had contributed to a chaotic and unsatisfactory lifestyle: David had been unable to pursue his acting career and was barely able to hang on to his current, relatively undemanding job. He was in debt both because of the cost in money of his sexual activities and the cost in time to earn income and attend to his financial affairs. His promiscuity had led his fiancee to end their relationship. He had narrowly escaped arrest for peeping on several occasions, and given the risks David was willing to take to engage in this activity (e.g., crawling through an air shaft to spy on a women's locker room), it seemed only a matter of time until he was caught.

I asked David to give me some background about himself. He told me that he had grown up in a large midwestern city in a blue-collar, Protestant family. He was the second of three sons and the only one to achieve anything educationally or vocationally. He described his father as rigid, dictatorial, and physically punitive; his mother as meek, too weak to serve as a counterweight to his father, and preoccupied with gambling on card games (so much so that she would sometimes be absent from the house for days at a time while she engaged in marathon card-playing sessions). David remembered beginning to masturbate as early as 5 or 6 years old and that he found the activity both exciting and calming. He started using drugs and alcohol when he was about 12 and his first sexual experience with a woman took place at age 14. In college, where he majored in theater, he was involved in a sexual relationship with a gay professor; although this was not David's sexual preference, he feared breaking off the relationship because the professor had the power to grant or withhold good grades and acting opportunities. (In telling this, David seemed not to condemn himself for what amounted to prostitution; he seemed somewhat annoyed at having to pay this price but not ashamed or guilty about it.) After college, David had some success acting in regional theater and commercials. He had been married for 3 years in his 20s but could say little about his ex-wife or their relationship. He currently considered himself engaged to a woman whose problems equaled his own; she, too, had work problems and large debts. In addition, she had been a lesbian until her relationship with David, a relationship she claimed to have undertaken because she wanted to get married and have children. David was unable to say what made him pursue this woman although he did believe that in some unspecified way he would be able to help her.

David's history has much in common with that of many other sexual addicts. Most report parents and other family members with addictions (such as David's mother's presumably compulsive gambling). While some of this reporting may be due to the addicted person's sensitivity, or even oversensitivity, to addictive behavior in others (classic are the alcoholics who see as similarly afflicted those who have even one cocktail on a daily basis), it probably does speak to a genuinely greater prevalence of such problems within addicts' families. This may be due to genetic predispositions and/or to learning; that is, a child growing up in such a home may learn that the way to get relief from unpleasant feelings is to engage in some consciousness-changing activity rather than to talk about the problem or seek real-world solutions.

David's history also has in common with that of other sexual addicts the early discovery of masturbation and its ability to bring not only pleasure but relief. One might speculate that sexually addicted people have an innately high sex drive, which facilitates their sexualizing tensions of whatever origin and gaining relief from them through orgasmic discharge. This, combined with the relative underdevelopment of more adaptive ways of handling life's problems, seems a formula for sexual addiction.

Like many other sex addicts, David had a history of addiction to other substances and activities as well. In David's case, the other addictions were to alcohol and drugs; other patients I have seen have reported problems with overeating, overspending, and gambling. David claimed that the worsening of his sexual addiction after he achieved sobriety from drugs and alcohol was an indication that sex was his "core addiction." My own understanding of this transition is that David got off drugs and alcohol but did not learn any more adaptive ways of coping; therefore, he moved on to a similar style of dealing with life with a theretofore relatively underutilized addictive behavior.

In common with many other sexual compulsives, David had a virtually impossible time talking about relationships, particularly about what it felt like to be in them and what differentiated one from another. The toll addiction takes in personal relationships generally seems greater than the toll it takes in vocational achievements; although David is not a particularly good example of this, many sexual addicts seem to have achieved a great deal in their careers despite the time, attention, and self-respect lost to the acting-out behavior.

I concurred with David's self-diagnosis of sexual addiction and told him that I believed the best way for him to deal with his problem would be to begin with an inpatient stay at a hospital specializing in treating this addiction. David did not object to my treatment plan on its merits— indeed it would have been his preference, too, as he knew how helpful such a stay had been for dealing with his drug and alcohol abuse—but because he had no insurance or other financial resources, it was out of the question. With a good deal of reluctance, which I conveyed to David, I agreed to try working with him on an outpatient basis.

Surely sexual addiction is the only problem a sex therapist confronts where hospitalization is a treatment modality to consider! But being willing to consider it and recommend it when necessary marks a watershed in the therapist's acceptance of the seriousness of the problem. I know that at first I certainly resisted the idea that a person might have to be hospitalized to stop his acting out. It was not as if there were physical consequences of withdrawal to monitor, as there were with detoxing from alcohol and drugs, and the person did not have a physical dependency on the substance (sex). That is how I thought back in the days when I considered sexual addiction an interesting metaphor for the problem but not its true nature. I now believe that it can be as wrenching for a sex addict to control his sexual activity as it is for someone else to control drug and alcohol use. Hospitalization can be a secure and supportive place to take the first step, an asylum (literally and figuratively) from the pressures and temptations that fuel sexual acting out. (The charge that there are hospitals that drum up business for themselves by encouraging such treatment when it is not required may be true, but that abuse of hospitalization does not invalidate the principle at stake—any more than the occurrence of unnecessary hysterectomies means that such surgery should not be performed for uterine cancer.)

I asked David to do two things before our next session: (1) to make an effort not to stop his sexual preoccupation but to postpone it by telling himself whenever an impulse or thought arose that he would attend to it between 8:00 and 9:00 that evening but not before; (2) to attend a meeting of one of the 12-step groups that focuses on sexual addiction.

Let me say at the outset that the first thing I asked David to do was just plain ridiculous and betrayed the limited understanding I had of sexual addiction at the time I worked with him. I now know that if someone is able to postpone sexual thoughts and acts as I asked David to do, he does not qualify as a sexual addict! (My assignment was equivalent to asking an alcoholic to stop after drinking two glasses of wine; if he could stop after drinking two glasses of wine, he would not be an alcoholic.) But I think my mistake is typical of the kind of error a sex therapist is prone to making in treating sexual addiction. We are used to dealing with sex therapy patients whose problems involve overcontrol of their sexual impulses and who are anxious, guilty, and ashamed about behavior that it is easy for us to reassure them is normal. Sexual addiction patients' problems stem from undercontrol of their sexual impulses, and they are anxious, guilty, and ashamed about sexual behavior usually with very good cause. Trained as we are, and personally inclined as we are, to foster and encourage sexual comfort and pleasure, it is difficult, for us to turn around and see sexuality as a problem. All our instincts are suddenly wrong. Treating sexual addiction requires sex therapists to reprogram themselves, to go from reflexively encouraging a patient's sexual expression to recognizing that some forms of sexual expression are genuinely harmful.

I have noticed that the errors I and other sex therapists make in treating sexual addiction fall under two main rubrics. One is the teach-the-sex-addict-to-have-sex-like-a-normal-person error, an example of which is the assignment I gave David at the end of our first session. The thinking is that since non-sex addicts can postpone their sexual activity to the proper time and place, the sex addict should just do the same. The problem is not with the goal itself but rather with the notion that a sex addict can make the transition in one smooth step without the need for an intervening period of "detoxification" and abstinence. Another common example of the teach-the-sex-addict-to-have-sex-like-a-normal-person approach is telling patients that they can think whatever sexual thoughts they like because fantasizing something is not the same as doing it. While this is true for most people, it is not true for sex addicts for whom "perverse" fantasy is not an alternative to forbidden sexual activity but rather a rehearsal for it. (We also sometimes reassure sex therapy patients that while they like their fantasies as fantasies, they probably would not actually enjoy participating in the activity itself if given the opportunity; sex addicts, on the contrary, enjoy the actual activity even more than the fantasy.)

The second category of error the sex therapist is apt to fall into when treating sexual addiction is what I call the "connoisseur approach," an approach that advocates substituting quality for quantity. The rationale here is that if the sex addict could experience really good sex—often defined by the sex therapist as sexual intimacy with a loved partner—he/she would not need so much of it.

Following this approach, the sex therapist will often work with the addict and his/her partner to expand sexual communication and the range of sexual activity. However, the approach is about as fruitful as advocating a wine appreciation course as a cure for alcoholism. The error in that case would be conceptualizing alcoholism as a problem of beverage selection; with sexual addiction, the error involves believing that sexual addiction is *about* sex rather than about dealing with problematic feelings and situations *through* sex. (Addictions specialists working with sex addicts make their own kinds of errors, ones that therapists with expertise in sexuality would never entertain. For example, several patients have told me that they had previously been instructed to reprogram their arousal patterns by masturbating with an acceptable sexual fantasy in mind, rather than with the ones they naturally invoke. Sex therapists would see this approach as doomed to failure because it does not acknowledge the psychodynamic imperative of a person's fantasy choice, the way in which a preferred sexual fantasy reinvokes and reworks past experience.)

At the beginning of our second session one week later, I asked David about his experience with the assignments. Not surprisingly, he told me that he had tried the postponement assignment but had not been able to do it. More surprisingly, he also told me that he had not attended a meeting of a 12-step group dealing with sexual addiction although he continued to attend AA meetings regularly. When I asked why he was avoiding a modality that had been so helpful to him with his other addictions, he at first made excuses about scheduling and then finally acknowledged that going to such a meeting would indicate a wholehearted commitment to ending his sexual addiction, a commitment he realized he was still not ready to make.

It was certainly humbling to realize that entering psychotherapy for David did not constitute the same kind of commitment to change that attending a 12-step meeting would. Many therapists, myself included (certainly at the time I was seeing David), think of self-help groups (or, better, "mutual help groups," in the coinage of my colleague Mic Hunter) as an adjunctive modality, with the therapy being the main engine of change. Some therapists are uncomfortable with 12-step groups because they are uneasy with the religious overtones or because they decry what they see as the promotion of uncritical acceptance of its tenets. Others claim that "it only substitutes one addiction [the 12-step meetings themselves] for another"—a phenomenon that I believe occurs only rarely. (I have in fact seen only one case of it, a man who lived off money from an insurance settlement and devoted his entire life to 12-step meetings, therapy sessions, weekend and weeklong workshops on addictive topics, and yearly stays at hospitals for one of his many addictive problems—until the staff of one of the hospitals told him it was time for him to go it alone.) Even less informed therapists will make even less valid critiques; for example, one therapist told me that Sexaholics Anonymous was nothing but a money-making scheme. (Sexaholics Anonymous, like all 12-step groups, is, of course, free.)

My own opinion is that the 12-step groups for sexual addiction vary in usefulness. They seem most useful for patients like David who have had positive experiences with 12-step groups for other addictions. They appear to work better in some parts of the country than in others because not all localities have a devoted corps of members with long-standing recovery (as AA groups everywhere have). The groups naturally work better when the therapist is a proponent and supporter of attendance at them. I generally do not push attendance at meetings unless it is clear that nonattendance constitutes a resistance to dealing with the addiction (as it did in David's case). I do not think such meetings are useful for patients whose backgrounds and patterns of addiction differ greatly from those of most who attend a particular meeting. (In this opinion, I would probably not be supported by a single therapist coming from an addictions—rather than from a sex therapy—background, all of whom would say that the differences I cited were meaningless and that I was colluding with the patient in his denial of a real addictive problem.)

I have alluded rather generally to "12-step groups for sexual addiction" rather than mentioning particular groups. There are four main fellowships dealing with sexual addiction—Sexaholics Anonymous, Sex Addicts Anonymous, Sexual Compulsives Anonymous, and Sex and Love Addicts Anonymous. The groups vary primarily in how they define sexual sobriety, but for purposes of this discussion, they can be lumped together. (The group whose meetings David intended to attend was Sex and Love Addicts Anonymous, generally referred to by its acronym SLAA.)

Much of the rest of the session was devoted to additional history taking. Near the end of the session, I once again asked David to attend an SLAA meeting. I also asked him what else he thought would be a helpful assignment. David said he would like to try prayer and meditation.

Not being religious myself, I never would have thought of the assignment David devised for himself. In truth, at first I thought David was putting me on, and then when I realized he was not, I felt somewhat ill at ease and embarrassed. But this experience and others like it have sensitized me to a dimension of the sexual compulsion problem that I had not before recognized: In addition to the many negative consequences of such behavior that I was aware of (monetary cost, loss of self-esteem, toll on relationships, etc.), there is for many patients a terrible sense of alienation from God. In fact, for many sexual addiction patients the desire to be back in harmony with God's law is one of the strongest motivators of change. This is especially true because what I myself (and most other sex therapists as well, I believe) would consider a paramount motivation for curbing the addictive behavior—to be able to have an intimate relationship with a loved partner—is in fact only a vague and theoretical concept for many sex addicts. Although many patients like David pay lip service to the notion that they want intimacy, further probing reveals that many have no idea what that means and have had no such experiences in their entire lives. What the pleasure of such an experience might be is inconceivable because the close relationships many such patients have actually experienced have been characterized by abuse and emptiness. In fact, intimacy comes to be understood by many patients as merely the absence of sexual excitement—to the point that achieving it seems more like one of the costs, rather than one of the benefits, of sobriety.

In the third session, David once again confessed he had not gone to an SLAA meeting. He "compromised" by going to AA and talking about his sexual addiction with someone after the formal meeting. The man he talked to told him that he wished he could be as "lucky" as David. David complained that no one in AA could understand that a person could be addicted to sex. I pointed out that David could have predicted this because he had had similar experiences in the past—while he complained about not being understood at AA, he was avoiding SLAA where his problem would be recognized. David also talked with a woman member after the AA meeting and told her all about his sexual problem in great detail. The woman got excited hearing about his exploits, and they ended up leaving together and having sex. David's positive accomplishments for the week had been meditating every morning and praying every night. He also hit upon the idea of taking his glasses off when he came into his apartment and keeping them off until 8:00 when he knew the woman he habitually peeped at across the way would be finished with her nightly disrobing performance; David said that he was too myopic to see her window without his glasses. In answer to my query, David reported that he had actually taken his glasses off only one night during the week.

This on-and-off pattern of attempting to abstain from problematic behavior is typical not only of David but of many other sexually compulsive patients. David's week demonstrates his shrewd knowledge of what he needs to do not to act out (e.g., go to SLAA, take off his glasses) and his unwillingness to act on the basis of this knowledge consistently. Although some patients affect surprise at the outcome of their decisions, when pressed, most recognize that the results were only to be expected because they had occurred time after time. Most patients know that because certain actions will inevitably lead to certain outcomes, a sequence needs to be inhibited at its outset if the control is to be effective. Thus, David knew that unless he mechanically prevented himself from looking at his neighbor (by closing the blinds, taking off his glasses, not being home at show time), he would peep at her; to claim to himself that *this time* what had always happened would not happen was simply to have decided to act out. (An analogy is the dieter who buys chocolate chip cookies in case company drops in; buying the cookies is really a decision to eat the cookies no matter what the rationalization.)

Why is it that David will not do the things he knows he needs to do to stop the behavior that he believes is ruining his life? Unfortunately, this question can be answered only generally in David's case because a precise answer is only learned when the incessant acting out is diminished to a point where one can access the consequences of *not* acting out. That is, it is assumed that a person acts out to shut off painful thoughts and feelings that occur in the absence of acting out. Because David is in a constant state of acting out (counting the thoughts, plans, and reveries about sex as acting out as well as the sexual acts themselves)—a sort of *status sexus*—it is impossible to know what affects and ideas he is managing with his behavior. (David actually once said that his ideal life would be a state of constant orgasm.) With a more in-control patient, it eventually becomes clear that he acts out in the service of a particular restitutive fantasy. For example, when another patient was ignored or mistreated by his wife or his boss (which reevoked for him a childhood of profound neglect and dismissal), he soothed himself by going to a massage parlor where he could fantasize that the woman's only desire was to cater to his needs. Another patient, who had a loving and sexually fulfilling relationship with his beautiful wife, had spent years being a sugar daddy to a retinue of call girls—giving them checks that went well beyond normal fees and tips and actually setting some of them up in business ventures—in a way he came to realize was an identification with his abusive and extremely powerful father, who behaved similarly though on a much grander scale. The behavior really took off for this man after his father humiliated him in a particularly spiteful way; it was a classic case of identification with the aggressor, with sex simply being the means of enactment. Both of these men began masturbating as young children, presumably entertaining childhood variants of these same fantasy themes. Learning what the sexual acting out is accomplishing for the patient allows the therapist to help the patient both to understand his/her childhood hurts and to develop noncompulsive ways of dealing with similar feelings as an adult. With David, there was no opportunity to accomplish this.

Although David believed in the generic way that most 12-step adherents do that he was acting out to "change his feelings," he never had the trust in me, the process, and himself that would be needed to allow space for the underlying feelings to surface. In addition to his acting out, David also employed a barrage of ideas and cliches to stand between him and his feelings, and, I believe, he would have been unable to identify feelings if they did emerge (at least initially). After all, he had had no instruction in feelings identification and management as a child, and through most of his adulthood he relied on first one and then another addictive behavior to obviate such need. As another patient asked, in classic addict style, when the issue of experiencing his feelings was broached, "How do you do that? I mean, is there a feelings pill you can take?"

Twelve-step programs can be very helpful to patients in the early stages of recovery because they provide ready-made, albeit nonspecific, explanations that at least allow the patient to believe that there is some method to his madness. However, as treatment progresses, it is important for patients to be able to replace these generic constructions with knowledge of their own individual motivations. This transition can be difficult, as the following interchange with a patient indicates:

THERAPIST: So why do you think you do this [exhibit yourself to teenage girls]?
PATIENT: Because I get high from it.
THERAPIST: Right. But why this specific pattern?
PATIENT: Well, I guess I must have tried it and found it worked and so I kept on doing it.
THERAPIST: What do you think led you to try it the first time?
PATIENT: I don't know. (*long pause*) When I was in _____ Hospital, they told me I did it because I'm angry with women.
THERAPIST: Do you think they were right?
PATIENT: I don't know.

(Lest it be thought that the sterility of this interchange is due to the patient's low intelligence, I should mention that he is a very bright physician.)

At the end of the third session, it seemed to me that David walked too close to me when leaving the office. When the same thing happened at the end of the fourth session, I vowed I would ask David about it at the outset of our next meeting. David replied that he had been testing me—and that I had failed his test by backing away from him both times. He had been assessing my sexual availability. He also cheerfully volunteered that that had also been the intent of his oddly out-of-context question the previous session: "Are you happily married?" David expanded on this by telling me that this is what he did with women in general. He gave as an example a situation the previous week when he had had to install a telephone at a coworker's workstation. The project involved his crawling under the woman's desk, and when the woman neither got up from her chair nor closed her legs together, David knew he had identified another potential partner. They in fact had sex later that day.

I was shocked! Not at what had happened between David and the woman in his office; I was certainly used to such tales. And not that David had had a sexual fantasy about me; that is certainly an admission that patients make on occasion to their therapists. I was shocked that David was actually assessing my availability in the here and now, for real. Our professional relationship posed no barrier to David's assessing me as a sex partner, and he did not believe that my being his therapist would necessarily pose any such barrier for me. I felt violated both as a psychologist and as a woman. I considered whether David's behavior constituted "acting in the transference"—a concept that would allow me to understand this within a familiar framework. But I finally had to admit that that was *my* attempt to change the situation through fantasy. This was not transference at all. David simply saw me as a sexual prospect in the same way he saw every other woman. It was at that moment that I finally recognized the full scope of David's sexual addiction. I became even less optimistic about the prognosis.

The next five sessions progressed in the same desultory, dispiriting fashion. David finally attended an SLAA meeting, but he did not go back. He made sincere although short-lived attempts to control his sexual behavior, but the overall pattern of his life stayed the same. We made little progress in understanding the specific triggers to his sexual acting out; indeed, it began to seem as if sex was being used as a panacea for all manner of ills, a way of distracting his attention from every aspect of his life. David seemed less distressed than merely irritated about this lack of progress; at times the irritation seemed directed at me for not being more helpful. He continued to miss days at work because he would be deflected on the way to his job by sexual opportunities. After the tenth session, David telephoned to say that he had been fired and could no longer afford to see me. Since David never let cost deter him from doing anything he wanted to do—viz., the huge debt he had accumulated—I could only assume that he did not see giving up treatment as much of a loss. Nonetheless, I gave David the name of a facility where the cost of his treatment would be on an ability-to-pay basis; I subsequently learned that he never contacted them. Six months later I attempted to reach David for a follow-up report and found that his telephone had been disconnected with no forwarding number given.

At the stage of my career when I worked with David, I used to ask myself a lot whether the dropout rate for my sexual addiction patients was greater than for my sex therapy and psychotherapy patients because of the nature of their problem or because of my lack of experience and expertise in treating it. (I asked my more experienced sexual addiction colleagues the same question, and all tactfully claimed not to know.) I now believe the major reason was the latter, that I was just not knowledgeable and practiced enough to be truly helpful. I believe this because as I have persevered in this line of work, the retention rate for sexual addiction patients is virtually the same as that for patients with other presenting problems. Not that that means that I now would be able to work successfully with David; in fact, I would now act on my initial assessment that David needed to be hospitalized and was not a candidate for outpatient treatment. I wince now at the combination of naivete and grandiosity that led me to go against my better judgment. (I have since refused to treat two patients as out of control as David, and both have contacted me months later, after hospital stays, to thank me.) It takes time and experience for a sex therapist to accept the reality of a problem so different from ones he/she traditionally encounters, and it takes additional time and experience to know how to to treat it. The endeavor is worthwhile, however, because it expands the therapist's understanding of the uses to which sex can be put and because it allows treatment of a deeply suffering, and currently underserved, patient population.

REFERENCES

American Psychiatric Association. (1994). *Diagnostic and statistical manual of mental disorders* (4th ed.). Washington, DC: Author.

Carnes, P. (1983). *Sexual addiction.* Minneapolis: CompCare.

Carnes, P. (1990). Sexual addiction: Progress, criticism, challenges. *American Journal of Preventive Psychiatry and Neurology, 2,* 1–8.

Coleman, E. (1990). The obsessive–compulsive model for describing compulsive sexual behavior. *American Journal of Preventive Psychiatry and Neurology, 2,* 9–14.

Goodman, A. (1992). Sexual addiction: Designation and treatment. *Journal of Sex and Marital Therapy, 18,* 303–314.

Levine, M., & Troiden, R. (1988). The myth of sexual compulsivity. *Journal of Sex Research, 25,* 347–363.

Moser, C. (1993). A response to Aviel Goodman's "Sexual addiction: Designation and treatment." *Journal of Sex and Marital Therapy, 19,* 220–224.

Quadland, M. (1985). Compulsive sexual behavior: Definition of a problem and an approach to treatment. *Journal of Sex and Marital Therapy, 11,* 121–132.

21

Professionals Who Sexually Offend: A Betrayal of Trust

CANDACE B. RISEN
STANLEY E. ALTHOF

INTRODUCTION

Two salient clinical themes intertwine in this presentation of a physician who engaged in atypical fetishistic exploits while seemingly ministering to the health concerns of his female patients. Our first theme, the evaluation of professionals accused of sexual misconduct, has forced its way into public consciousness via the profusion of disturbing headlines about sexual improprieties of professionals in positions of trust and authority. After much whitewashing, minimizing, and denying of the reality that an alarming number of professionals harm those in their charge, governmental agencies, school and hospital boards, and religious orders are now searching for protocols to manage these painful predicaments. Therapists with an expertise in sexuality have become a valuable resource because they are well versed in managing issues of boundaries and boundary crossing, intimacy disorders, and sexual compulsivity as well as the traditional psychological problems of depression, substance abuse, and personality disorder.

Our second theme concerns the vicissitudes of treatment as this paraphilic physician and his therapist struggled to maintain a relationship complicated by deception, denial, and avoidance. The intricacies of this therapy process and the conflicting responsibilities of the therapist to the patient, the hospital, and the community at large are illuminated. Vital aspects of treatment are presented that reveal the nature and meaning of the sexual behavior to both patient and therapist.

A diagnosis of sexual paraphilia is often viewed with skepticism or derision. Libertarians contend that it reflects the conservative, antisexual, or moralistic bias of the psychological community. Conservatives, or those who champion a law-and-order philosophy, perceive this diagnosis to be a contemptible construction of weak-minded, gullible clinicians who foolishly medicalize criminal conduct.

In addition, there is a great deal of semantic confusion on the topic. The terms "sexual offenders," "perpetrators," "paraphiliacs," "sexual deviants," "sexual addicts," "sexual compulsives," "incest offenders" and "perverts" are often used interchangeably for those whose sexual interests and activities contravene socially acceptable norms. Unfortunately, there is little professional consistency in their use (Levine, 1992). Yet, the nomenclature employed by a therapist reflects important theoretical assumptions that may affect the therapy process.

In prior editions of the *Diagnostic and Statistical Manual of Mental Disorders* of the American Psychiatric Association, unacceptable sexual patterns were diagnosed as perversions. Because of the moralistic connotations of this label, the third edition (DSM-III) substituted the term "paraphilia." The fourth edition (DSM-IV; American Psychiatric Associatio, 1994) characterizes paraphilias as

> recurrent, intense sexually arousing fantasies, sexual urges, or behaviors generally involving 1) nonhuman objects, 2) the suffering or humiliation of oneself or one's partner, or 3) children or other nonconsenting persons, that occur over a period of at least 6 months (Criterion A). For some individuals, paraphiliac fantasies or stimuli are obligatory for erotic arousal and are always included in sexual activity. In other cases, the paraphiliac preferences occur only episodically (e.g., perhaps during periods of stress), whereas at other times the person is able to function sexually without paraphiliac fantasies or stimuli. The behavior, sexual urges, or fantasies cause clinically significant distress or impairment in social, occupational, or other important areas of functioning (Criterion B). (p. 523)

DSM-IV lists (1) exhibitionism, (2) fetishism, (3) frotteurism, (4) pedophilia, (5) sexual masochism, (6) sexual sadism, (7) transvestic fetishism, and (8) voyeurism as examples. Few women are ever diagnosed as paraphiliac.

In our experience, the criteria of DSM-IV are overly restrictive— that is, we believe that individuals who have not acted upon their unusual sexual interests, or who are not markedly distressed, may still be diagnosed as paraphiliac. A more robust diagnosis can be made utilizing three criteria: (1) a long-standing unusual erotic preoccupation that is highly arousing, (2) a pressure to act upon the erotic fantasy, and (3) an inhibition of conventional sexual behavior (Levine, Risen, & Althof, 1990).

We believe that paraphilia in males is a disorder of masculine development; the fantasies and behaviors are attempts to restore the image of the self as an adequate and competent man—that is, a masculine person. The term "unmasculinity" is employed to describe this painful and often humiliating sense of oneself as not masculine. Masculinity is merely a metaphor for a man's personal sense of competence. Culture has stereotypical expectations for behaviors based on gender and age. Males impose these cultural standards to assess their competence beginning early in life. At all ages, masculinity is an evaluation of oneself constructed in comparison to peers along the activities that culture defines as masculine, that is, athleticism, strength, assertiveness, dating competence, vocational success, and the like (Althof, Risen & Levine, 1992).

We believe that optimal treatment of paraphilia combines a behavioral and psychodynamic approach. Early in therapy, behavioral strategies are used to target the current acting out, and later, to develop relapse prevention plans. The psychodynamic work focuses on identifying and exploring the various contributions to the man's sense of unmasculinity. This lack of adequacy renders him more vulnerable to using fantasy or acting out as an means to restore competency. Finding and cultivating object relationships and developing new mechanisms to nurture this fragile sense of masculinity constitute the working-through phase of treatment. If treatment is successful, patients experience themselves as more adequate, no longer in need of the old maladaptive ways of feeling good about themselves. Yet, we perceive paraphilia as a lifelong struggle, much akin to addiction, whereby the former mechanisms of coping are ever ready should the newer ones fail.

CASE PRESENTATION

I (CBR) met Dr. Z following a consultation between the medical and lay administrators of a community hospital and the Program for Professionals (PFP).[1] The hospital had received complaints from several female patients accusing Dr. Z of kissing them on the lips, massaging and strok-

[1]The Program for Professionals was established with a grant from the Sihler Mental Health Foundation to evaluate and treat professionals (e.g., priests, therapists, and teachers) who sexually offend in the context of their profession.

ing their stockinged feet and legs, and, on one occasion, masturbating to orgasm while holding a nylon stocking.

Two PFP staff members met with the hospital's Special Peer Review Committee to address their concerns and to formulate a treatment plan. At this meeting it became evident that certain committee members were denying and minimizing the problem through an identification with the accused physician: "He's such a fine doctor. . . . Surely his behavior is being misinterpreted. . . ." They were reluctant to restrict his practice until an investigation could take place. The committee prioritized its concerns as follows: (1) to protect the rights of the accused physician, (2) to ensure the safety of his patients, and (3) to maintain trust in the community. The PFP staff urged the hospital committee to reorder this list by placing the safety of patients first. Three decisions were then made: (1) to proceed with an evaluation, (2) to immediately institute a nursing chaperon for all contacts with patients, and (3) to contact the state medical board for further guidance.

The evaluation of Dr. Z, a 35-year-old married, Brazilian father of three, began 3 days later. He was 20 minutes late for the first session, nonchalantly blaming traffic. He had not read the literature on PFP because he was "a busy physician." Within minutes, his beeper went off. He warned me that this would happen frequently and that he needed access to a telephone. He projected an "I don't have time for this nonsense" impatience that belied an underlying anxiety.

Dr. Z readily admitted to having rubbed and kissed the feet of numerous patients, claiming that it was therapeutic because it was relaxing. He characterized himself as a warm, friendly, and physically affectionate man who had been lauded in a recent newspaper article for these very qualities. Well-known for treating impoverished and terminally ill patients, he was proud of his reputation and critical of U.S. physicians who were stiff, formal, and cold. He denied that there was anything sexual in his behavior and maintained that no patient had ever protested or pulled away. While admitting that he was "a leg man who perhaps has a foot fetish," he boasted that he had no need for sexual contact with patients: "I'm proud to say that my wife is multiply orgasmic."

As I had access to detailed victim statements and was familiar with the "I've been badly misunderstood" posture of those accused of sexual misconduct, Dr. Z's denial was relatively easy to confront. I calmly informed him that several of his patients had described similarly detailed graphic depictions of his arousal. His sexual overtures had clearly not relaxed his patients; on the contrary, their anxiety was heightened. I told Dr. Z that there was no question in anyone's mind that these events had occurred, that he was in serious trouble, and that I was talking with him not to debate the truth but to determine whether he could be helped. Dr. Z became tearful and said that stroking feet and legs was a turn-on for him and that he liked the feeling of nylons. He related that he had become concerned with his behavior and had tried to stop after, unbeknownst to the hospital, a patient had filed a complaint at the local police station 6 months earlier. When she found out about this, his wife screamed furiously, "How could you be so stupid?" Dr. Z had no response. Despite his brush with the law, he continued to engage in the behavior.

Patient Evaluation

The clinical evaluation of Dr. Z took 1 month to complete and consisted of several hours with me (CBR), an interview with a second therapist (SEA), psychological testing, and drug screening. Mrs. Z angrily refused to participate in the evaluation, stating, "This is your problem. You fix it."

Dr. Z responded defensively to the Minnesota Multiphasic Personality Inventory (MMPI-2), Millon Clinical Multiaxial Inventory (MCMI-II), Beck Depression Inventory (BDI), Dyadic Adjustment Scale (DAS), and Michigan Alcoholism Screening Test (MAST). His MMPI-2 suggested that he harbored chronic intense anger and that these feelings were generally expressed in an inappropriate fashion—temper tantrums, sexual misconduct, and/or alcohol/drug abuse. The MCMI-II supported the MMPI-2 findings and offered the Axis I diagnosis of Generalized Anxiety Disorder and Axis II diagnosis of Narcissistic Personality Disorder. Mild dysphoria was evident on the BDI and problems with substance abuse were denied on the MAST. Scores on the DAS indicated that he had a satisfying marital relationship.

During this period, Dr. Z began to form a trusting relationship with me and was able to talk more openly. His initial defensive, arrogant posture shifted to one of vulnerability and shame as he gradually revealed his story. He repeatedly begged to be allowed to continue his medical practice and stated that he was willing to go to any lengths to do so. A treatment plan was formulated that included (1) ongoing chaperoning at both hospital and private office at his expense, (2) weekly psychotherapy, (3) monthly meetings with the hospital's Special Peer Review Committee, and (4) quarterly monitoring by an independent clinician to review his progress and to make necessary modifications and recommendations to the treatment plan.[2] Dr. Z, grateful that he could con-

----

[2]This signified the end of the evaluation and the beginning of treatment. A shift occurred from an investigation, whereby the clinical material was available to the hospital for its administrative purposes, to a confidential therapeutic relationship. Dr. Z understood that I would not hereafter report his revelations to the hospital or state board.

tinue practicing medicine, agreed to follow the plan although he was worried about shouldering the financial burden of a nurse chaperone.

Family Background

Dr. Z was born in Brazil but moved to the United States at an early age. He was the middle child of three, with a sister 9 years older and a brother 2 years younger. His mother was described as a beautiful, fashionably dressed lady; a beautician for the rich who pursued singing lessons on the side. She was away from home for much of the time, either working or singing, and the patient and his brother were cared for by their older sister and a series of housekeepers. When Mother was home, she was affectionate and demonstrative.

Father was described as a hard worker who held two factory jobs and was rarely home. When he was home, he was withdrawn and aloof. He was critical of both sons, driving them to succeed because he felt they would have to prove themselves to overcome discrimination against South Americans. He was often physically punishing; Dr. Z remembered being whipped "for so long, I would collapse from crying so hard." Father valued intellect and academic achievement. He was the eldest of several boys; the only one not to attend college because of working to put his brothers through. Both Dr. Z and his brother were excellent students and Father encouraged and supported all their academic endeavors.

Dr. Z's parents had physically violent arguments centered around Father's jealous suspicions about Mother's wish to become an opera singer. "Any woman in the arts has to prostitute herself to get ahead." He forbade her to have male voice coaches. Mother, in turn, accused him of being unfaithful. Although not aware of his father's infidelity, Dr. Z knew that his paternal uncles were promiscuous.

Dr. Z had vivid memories from ages 6 to 9 of lying in bed or sitting on the floor next to his mother with his head in her lap, stroking her stockinged legs. He initially described this interaction as loving and affectionate and denied that it might in any way have been wrong. With some prodding, however, he acknowledged being aroused. He recalled a time when his father walked in and his mother abruptly pushed him away. That night he retreated to bed feeling confused and upset.

When Dr. Z was 9 years old, his mother was diagnosed with lung cancer. Over the next 3 years, as her health deteriorated, she was forced to relinquish her work and singing career. Dr. Z sought to assist his mother by taking on the burden of running the household. When he was 12, the family returned to Brazil hoping the climate would be better for his mother's health. Unfortunately, she died 11 months later.

Adolescence and Early Adulthood

After the death of his mother, Dr. Z spent his adolescence in Brazil, never sharing his grief or other feelings of neediness and dependency. Father took her death hard. He drank heavily and was more abusive and threatening until he met and married a widow 18 months later. Dr. Z got along well with his stepmother although he remained emotionally independent. He continued to clean and care for the household as he had before. He was popular and active in high school but did not date until his late teens because of severe acne.

His early masturbatory fantasies involved his mother's legs. Thereafter, he used the images of feet, legs, and stockings of other women as the major source of his arousal. He began to date and became sexually active when he attended college in the United States. He always urged his partners to dress in stockings, garters, and high heels. He relished buying these items and became proficient in doing so, priding himself on knowing every lingerie shop in the community "better than the women did." Dr. Z maintained that none of his partners had objected to these practices. Most seemed to delight in it.

Dr. Z had a serious 5-year relationship with an American woman spanning college and medical school. When she broke it off, ostensibly because of her parents' objections to his ethnicity, he became severely depressed and was urged to seek psychiatric care. He saw a psychiatrist for six sessions but could not afford to continue.

Marital Relationship

Over the next 3 years, Dr. Z dated and bedded many women before meeting and marrying his wife. At the time of the evaluation, Dr. Z had been married for 7 years. He described his marriage as "wonderful"; however, I had been told by the hospital that his wife had hired a detective because of her repeated suspicions of his infidelity. Indeed, he had been unfaithful in at least one instance. In the first years of their marriage, he had a protracted affair with a Brazilian hospital employee who reminded him of his mother. She, too, dressed elegantly and wanted to become a beautician. This relationship ended when Mrs. Z found them in her bedroom. Dr. Z insisted that this was the only transgression.

While professing how "wonderful" his marriage was and how much he loved his wife, Dr. Z hinted strongly about conflict. He arrived for one session with a black eye, confessing that his wife had physically assaulted him. He denied ever striking back, was surprisingly tolerant of her anger, but wished she would not attack him in front of the children. His account of the scenario was punctuated with words of endearment: "I said, 'Honey, please don't do this now. Sweetheart, please come into the bedroom if you want to yell at me.'" These scenes were apparently quite common. On another occasion, he described performing all the cooking, cleaning, and most of the bathing and dressing of the children, despite his busy practice and his wife's full-time presence in the home. He complained of exhaustion yet seemed curiously proud and comfortable with their arrangement.

The Nature of the Paraphilia

The early months of psychotherapy focused on the nature and meaning of Dr. Z's fetishistic interest in stockings. At this time, neither Dr. Z nor I had any immediate concerns about his acting out these interests with patients due to the presence of the nurse chaperone. Dr. Z's initial description of his behavior as impulsively sparked by a sudden and unexpected sexual urge gradually gave way to the emergence of a premeditated, elaborate, and repetitive script. He revealed his selection of "victims" by their youth and appearance and described how easily he managed to cultivate a trusting relationship. The actual stroking of legs and feet emerged only after several visits during the course of which there was friendly banter and eliciting of increasingly personal information under the guise of a medical history. "I asked all kinds of questions about their marriage and sex life that really had nothing to do with why they were coming to see me. I especially listened for marital or personal troubles because those women welcomed sharing their problems and might then look to me as a confidant."

Dr. Z kept a cache of silk stockings in a locked drawer for those patients who did not wear them or whose stockings were of a rougher texture than what he found erotic. He introduced the foot and leg massage as a relaxation technique, and the stockings as a means to facilitate the process. He maintained that his arousal had been largely disguised from his patients and was anxious and upset to discover how obvious his sexual excitement had been to his victims. Dr. Z became cognizant that his heightened arousal had resulted in alternations in his level of consciousness. He appeared to have lapsed in and out of dissociative states, so much so that he could not clearly recall the details of how these exploits had ended.

With great shame, Dr. Z acknowledged and examined the detailed progression of his activities. He was appalled by the extent of his manipulation and exploitation of his patients' trust. "This sounds so horrible," he would often exclaim. From these discussions, however, grew the realization that his acting out was not a product of sudden "horniness" or impulsive affection. It was part of a premeditated script and was conceived in a predatory manner that suggested an aggression and control of which he was only vaguely aware.[3]

While Dr. Z acknowledged that the origin of his fetishistic interest dated back to sexual contacts with his mother, he could not comprehend the extent of his paraphiliac desires. Up to this point, Dr. Z spoke of these early memories only in positive terms. However, one day he announced suddenly that there was something he had not revealed as it would reflect badly on his mother. He related an incident when she called him into the bedroom to stroke her feet. This was the only time Dr. Z remembered words being spoken about the behavior. This verbal exchange made him anxious and uneasy. He refused to enter the bedroom, and from that moment, his mother never allowed him to touch or sit near her again. He was confused and angry with her for rejecting him and with himself for having denied her, thereafter forfeiting the opportunity to be with her. Dr. Z was deeply troubled by this memory; to him it meant that as a boy he had already known that something was amiss with this behavior. He now believed that his mother had been aware of his arousal and that perhaps she had been aroused herself. For the first time he used the word "incest" to describe their interaction and said, "she introduced me to the pleasures of that contact for whatever reasons of her own, and then she took it away from me and left me feeling bereft. . . . It wasn't fair to me . . . by then I longed for it and I was denied it." This was the first crack in his professed vision of his mother as a "saint."

As this theme was discussed, Dr. Z became aware of his anger toward his mother. He wondered whether he was retaliating against her by manipulating other women to provide what his mother had denied him. The theme of revenge was a powerful one to contemplate. "My patients are as vulnerable to me as children are to their parents. I can make them do whatever I want because they need and trust me. I made these women comply. They were probably experiencing the same mixture of confusion and anxiety as I was with my mother. I turned the tables, didn't I?"

Anger at his mother manifested itself in other ways. Dr. Z recalled that as her health deteriorated, he took on more and more of the housekeeping tasks. He approached these tasks with a vengeance and learned to do them "better than my sister, better than my mother, better than

---

[3]Only when the paraphiliac patient abandons the notion that behavior was something that "came over" him and acknowledges the elaborate thinking and planning that generates and maintains it can true progress be made. Relapse prevention strategies depend on the knowledge and recognition of these early affects and cognitions before they result in paraphiliac fantasy and behavior.

any female." Only in retrospect could he see that this had been his way of coping with the loss of all maternal support and caring. "I was determined to need no one. I would do it as well as them and even better." This drive to be better than any woman proved to be a major source of conflict in his marriage and a central theme in therapy. Repeatedly he enumerated the household chores he currently undertook because of his wife's illnesses, depression, exhaustion, or laziness. Gradually what had been portrayed as his wife's failure to keep the household running smoothly was reframed as his need to render her less effective than he. He recognized his attempts to undermine her, constantly "showing" her how to do things right, rushing in to perform tasks faster and better, and then complaining about how exhausted he was by doing the jobs of two people. His underlying contempt for her mirrored his contempt for women in general as expressed in the paraphiliac behavior. This was difficult for him to accept because, on the surface, Dr. Z professed an adoration for his wife and for women in general.

Further Revelations

Eight months into treatment, Dr. Z tearfully related that he was being sued by a former patient for having had a sexual affair with her. He then confessed to having had sexual relations with 11 other patients prior to entering psychotherapy. The encounters took place in a motel; he supplied the garters, stockings, and so on, and took great pleasure in the elaborate ritual of dressing the women and stroking their legs. His contempt toward women was now obvious to him. "I regarded them as whores . . . women who betray their husbands as my mother did. . . . She betrayed my father when she let me stroke her legs . . . it was our secret against him."[4]

The lawsuit was eventually dismissed; however, it had been reported to the state medical board. Although the board had not responded to the hospital's early inquiries, it now began a formal investigation into both the early complaints and this latest charge. Dr. Z's anxiety again escalated, as did his wife's anger. Both were reminded of the potential consequences of this behavior.

At this point in treatment, Dr. Z was prepared to acknowledge how much his paraphiliac behavior had cost him in the past. He returned to talking about his first love, the woman he had dated in college and medical school. He revealed that the reason for their breakup had not been

---

[4]Dr. Z's confession was a somber reminder to me of how much paraphiliac patients lie and deceive to avoid the shame of disclosure and to maintain the behaviors, all the time protesting that "this time, doctor, I'm telling you the whole story."

because of her family's objections to his ethnicity but because she discovered he was sexually involved with another woman. When asked why he had involved himself with another woman, he reluctantly admitted that his girlfriend had begun to express her discomfort with his ritualization of their lovemaking. This was the first admission that a woman had ever protested about his fetishistic behaviors. In the past, he had always asserted that "women love it."

At the 1-year mark, Dr. Z and I felt that he was ready to practice without a chaperone. The external constraints that had contained him early on (i.e., the chaperone, the fear of losing his license, or the fear of being prosecuted) had gradually given way to an internalized restraint stemming from an understanding of the dynamics of the behavior. He could now acknowledge the real harm he had inflicted on patients, which was in direct conflict with his wish to "be a good person and a good doctor; not someone who hurts people." He now easily identified and acknowledged the urge to sexualize a contact with a patient. It occurred infrequently, usually after a particularly frustrating encounter with Mrs. Z. As Dr. Z felt stronger and more in control of his life, the focus of therapy shifted to his increasing discontentment with his marriage. Conflicts that he had alluded to early on now came to the forefront. Mrs. Z's inability or unwillingness to manage the household was coupled with her compulsion to spend money faster than he earned it.

Only when Dr. Z could no longer afford to pay his office staff and was threatened with their home utilities being turned off was he able to face the reality of his wife's compulsive spending. He was encouraged to use what he had learned about his own compulsivity to take action—that is, confront his wife, remove all credit cards and access to bank accounts, and insist that she enter treatment. He bitterly stated, "I deserve this. I knew when I dated my wife that she was a slob and spent money like crazy. Her parents bailed her out. I ignored these issues and married her for sex. She wanted sex as much as I did and liked our games. She told me she had been inordinately interested in stockings and high heels since she was a little girl. She loved that I dressed her up in them. She never grew tired of it. I put blinders on about the rest of it and married her to indulge my sickness. And now we have three babies and I feel trapped."

COMMENTARY AND DISCUSSION

Eighteen months into psychotherapy, the Special Peer Review Committee has granted Dr. Z.'s request to see patients at the hospital without a chaperone. His private practice work continues to be supervised, however. Mrs. Z is in therapy to address her issues and both Dr. and Mrs. Z have considered entering marital therapy. The state board's investigation inexplicably continues to drag on, and Dr. Z still faces the possible loss of his license.

Dr. Z's psychotherapy will likely continue for several years. He is just beginning to acknowledge his feelings for me; how much he has had to see me as "a therapist . . . not a woman," because to see me as a woman evokes the desire to cross some boundary, to personalize and sexualize the relationship so as to gain control. He professes appreciation and gratitude for my help. Negative feelings—ambivalence about dependency, loss of control, exposure of shame, etc.—have yet to be acknowledged.

Effective treatment of the paraphiliac patient rests on the appreciation of this disorder as chronic and tenacious. Patients' conscious pleas for help in relinquishing these behaviors are often overshadowed by their less conscious needs to maintain them. The deceptions and distortions of paraphiliac men greatly complicate the alliance between patient and therapist. Relapses often occur and have profound consequences for both those who offend and their unfortunate victims. For these reasons, mandated, long-term treatment, coupled with external constraints, is likely to be the most effective. Such treatment requires that the therapist be skillfully active, frequently confrontative, and able to withstand the artifice inherent in the process.

It is clear to us that professional organizations remain in a quandary as to their role in the investigation and management of sexual complaints. Their fear of violating the rights of the accused and their tendency to identify with the professionals in their charge often render them ineffective. Some organizations have actively responded to the challenge, while others continue to hide their head in the sand and hope that they are never directly confronted with the problem.

As sexual complaints against professionals escalate and the demand for action intensifies, many professional organizations are searching for guidance and instruction. Programs such as ours assist in developing rational and compassionate protocols that seek to protect victims and offer help to impaired professionals.

REFERENCES

Althof, S., Risen, C., & Levine, S. (1992, March). *Understanding paraphilia as a disorder of masculine development.* Paper presented at the annual meeting of the Society for Sex Therapy and Research, Montreal.

American Psychiatric Association. (1994). *Diagnostic and statistical manual of mental disorders* (4th ed.). Washington, DC: Author.

Levine, S. (1992). *Sexual life: A clinician's guide.* New York: Plenum Press.

Levine, S., Risen, C., & Althof, S. (1990). An essay on the diagnosis and nature of paraphilia. *Journal of Sex and Marital Therapy, 16*(2), 89–102.

22

Marital Discord and Sexual Dysfunction Associated with a Male Partner's "Sexual Addiction"

JOHN P. WINCZE

INTRODUCTION

Since the publication of *Out of the Shadows: Understanding Sexual Addiction* (Carnes, 1983), there has been much debate in the scientific literature as to the existence, validity, and usefulness of such a diagnostic category (Goodman, 1992; Levine & Troiden, 1988). The essence of the argument against such a categorization has been stated as follows: "We argue that sexual addiction and compulsion represent pseudoscientific codifications of prevailing erotic values rather than bona fide clinical entities. The concepts of sexual addiction and compulsion constitute an attempt to repathologize forms of erotic behavior that became acceptable in the 1960s and 1970s" (Levine & Troiden, 1988, p. 349).

This point of view may be bolstered by a historical look at other sexual behaviors, such as homosexuality and masturbation, which were classified previously as pathological until social pressures dictated otherwise. While Levine and Troiden (1988) point to social pressures or "prevailing erotic values" as the force behind the cycle of normalization or pathologization of certain sexual behaviors, they do not address the fact that change also results from increased scientific knowledge. For example, the work of Kinsey and associates (Kinsey, Pomeroy, & Martin, 1948; Kinsey, Pomeroy, Martin, & Gebhard, 1953) provided knowledge about the universality of masturbation in men and women and defused previous arguments that masturbation was physically and psychologically harmful. More recently the idea that sexual relations between therapist and patient might be beneficial to the patient (which was endorsed by some therapists of the 1960s and 1970s; *Ob-Gyn News*, 1976, cited in Schoener, Milgram, Gonsiorek, Luepker, & Conroe, 1989) has been strongly challenged by numerous research studies that have documented near universal harmful effects of therapist–patient sexual relations (Pope, 1988; Schoener et al., 1989).

Whether as a result of social–political pressures or of scientific knowledge, it is clear that sexual values have changed markedly over time, and that we should be cautious about readily identifying any sexual behavior as normal or abnormal, and in using diagnostic labels to support our contentions (Levine & Troiden, 1988). The use of the label "sexual addiction," in particular, remains controversial despite compelling arguments for such a diagnosis. Goodman (1992) favors the use of the "sexual addiction" diagnostic label but qualifies it as follows: "It is not the type of behavior, its object, its frequency, or its social acceptability that determines whether a pattern of sexual behavior qualifies as sexual addiction: it is how this behavior pattern relates to and affects the individual's life, as specified by the diagnostic criteria" (p. 231).

Whether or not the term "sexual addiction" is used, it is obvious to therapists who treat sexual problems that there are individuals who have difficulty controlling their sexual behavior. Such uncontrollable sexual behavior may be destructive to the individual or unacceptable to a partner. Goodman (1992, p. 230) has outlined the common ingredients he feels compose the sexual problem labeled "sexual addiction":

A. Recurrent failure to resist impulses to engage in a specified sexual behavior.
B. Increasing sense of tension immediately prior to initiating the sexual behavior.
C. Pleasure or relief at the time of engaging in the sexual behavior.
D. At least five of the following:
   1) frequent preoccupation with the sexual behavior or with activity that is preparatory to the sexual behavior.
   2) frequent engaging in the sexual behavior to a greater extent or over a longer period than intended.
   3) repeated efforts to reduce, control, or stop the sexual behavior.
   4) a great deal of time spent in activities necessary for the sexual behavior, engaging in the sexual behavior, or recovering from its effects.
   5) frequent engaging in the sexual behavior when expected to fulfill occupational, academic, domestic, or social obligations.

      6) important social, occupational, or recreational activities given up or reduced because of sexual behavior.

      7) continuation of the sexual behavior despite knowledge of having a persistent or recurrent social, financial, psychological, or physical problem that is caused or exacerbated by the sexual behavior.

      8) tolerance: need to increase the intensity or frequency of the sexual behavior in order to achieve the desired effect, or diminished effect with continued sexual behavior of the same intensity.

      9) restlessness or irritability if unable to engage in the sexual behavior.

  E. Some symptoms of the disturbance have persisted for at least one month, or have occurred repeatedly over a longer period of time.

It is not the purpose of this chapter to argue for or against the use of the diagnostic category of sexual addiction. Rather, my purpose is to sensitize the reader to the issues involved and to present a case study that illustrates the complexity of problems faced by clinicians treating such individuals.

Individuals evidencing sexual behavior labeled "addictive" typically seek treatment only at the request or coercion of a partner or when they have lost a job or have been threatened with arrest. Without external pressure, such individuals rarely are willing to abandon the behavior, or even to modify it. It is intrinsically rewarding to such individuals and often serves an important psychological role in reducing dysphoric states. The lack of "internal" motivation for change is often present in treatment and is difficult to overcome. Because individuals do not typically identify their sexual addiction as a problem, they may have repeatedly engaged in the behavior over many years, making it a highly reinforced behavior that is very resistant to change.

Sexual addiction falls under the more general category of paraphilia or atypical sexual behavior. In addition to sexual addiction, numerous other categories of sexual behavior may be classified as paraphilias, including exhibitionism, fetishism, frotteurism, pedophilia, sexual sadism and masochism, and voyeurism. The presence of more than one paraphiliac behavior is often found in these individuals and may further complicate the treatment picture.

The case presented in this chapter represents a complicated interaction of sexual addiction, fetishism, sexual dysfunction, and marital discord. Treatment involved helping the couple to work toward resolving their collective and individual problems and to gain a clearer understanding of the underlying difficulties.

PRESENTING PROBLEM

Reverend and Mrs. J were referred by a marriage therapist who felt that the couple's problems were too complex for traditional marriage therapy. The presenting complaint was lack of sexual frequency. The couple had been married for 30 years and had three adult children who were no longer living at home. During the intake interview with both present, Rev. J expressed an interest in sexual activity with his wife but complained of being spurned by her anger and frustrated by her chronic lack of sexual interest. In fact, the couple had not had successful sexual relations for more than 5 years. They sought out treatment when their third child left home, leaving them to focus on a marital relationship that was lacking in intimacy and imbued with anger.

On rare occasions when Mrs. J "allowed" sexual relations to occur, Rev. J experienced erectile failure. This would launch an angry response from Mrs. J and convince her that her husband was homosexual.

He was able to obtain an erection at times but would always lose his erection after a few moments. On most occasions when he approached his wife for sexual relations, he was unable to obtain an erection. His sexual difficulties appeared to be more a result of an overall lack of compatibility and lack of sexual enthusiasm on Mrs. J's part than competing homosexual or fetish interests.

ASSESSMENT PROCEDURE

The assessment procedure involved separate interviews with each partner as well as completion of the Derogatis Sexual Functioning Inventory (DSFI). During the individual interview with Rev. J, he openly revealed that he had had several affairs with women during the course of their marriage. He also stated that he had been interested in homosexual videotapes, but had never acted out his homosexual fantasies with a partner. He had, however, always maintained a secret post-office box in order to receive catalogs and items of male clothing that he knew were objectionable to his wife. The clothing ranged from skimpy and sexually provocative underwear to traditional fashion items found in catalogs like J. Crew. He claimed that his wife disapproved of all but the most conservative older men's clothing.

There was a sense of "addiction" to ordering and wearing the clothing because he derived great pleasure and arousal from dressing up yet knew that being seen in the clothing by his wife would evoke considerable anger and upset. He often masturbated while wearing certain items of clothing and making "900" telephone calls. Rev. J stated that he did not wish to leave the marriage, but this was expressed more out of a sense of loss of comfort and convenience than a genuine appreciation of the relationship.

The results of Rev. J's DSFI revealed an endorsement of homosexual fantasies and the use of masturbation several times per week as his only sexual outlet. He also showed very liberal-minded sexual attitudes. The only other noteworthy information from the DSFI was that he rated being seen in a bathing suit as "extremely" enjoyable. He denied exhibitionism but said he would not be upset if he was seen nude by strangers; in fact, he frequented a nude beach during summer months and wore genital jewelry to attract attention.

Overall, Rev. J's homosexual interests appeared to be mildly to moderately strong. He was capable of going for weeks without acting on any component of this interest. When he made "900" phone calls and viewed homosexually oriented videos he felt sexually aroused and obtained erections and masturbated to orgasm. These behaviors, however, seemed to occur sporadically and only when Mrs. J was absent from the house for an extended length of time.

Rev. J wore "skimpy" clothing and shaved his body more consistently, but he claimed these behaviors were not usually sexually driven. He claimed that he masturbated while wearing "skimpy" underwear only rarely and he never felt aroused while shaving his body; he merely "felt better" while doing it. He conceptualized viewing homosexual videos and making "900" phone calls as "wrong" and under his control. Wearing "objectionable" clothing and shaving his body were not viewed as wrong and he was less motivated to change these behaviors but passively stated he would try to change for the sake of the marriage.

Mrs. J revealed in her interview that she was angry with her husband for his extramarital affairs and could not forgive him. As it turned out, the affairs were two "one-night stands" 15 years earlier; both were heterosexual. In addition, she was most concerned about his "gay" behavior. She displayed his "gay clothing" in the session, which consisted of a T-shirt and a pair of loose-fitting pants with an African design. She also mentioned the catalogs of "homosexual" clothing and that he shaved his body and, on one occasion several years ago, wore shorts that exposed his penis when bending over.

Mrs. J came from a family in which her father was verbally and physically abusive and her mother was completely subservient. Mrs. J had very poor self-esteem and it is quite likely that her relationship with her father prepared her for accepting a nonloving and exploitive marriage. Furthermore, sexual expression was actively suppressed and she was highly conservative in her views of sexuality. This was substantiated by her response to the DSFI in which she endorsed a very restricted and conservative view of sexual behavior. Heterosexual kissing, hugging, and intercourse were the only behaviors she found acceptable.

ASSESSMENT RESULTS AND DEVELOPMENT OF TREATMENT PLAN

The assessment process revealed that this couple was entering therapy with a high degree of marital dissatisfaction. Miscommunication, lack of mutual interests and goals, and extremely different views of sexuality were only some of their problems. In spite of these enormous differences, the couple wished to give therapy a try to "help make their final years together satisfying."

Because concern about Rev. J's homosexuality was a key issue, it was important to discuss this topic in the treatment plan. Also, the issue of homosexuality had to be distinguished from his fetishistic behavior. I felt that no progress could be made unless the following specific areas were addressed:

1. Homosexual concerns and misunderstandings;
2. Full disclosure of fetishistic behavior by Rev. J leading to a discussion and agreement by the couple regarding the inclusion or exclusion of such behavior in their future relationship;
3. Building trust and openness in communication;
4. Working together to find common interests and activities; and
5. Building intimacy and sexuality.

The treatment plan was developed with goals and strategies in each of the above five areas, and the major interventions were derived from a cognitive-behavioral therapeutic model (Wincze & Carey, 1991).

TREATMENT GOALS AND STRATEGIES

Goal I

The aim was to provide information to the couple about the etiology of sexual orientation and variety of sexual experiences, attitudes, and values.

I hoped that in the process of this discussion, the couple would develop greater appreciation and acceptance of each other's sexual patterns. The strategy for accomplishing this goal was to begin by acknowledging differences in beliefs about sexual orientation and by asking the couple to describe how their beliefs originated. Following this discussion, I planned to provide normative information along with a cognitive-behavioral conceptualization of the etiology of sexual orientation. I felt that this issue was the source of major conflict for the couple and had to be confronted directly before progress could be made in any other area.

Goal 2

Here my aim was to encourage Rev. J to fully disclose the extent of his fetishic behavior and assist the couple in understanding how such behavior impacted on their relationship. Additionally, I wished to develop control mechanisms for Rev. J that would include directly addressing the reinforcing characteristics and stress reduction/escape functions of the behavior.

My strategy for working on this goal was to begin by sensitizing Rev. J to the destructive nature of his fetish. It was first necessary for him to describe all the variants of the behavior and how he felt about his participation in each aspect . Next, it was important for Mrs. J to describe how Rev. J's behavior made her feel. Although she had expressed her anger in the past, she had not expressed her sadness, embarrassment, and humiliation.

The strategy for helping Rev. J to control his behavior was to have him keep a behavioral record of urges and incidents to help identify antecedents and patterns. Next, stress-reduction strategies (e.g., relaxation training, engaging in alternative activities, and relabeling emotions) would be applied to help reduce sexual acting out that was associated with stress. Finally, I used covert sensitization (Cautela, 1967) to help reduce the reinforcing consequences of the sexual behavior.

Goal 3

The aim here was to direct Rev. J to cease all secretive behaviors including canceling his secret post-office box and becoming more open about his feelings.

My treatment strategy for this goal was to enlist a commitment from Rev. J to express his feelings more openly in interacting with his wife. Once this agreement was made, couple communication sessions could be planned. These sessions would involve setting aside prearranged time during the week for the couple to meet and discuss various relationship and family issues. I planned to address disagreements and faulty communication patterns by providing a written communication guide and through discussion and feedback in therapy sessions.

Goal 4

The strategy here was to encourage the couple to build reinforcing activities together.

Their relationship had been characterized by separate activities throughout most of their marriage. Neither partner was able to identify "couple" activities that were mutually enjoyable. I could not apply the strategy to achieve this goal until the first three goals were reasonably fulfilled. Even if the couple could have identified mutually enjoyable plans, Mrs. J was so angry at Rev. J that she would not have been motivated to work on these plans. Assuming accomplishment of the first three goals, the strategy for attacking the fourth goal was to jointly create a list and then begin to carry out plans on a weekly basis. A designated time slot would be identified as "couple activity time" and this weekly time slot would be established as "protected highest priority time." Both Rev. and Mrs. J would be responsible for generating a desired list and each would alternate in choosing the activity for the week. Therapy sessions would be used to help review and process these experiences.

Goal 5

The aim was to help Rev. and Mrs. J to establish a comfortable and pleasurable intimate/sexual relationship.

The strategy for this goal, as in the case of previous goals, could only be implemented when progress was achieved in other areas. The strategy would address both the conceptual and the behavioral level of sexual intimacy. On the conceptual level, it would be important for the couple to think about sex as a continuum of behaviors rather than "all or none." Many couples, including Rev. and Mrs. J, believe that if "I start something sexual, I have to finish it."

Letting a couple know that they have options and that they may "pick and choose" what behaviors to participate in is usually helpful in taking the pressure off performance (Wincze & Carey, 1991). In addition to addressing the cognitive aspects of intimacy through discussion, I often assign readings to further understanding (McCarthy, 1988; Zilbergeld, 1978).

The behavioral component to this strategy would be to discuss sensate focus exercises (Kaplan, 1974; Masters & Johnson, 1970; Wincze & Carey, 1991) and to establish times for carrying out the exercises. Therapy would then monitor progress and adjust the procedure as needed.

TREATMENT OUTCOME

Every experienced therapist knows that the best laid plans do not necessarily come to fruition. In this case, the couple initially seemed to respond to the treatment plan. Both seemed to understand and accept information about homosexuality and patterns of sexual behavior, although Mrs. J did so somewhat reluctantly. She seemed to have difficulty in not being able to place her husband in a neatly labeled category. Nonetheless, she stated that she was willing to continue living with Rev. J and working on their relationship if he was able to control his sexual acting out. In turn, Rev. J stated he would make every effort to do so. To make good on this promise, he threw away all objectionable clothing, catalogs, and videos and discontinued his secretive post-office box. He also stated that he would no longer make phone calls to the "900" gay sex line.

I met with Rev. J individually for 10 sessions, working specifically on the control of his "objectionable" behavior. During the 10 individual sessions, he was cooperative, more friendly, and seemingly more relaxed than in the joint sessions with his wife. On a daily basis, he recorded the frequency of the following behaviors: shaving body, dressing in objectionable clothing, "900" phone calls, and masturbation to homosexual videos. In addition, he recorded his mood on an 9-point Likert scale (0 = not at all upset to 8 = extremely upset). He responded well to identifying the antecedents and visualizing aversive consequences. During this period, he reported that he and his wife were getting along better and not arguing. He agreed to attempt to control his atypical behavior because he recognized how destructive the behavior had become to his marriage. He did not believe, however, that there was anything intrinsically wrong with what he had been doing.

Rev. J's behavioral record indicated no incidents of body shaving, "900" phone calls, or masturbation to homosexual videos. There were a few incidents of wearing objectionable clothing, which included turtleneck jerseys and jeans but no silky underwear. Although he considered his clothing "normal," he was fully aware of his wife's objections. In fact, the only increase in recorded anxiety occurred following disagreements about his clothing (from an anxiety level of 1 or 2 to an anxiety level of 5).

Following this phase of the therapy, I received an "emergency" call from Mrs. J. She said she had left her husband because she discovered that her "husband had shaved his shoulders." She said this was gay behavior and she assumed he did this to attract other gay men at the beach. She was unwavering in her belief and felt duped and deceived by her husband. She refused to consider continuing in therapy to discuss this issue.

Rev. J contacted me and agreed to attend a session alone. In the session that followed, he stated that he had used tweezers to extract hair from his shoulders for the purposed of enhancing his self-image, as "the hairs were wiry and gray." He did admit that he knew such behavior might upset his wife but assumed she would accept it. This was, in fact, the pattern of his past behavior, and he failed to judge the seriousness of her ultimatum. He denied that he had used this as a ploy to terminate the relationship.

Following his rejection by Mrs. J, he continued in therapy on an individual basis and reported dropping over repeatedly to Mrs. J's home and trying to cajole her into taking him back. She did not waver, however, and it became clearer that Rev. J was more interested in pursuing a comfortable lifestyle and acting out his sexual fantasies, than in establishing a close or meaningful relationship with his wife. He finally accepted the fact that his wife was determined not to reconcile. At this point he announced his decision to terminate treatment as he saw no need for individual therapy.

Rev. J professed not to really understanding that using tweezers to "pluck" his shoulder hair was similar to shaving hair. He was quite sure that his wife objected to his shaving hair from his body, but he said he did not think that it would really matter if he tweezed a few gray hairs from his shoulders.

DISCUSSION

This case presented a major therapeutic challenge in attempting to distinguish real differences from simple misunderstandings. The case also illustrates that despite presentation of compelling evidence to the contrary, many individuals have fixed beliefs about sexuality that are highly resistant to change. For example, Mrs. J had a preconception about what constituted homosexuality and what the term implied. Despite her initial acceptance of normative information about homosexuality, she could not shake her deep-seated attitudes and prejudices, nor could she focus on the more fundamental problem: her husband's insensitivity and lack of love toward her. Her focus on a need to specify a diagnosis of homosexuality not only detracted from these underlying problems but also from the "addictive" nature of his sexual behavior. In contrast, Rev. J was a bright, well-informed man and readily identified his wife's misunderstandings about homosexuality. Because of her ignorance and sexual conservatism, Rev. J was able to downplay his need to address the above problems as they affected his relationship.

This case presents atypical sexual behavior which could fit the definition of sexual addiction, as outlined by Goodman (1992, 1993) and presented earlier in this chapter. In this case, Rev. J demonstrated a recurrent failure to control his sexual behavior, and a continuation of the behavior despite significant harmful consequences. Both of these components are essential to my conceptualization of sexual addiction. For Goodman (1993), sexual addiction is not behaviorally specific; rather, sexual addiction represents how a behavior relates to a person's life. Therefore, all fetishes are not necessarily representative of an addictive process. A fetish only becomes a sexual addiction if it meets the criteria outlined earlier.

From the perspective of Levine and Troiden (1988), however, it could be argued that Rev. J's sexual behavior merely represents a variation that is not acceptable to society as a whole. Because there was no victim, his behavior was disturbing only to Mrs. J.

Whether labeled "addictive" or not, this case presents a significant challenge to our understanding of the nature of paraphilias, as well as the interaction with sexual dysfunction. While I am relatively experienced in both these areas, and the case conceptualization and treatment approach were generally adequate, I could have devoted more attention to defining the couple's interest in therapy and delineation of the couple's differences. The overall goal of helping this couple to decide whether or not to live together could have been emphasized more from the outset.

It appeared that Rev. J's motivation for engaging in therapy was to maintain his status quo. For him, this meant living in a comfortable home with the appearance of a socially acceptable marriage but without the substance of psychological or sexual intimacy. I do not believe that he purposely excluded intimacy but rather that such intimacy was unimportant to him or unknown to him.

Mrs. J, on the other hand, entered therapy because she could no longer tolerate a relationship that lacked intimacy, nor could she tolerate a relationship imbued with what she saw as sexual "perversions." She was clearly more focused on the perversions. The lack of intimacy and Rev. J's sexual dysfunction were, in her mind, evidence of his perversion.

Thus, the clients' goals, simply stated, were as follows: Rev. J's goal was to placate his wife and establish his normality. Mrs. J's goal was to declare her husband perverted and "cure" him of this. The established goals for therapy, however, were to work on improving psychological and sexual intimacy. Although both Rev. and Mrs. J agreed on these seemingly logical and desirable goals, in retrospect these goals were in conflict with this couple's hidden agenda. Therapy may have been more successful if these hidden goals could have been identified early on and thoroughly discussed until goals truly agreed on by all (therapist included) were established.

In retrospect, the marriage had always been lacking in positive concern and mutual attraction. Rev. J was a highly self-centered individual who was adept at impression management but had a great deal of difficulty in putting aside his needs for others. For him, the marriage provided necessary comforts but little else. Because Mrs. J had grown up with a cold and abusive father, she seemed to expect little from her marital relationship. Compared to her father, Rev. J was attentive and loving. For this reason, she focused on the sexual issues rather than on overall relationship issues. In fact, she never clearly articulated a lack of a emotional connection, but to the end she focused exclusively on her husband's sexual behavior.

Finally, this case illustrates the complex interaction between sexual dysfunction and paraphiliac issues. The presenting problem was lack of sexual desire and arousal. The presence of paraphiliac behavior in one or both partners does not necessarily result in, or even contribute to, sexual dysfunction. I have treated a number of cases in which the paraphiliac behavior of one partner was accepted and incorporated into a couple's ongoing sexual script. In order for the paraphilia not to interfere with a couple's sexual relationship, however, the following ingredients should be present:

1. Nonsexual aspects of the relationship should be mutually rewarding.
2. The couple should communicate openly and effectively.
3. There should be a liberal attitude toward sexual behavior.
4. The paraphilia should be expressed judiciously so that it is balanced with other nonparaphiliac sexual expressions.

Unfortunately, none of these elements or conditions were present in this case. When these conditions are lacking, in my experience, there is little likelihood of a successful outcome. In such instances, the role of the therapist should be to assist the couple in delineating the issues and in deciding whether or not to dissolve the relationship. In all such cases, the therapist should attempt to carefully assess the paraphiliac behavior and avoid a priori assumptions that it is the source of all relationship difficulties or sexual dysfunctions

The case of Rev. and Mrs. J is unusual perhaps because of the nature of some of the behaviors involved (body shaving, genital jewelry, gay clothing) but not unusual in the sense that one partner's sexual interests were objected to by the other partner. A common example of this, which often does not come to treatment, is when a male partner enjoys looking at pornography and the female partner objects. In cases of conflict that do end up in therapy, the therapist should help a couple define the problem in terms of the expenditure of time, energy, money, and interpersonal stress rather than in terms of right or wrong, moral turpitude, or psychopathology. This approach helps maintain a therapist's objectivity and influence. Problems arise, as they did in this case, when each partner attempts to use the therapist and the process of therapy against the other partner. In such instances (including this case), the couple may best be served by a course of individual therapy for each until goals are more openly defined and agreed upon.

REFERENCES

Carnes, P. (1983). *Out of the shadows: Understanding sexual addiction*. Minneapolis: CompCare.
Cautela, J. R. (1967). Covert sensitization. *Psychological Reports, 20*, 459–468.
Goodman, A. (1992). Sexual addiction: Designation and treatment. *Journal of Sex and Marital Therapy, 18*, 303–314.
Goodman, A. (1993). Diagnosis and treatment of sexual addiction. *Journal of Sex and Marital Therapy, 19*, 225–251.
Kaplan, H. S. (1974). *The new sex therapy: Active treatment of sexual dysfunction*. New York: Brunner/Mazel.
Kinsey, A., Pomeroy, W., & Martin, C. (1948). *Sexual behavior in the human male*. Philadelphia: Saunders.
Kinsey, A., Pomeroy, W., Martin, C., & Gebhard, P. (1953). *Sexual behavior in the human female*. Philadelphia: Saunders.
Levine, M., & Troiden, R. (1988). The myth of sexual compulsivity. *Journal of Sex Research, 25*, 347–363.
Masters, W. H., & Johnson, V. E. (1970). *Human sexual inadequacy*. Boston: Little, Brown.
McCarthy, B. (1988). *Male sexual awareness*. New York: Caroll & Graf.
Pope, K. (1988). How clients are harmed by sexual contact with mental health professionals: The syndrome and its prevalence. *Journal of Counseling and Development, 67*, 222–226.
Schoener, G., Milgram, J., Gonsiorek, J., Luepker, E., & Conroe, R. (1989). *Psychotherapists' sexual involvement with clients*. Minneapolis: Walk-In Counseling Center.
Wincze, J. P., & Carey, M. P. (1991). *Sexual dysfunction: A guide for assessment and treatment*. New York: Guilford Press.
Zilbergeld, B. (1978). *Male sexuality: A guide to sexual fulfillment*. Boston: Little, Brown.

Index

CPSIA information can be obtained at www.ICGtesting.com
Printed in the USA
LVOW12*2124270314

379294LV00004B/27/A

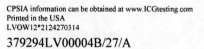

9 780898 628487